WAKING THE WARRIOR GODDESS

Dr. Horner has assembled a great deal of useful information about the prevention and treatment of breast cancer. I will recommend this book to patients and families of all people concerned with this dreadful disease and its increasing frequency.

> —Andrew Weil, M.D., Founder and Director of the Program for Integrative Medicine, and Clinical Professor of Internal Medicine University of Arizona; Best-selling author of *Spontaneous Healing, 8 Weeks to Optimum Health, Eating Well for Optimum Health,* and *The Healthy Kitchen*

This book is a significant resource for women who feel inspired and desire to participate in their life and health. When you combine inspiration with information you have the potential to alter the physical world, health, your life, and derive the associated physical benefits. Without information, women have no choice about their health.

> —Bernie Siegel, M.D., Founder of Exceptional Cancer Patients; Best-selling author of *Love, Medicine, and Miracles: Lessons Learned about Self-Healing from a Surgeon's Experience with Exceptional Patients; 365 Prescriptions for the Soul: Daily Messages of Inspiration, Hope, and Love* and *Help Me to Heal*

Christine Horner, M.D., presents a powerful and comprehensive approach to achieving the very best of health. This is a prescription every doctor should write.

> —Neal Barnard, M.D., President of Physicians Committee for Responsible Medicine; Adjunct Associate Professor at the George Washington University School of Medicine; Author of *Breaking The Food Seduction; Turn Off the Fat Gene; Eat Right, Live Longer;* and *Food for Life: How the New Four Food Groups Can Save Your Life*

Dr. Christine Horner has done every woman a great favor by compiling under one cover all the essential knowledge for achieving breast health naturally. *Waking the Warrior Goddess* is enchantingly scripted, rich in practical tips and profoundly empowering. Read this book and follow its recommendations now, and you will create not only healthy breasts, but a healthy, fulfilling life!

> —Nancy Lonsdorf, M.D., Medical Director of The Raj Ayurveda
> Health Center; Author of *A Woman's Best Medicine* and *A Woman's
> Best Medicine for Menopause*

For most women, breast cancer remains the most threatening disease possible. Christine Horner's book offers the best available knowledge to prevent this dreaded illness. All women and their husbands should heed this advice.

> —C. Norman Shealy, M.D., Ph.D., President of Holos University
> Graduate Seminary; Founding President of American Holistic
> Medical Association; Author of *Miracles Do Happen, 90 Days
> to Stress-Free Living,* and *The Creation of Health*

This book is a paradigm shifter! I recommend that all women read it. You'll never think the same about your body or your health again.

> —Marci Shimoff, Coauthor of *Chicken Soup for a Woman's Soul, Happiness
> for No Reason,* and *Love for No Reason*

This may be one of the most important books of our time for women. The information in this book can help stop the epidemic of breast cancer.

> —Jennifer Read Hawthorne, Coauthor of *Chicken Soup for the Woman's
> Soul;* Author of *The Soul of Success: A Woman's Guide to Authentic Power*

An important contribution to understanding and preventing breast cancer. Dr. Horner's sensitivity to ancient healing sciences is particularly valuable to patients and practitioners alike.

> —Tom Newmark, President of New Chapter Herbs; Coauthor of
> *Beyond Aspirin* and *Life Bridge*

THIRD EDITION—UPDATED AND EXPANDED

WAKING THE WARRIOR GODDESS

DR. CHRISTINE HORNER'S PROGRAM TO PROTECT AGAINST & FIGHT BREAST CANCER

Christine Horner, M.D., F.A.C.S.

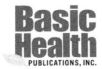

Basic Health
PUBLICATIONS, INC.

The information contained in this book is based upon the research and personal and professional experiences of the author. It is not intended as a substitute for consulting with your physician or other healthcare provider. Any attempt to diagnose and treat an illness should be done under the direction of a healthcare professional.

The publisher does not advocate the use of any particular healthcare protocol but believes the information in this book should be available to the public. The publisher and author are not responsible for any adverse effects or consequences resulting from the use of the suggestions, preparations, or procedures discussed in this book. Should the reader have any questions concerning the appropriateness of any procedures or preparation mentioned, the author and the publisher strongly suggest consulting a professional healthcare advisor.

The author of this book has a financial interest in the product Protective Breast Formula. This does not constitute an endorsement by Basic Health Publications, Inc.

Basic Health Publications, Inc.
28812 Top of the World Drive
Laguna Beach, CA 92651
Phone: 949-715-7327 • www.basichealthpub.com

Library of Congress Cataloging-in-Publication Data

Horner, Christine.
  Waking the warrior goddess : Dr. Christine Horner's program to protect against & fight breast cancer / Christine Horner. — 3rd ed.
    p. cm.
  Includes bibliographical references and index.
  ISBN 978-1-59120-363-6
 1. Breast—Cancer—Popular works. I. Title.

  RC280.B8H665   2007
  616.99'449—dc22

                                                    2007021971

Editor: Jane E. Morrill
Copyeditor: Carol Rosenberg
Typesetting: Gary A. Rosenberg / Theresa Wiscovitch
Cover design: Mike Stromberg
Illustrator: Skye Gibbins

Printed in the United States of America

10   9   8   7   6   5   4   3

Contents

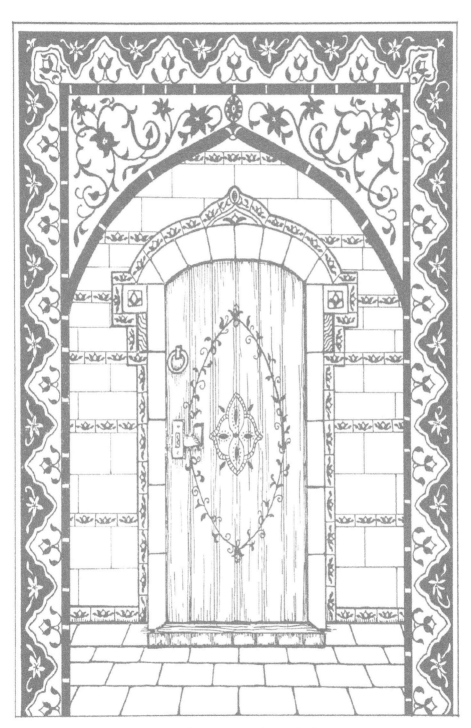

Open the doorway to knowledge . . .

To my mother
and all the women
who have fought battles
with breast cancer

Acknowledgments

The process of writing a book is invariably a personally challenging journey—and one that cannot be done alone. The greatest gift of this process was the reminder that I am blessed to walk this Earth with the support of many friends who are extraordinarily talented, tremendously loving, and generous.

There are many kind and remarkable people who gave me valuable feedback and donated their time and talents to editing the proposal for this book: Paula Sellars, Linda Naylor, Antoinette Asimus, Mackey McNeill, Jayn Meinhardt, and Chris Conlan. Heartfelt thanks to Julie Silver, M.D., for believing in me and this book so much that despite her extremely busy schedule as a physician, author, wife, and mother of three young children she made the time to take me under her wing and share her comprehensive wisdom and experience.

I have enormous appreciation for the generosity and expert editing skills of my sister, Carolyn Horner, and her heroic down-to-the-wire effort to help me edit the final version of the manuscript.

Thanks and praise go to the late Janet Greene, M.D.; my niece, Adrienne Horner; Paul Schaefer; and my dear friends Dotti Posillico, Bette Craig, Joan Zenker, and Jay White, who donated their time and expertise during the editing process.

My gratitude goes to Skye Gibbins and her artistic talent in creating the illustrations for this book.

I am also indebted to Lisa Curry Gray for her feedback, support, and legal advice.

There are many other people who deserve acknowledgment for a variety of contributions: Cindy Meehan-Patton for sharing her knowledge about nontoxic products for the home; Sandra Ingerman and Chris Kilham for their friendship and generous expert advice as experienced authors; Jade Beutler and Tom Newmark for their support and networking; Vivien and Neil Schapera for helping me with the spiritual work I needed to do before I began the first draft; and Andrew Weil, M.D., Bernie Siegel, M.D., Norman Shealy, M.D., Neal Barnard, M.D., Nancy Lonsdorf, M.D., Jennifer Hawthorne, Marci Shimoff, and Tom Newmark for their endorsements.

Thanks to my agent, Jeanne Fredericks, for "getting" my book and having absolute faith in it and me, and also for her extraordinary professionalism, excellent communication, experienced advice, deep devotion, hard work, and superb negotiating abilities. She deserves additional accolades for her patience and the time that she cheerfully offered to thoroughly answer all my questions. You'll find my name on the *long* list of her author/clients who "can't say enough good things about her."

I have an immense amount of gratitude to all the talented folks at Basic Health Publications, Inc., especially publisher Norman Goldfind for his belief in my book and for allowing me full creative expression; managing editor Carol Rosenberg for her masterful copyediting; editors Jane Morrill and Cheryl Hirsch for all their hard work; Gary Rosenberg for the book design and typesetting; and Mike Stromberg for the cover design.

Finally, I'd like to thank my mother, Beulah Horner. My mother's courageous battle with breast cancer sparked and fueled my passion and commitment to help stop this epidemic. Her tragic death from this disease was the inspiration for this book. She also was the one who taught me to believe in the message from an old Les Brown tune, "Shoot for the moon. Even if you miss, you'll land among the stars."

Thank you, Mom!

My Journey

hen I heard the news on October 21, 1998, that President Clinton had signed the Woman's Health and Cancer Rights Act into law, I wiped the tears from my eyes and gave my mom in heaven a high-five. "We did it, Mom!" I exulted.

It had been a tough five-year battle to get this legislation passed, but worth every frustration, every heartache, every late night, every dime. The new law meant that if a woman had to have a mastectomy, her insurance company would have to cover reconstructive breast surgery. In the early 1990s many insurance companies, in a misguided effort to save money, had decided to stop paying for this essential restorative operation. Now, coverage would be required, and every patient would have the chance to be made whole again.

This story begins seven years earlier, in the fall of 1991, when I opened my solo plastic surgery practice in the greater Cincinnati, Ohio area. At age thirty-three, I had finally completed twenty-seven years of intense training and education to realize my childhood dream of becoming a surgeon. It was extremely fulfilling to finally be able to help people with my surgical skills.

As I developed my practice over the next two years, I felt a special passion for serving a particular group of patients. They struck a deep personal chord within me because my mother was one of them. These were women with breast cancer.

One day in 1993, a young woman in her thirties sat anxiously in my office as she told me that the treatment of her breast cancer required mastectomies of both of her breasts. She wanted me to reconstruct them. Following her consultation, as required, I sent a letter to her insurer, Indiana Medicaid, requesting authorization to perform the reconstructive surgery. I thought the letter was a mere formality because insurance companies had always routinely paid for breast reconstruction after a mastectomy. But several weeks later, I received a reply saying that the surgery was "not medically indicated." Those words are insurance jargon that usually means, "There's no real reason to deny this surgery, but to cut costs so that we can protect corporate profits and our CEO's huge salary, and we're not paying for it."

I thought their decision was an administrative error and wrote to them again. It was not an error. The Medicaid insurance executive was unrelenting. This businessman declared again that the surgery was "not medically necessary."

Outraged, I decided that, no matter what it took, I would fight this horrendous ruling that prohibited my patient from being able to have a normal female form. The appeals process required that I first write several letters and participate in a series of telephone conference calls with various insurance company bureaucrats. The calls continued until I had worked up the entire ranks of Medicaid officials. At each step, their decision was always the same: "No."

Finally, I reached the top rung on the appeals process ladder. The only option I had left was to present the case before a judge at a state Medicaid hearing—the "supreme court" of the state-run Medicaid program. As I was driving to the hearing in a small rural town in Indiana about an hour and a half away from my office, it struck me that the appeals process was intentionally designed to be difficult, time-consuming, and financially costly, so that few, if any, doctors would follow it this far. But I didn't let that stop me. I wouldn't abandon my patient. I could relate too well to what she was going through.

Just imagine being told you have breast cancer. That news alone is horrific enough. But then, you're told you must have one or both of your breasts surgically removed. You're also told you'll be treated with poisonous chemicals that will make you very sick, cause all your hair to fall out, and possibly damage your vital organs. Your mind begins to race with questions that strike terror in your heart. Will this disease kill you? Will the side effects of the treatments make you wish you were dead? Will the postoperative pain be agonizing? Will your significant other still love you and find you sexually attractive? The only comforting news you hear is that you can be restored to physical wholeness with reconstructive breast surgery. A little patch of blue in the stormy sky. But shortly after this, you find out that your insurance company refuses to pay for this surgery. Your world caves in. Imagine.

That much bad news, in my experience as a physician, is too much for most women to bear. That an insurance company could deny a woman the opportunity to be made physically whole again after mutilating and defeminizing surgery strikes me as so incredibly heartless—it seems criminally inhumane. The thought of this injustice lit a fire in me and fueled my ability to persevere through any challenge.

Armed with stacks of published research, I pleaded my case to the judge. I presented studies documenting the enormously beneficial effects of breast reconstruction. They all showed that when women undergo breast reconstruction in the same operation as the mastectomy, they suffer far less emotional trauma. The judge—a woman—agreed, and I won my case.

During the appeals process, I'd realized that denying insurance coverage for breast reconstruction was an appalling symptom of a much larger problem: the widespread insurance-coverage discrimination against women. For example, in one of my appeal letters, I'd asked a simple pointed question: "Does Indiana Medicaid pay for penile reconstruction?" If they do, I'd argued, this was clearly a case of sexual discrimination. The written reply was, "Young lady, you are completely out of line!" That defensive and predictable response confirmed my suspicions.

As I was leaving the hearing, one of Medicaid's representatives, a woman, stopped me in the hall and said, "I'm so glad you won. You were right. Medicaid pays for penile reconstruction. They also pay for penile implants for sexual dysfunction. In fact, Medicaid pays more money every year for that procedure than for any other!"

Winning this case, however, wasn't the end of my battle for breast cancer patients—far from it. A short time later, I was shocked to discover that this case did not set a precedent and had no bearing on any future cases. Every Medicaid case is evaluated separately. That meant I would have to go through the same draining, time-consuming, costly, administrative slugfest for every single Medicaid patient who needed breast reconstruction!

Worse still, Medicaid suddenly wasn't the only insurance company denying breast reconstruction. Private insurers started jumping on the bandwagon. If Medicaid could save money this way and get away with it, they thought they could too. Then one day, a letter from Blue Cross and Blue Shield of Kentucky arrived that proclaimed that breast reconstruction for my thirty-three-year-old patient was unnecessary because there was no medical need to reconstruct "an organ with *no function*."

My eyes fixated on those five words: *an organ with no function.* "An organ with *no function*?" I yelled. "What kind of callous, cold-hearted idiot could say such a thing?" Waving the offensive letter in my hand, I stormed down my office hall, seething "You just said that to the wrong person. You will pay, and every insurer will pay!"

At the time, by no cosmic coincidence or accident, I was taking a series of courses designed to teach people how to live life more powerfully. I was in the third of a series of three courses called the "Curriculum for Living" sponsored by Landmark Education Corporation. The course was called "Self Expression and Leadership." Our assignment was to use all the skills we had learned to create and lead a project that would benefit others.

Instantly, I knew the goal for my project: Insurance coverage for reconstructive breast surgery for every woman who must have a mastectomy.

I knew this was no simple task because laws would have to be passed. To make matters even more challenging, I was working eighty hours a week in my surgical practice and I knew absolutely nothing about the political process. Worse yet, even with a doctorate, I had always been a little hesitant to speak up because I was afraid of sounding stupid. But I knew that if I kept following my heart, somehow I could make this happen.

And so the adventure began. And what an adventure it was—awe-inspiring, magical, and profoundly spiritual. On the other hand, it was also filled with extraordinarily difficult, frustrating, sometimes shocking experiences that required enormous perseverance, growth, and strength. But the miracles outweighed the obstacles. It seemed like everything and everyone I needed for the project magically fell into my lap. For example, deep into the project, I realized that Senator Ted Kennedy was the best person to sponsor the federal bill because of his success at getting health bills through Congress. I hadn't taken any action or spoken to anyone about this idea. A week later, out of the blue, a visiting plastic surgeon from Boston walked up to me at a state medical meeting and said, "I'm meeting with Ted Kennedy next week. Do you want me to ask him to sponsor your bill?"

From the moment I started this project, seemingly random offers of help and perfectly timed meetings and events like this happened so routinely, I came to expect it. It seemed like I had a direct line to God. "Ask and ye shall receive"— no kidding!

But, there were also many challenges—some seemingly insurmountable. When I launched the project, it made sense to focus on passing one federal law, rather than attempting to pass fifty separate state laws. Unfortunately, my legislative initiative came on the heels of the Clintons' failed National Healthcare Plan. The word in Washington was that *no* federal healthcare bills would even be considered. The news was a nightmare. Now, I *had* to pass fifty individual state laws. So, I took a deep breath and began planning, organizing, calling, and writing. Within a year, I had enrolled the help of plastic surgeons, breast cancer survivors, and numerous organizations in every state. And one by one, state laws began to pass.

Then, one morning in 1994, I got the darkest news yet. I learned that our successes in the states basically meant nothing, thanks to a loophole. A law called ERISA—the Employee Retirement Income Securities Act—contains language that excludes most people from the protection of state healthcare laws. To fulfill my commitment, I realized that a federal law would have to be passed, after all.

The challenge and chances of success seemed as intimidating as climbing Mt. Everest shoeless. But something personal and tragic happened in 1994 that cemented my resolve. My mother, the vibrant extraordinary woman who taught me to reach for the stars, was diagnosed with metastatic breast cancer in her bones. She had been treated for "early stage" breast cancer five years earlier. Everyone—her doctors, my dad, my brothers and sister, and I—thought that she was going to be fine. But she wasn't. Nine months later in the hospice, I held her hand and felt her spirit go free as she took her last breath.

She was seventy-five. She shouldn't have died that young. She was a Mac-Dougall—a Scottish clan known for their extraordinary strength, good health, and longevity. Virtually everyone in the family who preceded her had lived to be at least 100. My mom was in perfect health—that is, until she got cancer. She had done all the right things—yearly mammograms and breast self-exams (BSEs). Like me, she believed in Western medicine's advice and reassurance that if we do these "right" things, we can catch breast cancer "early" enough to save our lives. This isn't true for everyone—certainly not my mom. In some cases, it's only wishful thinking. The truth is, with this approach, there's absolutely no guarantee that we can catch breast cancer early enough to stop this killer and save lives.

I didn't want my mother's death from breast cancer to be another meaning-less statistic, a faceless number in the loss column. This abhorrent disease had stripped her of her dignity and cut her life short. I wanted her life, suffering, and untimely death to mean something for the world. Generally, I like to believe that everything happens for a reason. So, I decided my mother died of breast cancer to be a beacon of change for the world—through me. I pledged to myself that her untimely death would be a pivotal event in the worldwide fight against this disease. In addition, it fueled my commitment to get breast-reconstruction leg-islation passed. I decided no matter what it took, or how long it took, I would never give up. I would do it for her. I dedicated the project, now called the Breast Reconstruction Advocacy Project (BRA Project), to her memory.

By the time I faced the monumental task of achieving a federal bill, I had grown more politically savvy. I decided to go straight to the top, instead of work-ing up from the bottom. That meant I had to meet the President of the United States, Bill Clinton. I'd heard it said that we are only three people away from meeting anyone, so everywhere I went I started asking everyone, "Do you know how I can meet President Clinton?" Within two weeks, a friend introduced me to David, a member of the Federal Trade Commission. A few days later, I met David for lunch and told him about my plans. He told me he went to Wash-ington to meet with the President four times a year, and the next time he went, I could go with him.

Two days later, he called me and announced, "We're going on Tuesday."

"What?" I said, looking at my packed calendar with about forty patients scheduled for the office that day.

"Your patients will understand," he explained, "You're meeting *the President*. Oh, and by the way," he added, "there's one other thing. It will cost you $10,000. It's a fundraiser for the 1996 election and that's the minimum contribution."

Incredulous shock paralyzed me for a moment. "There's no way!" I yelped. "I can't do that."

"Look," he reasoned, "you don't understand. This is a once-in-a-lifetime opportunity. You can fundraise from your friends. It's for a good cause."

Suddenly, I had a strong feeling in my gut that said, "Do it." Because my gut rarely fails me, I listened. And so, a few days later, I was in Washington to meet the President.

A vague memory of a picture of Jacqueline Kennedy Onassis in *Life* magazine decades before completely shaped my decision to wear a perfect, black, strapless evening gown and elbow-length, black velvet gloves. I felt like a million bucks as I left my room at the Mayflower Hotel. After waltzing through the metal detector, I gave one final check and adjustment to my gown and gloves and entered the room—where everyone was wearing a business suit!

When I stopped to get my seat assignment, I was told that the President's table was short one woman and that I'd been moved there. The attendant wanted to know if that was okay. Without a moment's hesitation, I responded, "Absolutely!"

As I headed for my table, my embarrassment intensified as heads swiveled in my direction.

"Thanks for dressing for us," one of David's friends quipped as I walked by.

"Oh, you're welcome," I said with a genuine smile, my embarrassment fading. "It was really no trouble at all." I realized I might as well make the best of my faux pas and enjoy myself.

An hour later, the President arrived. He was taller than I had imagined, with a ruddy complexion and gray hair—and yes, he is as charming and charismatic as legend says.

I waited patiently on the receiving line to meet him. When I finally made it to the front, I reached out to shake his hand. "I'm Dr. Christine Horner," I said.

"Yes, I know who you are," he replied, grasping my hand with a firm shake. "You live across the river from Cincinnati and you're working on legislation about breast cancer. And I believe you are sitting at my table tonight, aren't you?"

"Why, yes, I am," I answered, trying to hide my astonishment. He really was amazing! I had been asked to send information about myself before the event because the President liked to be briefed about everyone he would be meeting. I had heard that he never forgot a name or a face, but still, I was impressed.

"I'll see you later at the table," he said as the next person in line moved up to shake his hand.

My place at the large round table was directly across from the President's. The twelve feet between us made it too difficult to have a conversation. Endless streams of people came up to speak to him throughout the meal. As the evening passed and the time for him to give his speech rapidly approached, I was struck with the thought that I had just spent $10,000 to talk to the President, and I might not get to do it. In a mild panic, I leaned as far across the table as I could, caught his eye, and shouted, "I want to talk to you!" He jumped a little and called back across the expanse, "Okay. I'll come and get you after my speech and we can talk."

After giving his twenty-minute speech, he left the podium and, as promised, came by the table and signaled to me to follow him. I rose from my chair and walked behind him. He shook hands, smiled, and bid good-bye to everyone with sweet, laid-back Southern charm. I followed him into the hallway, and the doors closed behind us.

Swarms of Secret Service descended upon him. He began snapping his fingers at his assistants. "Give it to me now," the President demanded. Papers were thrust at him from all directions, and he began signing them with rapid-fire dedication. At the same time, streams of young men updated him on the latest happenings in quick sound bites. Tension was high, and he was working at lightning speed. I looked on in amazement.

Suddenly, he turned to me. "Now, what is it you want to say?" he asked in a relaxed tone that contradicted the chaos.

I was still reeling from the urgency and pressure of moments ago, and my knees felt weak. I felt like Dorothy trembling before the Wizard of Oz. One minute of presidential time seemed equivalent to an hour, so I quickly regained my composure and started speaking as fast as I could. I told him about the problems with insurance companies denying coverage for breast reconstruction and our efforts to get a bill to Congress. He jotted down a few notes and seemed genuinely interested. Then he told me he would look into it and see what he could do. Moments later, he and his entourage left the building.

Three days later, I received a call from a member of the Democratic National Committee. "We like your spunk," he said. "Normally a $10,000 contribution is the cost for two people to attend a fundraising event. Since you came by yourself, we'd like to invite you to meet with the President again when he comes to Cincinnati in two days."

Wearing just the right business suit this time, I listened intently as the President gave his speech at the private luncheon. When he turned to leave, I sprang from my chair. I leaped in front of him, blocking his path up the stairs to the men's room. Dorothy was gone, and Xena the Warrior Princess had taken her place! With less than a half a foot between us, I met his eyes directly and said, "My mother died of breast cancer, and so did yours. We can make a tribute to our mothers' lives by passing breast-reconstruction legislation!"

He snapped his fingers at an assistant and asked for his business card—the one with his private address at the Oval Office printed on it. Handing it to me, he said, "Send me a packet of information at this address."

I did. A few weeks later, I received a letter on White House stationery, personally signed by the President, thanking me for the information and promising he would look into the matter.

That meeting led to more meetings, including several with First Lady Hillary Clinton and her staff in the West Wing of the White House. Suddenly doors began to open. Media coverage for the project exploded. Several major women's magazines called for interviews, including *Glamour, Allure, Elle,* and *Ms.* There were dozens of television, radio, and newspaper interviews. It seemed like everyone across the country wanted to get on board.

I was buoyed with optimism when the bill was introduced to Congress in 1997. Then, it stalled. It was promptly put into legislative committee—"a black hole," as it's also known—where it sat for two years, seemingly dead. I knew that bills rarely, if ever, pass on their own merit; they only make it through by being tagged on to a larger, "moving" bill. But even that wasn't working. The reconstruction legislation was tagged on to every moving bill, but none passed. With only a day left of the 1998 Congressional session, it looked as if the situation were hopeless. Sure enough, I received a phone call that day from a staff liaison for the American Society of Plastic Surgeons. His words cut through me like a knife. "Bad news, Christine; it's all over. There aren't any other bills to tag it on to."

My heart sank. I couldn't believe that all those years of hard work with such clear divine support could end like this. We had come so close!

The next day, my secretary knocked on the door while I was examining a patient. She rarely interrupted me, and I thought something must be terribly wrong.

"You have an urgent phone call you must take now," she said. My heart raced as I picked up the phone. Then I heard the voice of the same staffer, but his tone was entirely different. He sounded elated.

"It passed!" he said.

"What?" I said. "What did you say?"

"It got tagged on to the budget bill at the last minute and it passed!" he exclaimed.

In a daze I thanked him and hung up the phone. Then I burst into tears, and gave my mom a high-five. My heart spoke the words, "We did it, Mom!" and her spirit filled the room. My mother's great sacrifice *had* made a difference. Her life and death would help millions of women. At least now they could be spared the trauma of not being able to have reconstructive surgery.

During this campaign I met with many powerful, creative, and amazing people: the President, senators, congressmen, and governors. To every one of the elected officials who supported the legislation I give my undying gratitude: President Clinton, First Lady Hillary Clinton, Senator Ted Kennedy, Senator Alfonse D'Amato, Congresswoman Anna Eshoo, Congresswoman Sue Kelly, Kentucky Governor Patton and his wife, Judy Patton, and a whole host of other dignitaries. I also had the pleasure of working with fifty wonderful plastic surgeons who took on leadership roles to pass the legislation in their own states. There was an enormous number of remarkable people who helped along the way. Without every one of them, the legislative project would never have succeeded the way that it did.

But deep within, at the moment of this great victory, something troubled me. One problem was solved, but another, much greater problem remained and clouded the celebration—the growing *epidemic* of breast cancer. In the United States, breast cancer strikes an appalling, ever-increasing number of women. Why was it still growing? How could we stop it? I knew there had to be answers. So began a new and far more important mission: to trace the tracks of this killer back to its root causes and help protect women from developing breast cancer in the first place.

My search began with the collection of all the published medical research, and what I found inspired me, gave me hope, and then outraged me. I found *many* research-proven "natural" ways women can significantly lower their risk of breast cancer. Not only can these foods, herbs, spices, supplements, and lifestyle choices lower the risk, but good solid research published in peer-reviewed journals shows that they can also help women already diagnosed with breast cancer by slowing down tumor growth, preventing metastasis, and even shrinking the size of their tumors. Many of these natural techniques have been found to increase the effectiveness of Western medical treatments (chemotherapy and radiation) and protect against their harmful side effects.

But most doctors, as well as most women, are completely unaware of this lifesaving information. One explanation could be that these techniques—most having roots in ancient traditional systems of medicine—are nonpharmaceutical and nonsurgical. In other words, these techniques are not generally included in Western medicine and won't create any significant financial rewards. So, tragically, our economically driven system of medicine has no incentive to get this information out.

I, however, do.

In 1999, I helped create the first syndicated television news segment devoted to teaching people how to prevent common diseases and stay healthy using the research-proven techniques of complementary and alternative medicine. I was also the host and medical editor of the segment, which aired in Cincinnati on the ABC and NBC affiliates and was then syndicated to the Wisdom Television Network.

In 2002, my passion for teaching natural preventative medicine led me to jump off another professional cliff. I left my plastic surgery practice to dedicate my life full-time to writing and teaching. First on my agenda was to write this book.

Waking the Warrior Goddess: Dr. Christine Horner's Program to Protect Against & Fight Breast Cancer reveals all the best, research-proven, natural approaches scientists have found that substantially lower the risk of breast cancer. When used in conjunction with standard medical treatments for women with breast cancer, these same techniques can help to improve their chances of survival.

From my work on the legislative project, I learned that powerful and magical things happen when you envision a better life for the future and enroll other people into that vision. With this book I declare the following vision for the world: All women experience perfect health because they recognize and use their powerful inner ability to heal themselves.

How to Use This Book

ou have the power and ability to influence your state of health more than you ever imagined. Your choices every day significantly influence your chances of staying healthy or developing a terrible disease such as breast cancer. Genetics and luck have very little to do with your risk of developing most chronic disorders, including breast cancer. This book will teach you how to protect your breasts and your overall health. It includes more than fifty different research-proven ways to lower your risk of breast cancer, and if you have breast cancer, these same techniques—when done in conjunction with Western medical treatments—improve your chances of survival. Chapter 29 puts all of the risk-lowering techniques together in an easy thirty-step program.

If you are eager to do everything you can to protect yourself quickly, you can complete the program in thirty days. But don't pressure yourself to adopt all the new habits in thirty days if it's not comfortable. The program can be completed in thirty weeks or thirty months if that works better for you. Each day, week, or month you start doing something new will make a substantial difference in lowering your risk. By the end of the month or year, you'll be doing everything science knows how to do to lower your risk of breast cancer. When added up, the amount of risk reduction you'll enjoy won't simply be the sum of all the parts—it will increase exponentially.

In preparing to write this book, I conducted an exhaustive study of the medical literature on breast cancer. I pulled out all the articles on anything and everything that showed a statistically significant benefit in lowering your risk of this disease. To my knowledge, virtually everything we know to date about lowering the risk of breast cancer is covered in this book. Keep in mind, research shows that almost everything that can help to lower your risk of breast cancer can *also* improve your chance of survival if you already have the disease. These techniques and recommendations should not be used as a replacement for Western medicine, but rather as support for the treatments. We will undoubtedly know much more in the near future. For example, scientists have found that nearly all vegetables and fruits have a variety of cancer-fighting properties. As researchers begin to analyze individual plants—vegetables, fruits, herbs, and spices—I'm sure many of them will prove helpful in preventing and fighting breast cancer.

Reading a research-based book can sometimes be a little dry and boring. For that reason, I wrote this book from a slightly different angle. First, I use principles of *Ayurveda,* the oldest and most complete system of prevention-oriented holistic health still practiced today, as a basis for many of the recommendations for natural approaches that protect against breast cancer. Second, I use a metaphor—the Warrior Goddess—for the body's internal healing intelligence.

Ayurveda originated in the *Vedic* culture—an advanced culture that thrived more than 5,000 years ago in the area of the world that is now India. Today, various fragmented forms of *Ayurveda* are practiced in India, Sri Lanka, and southern Asia. About one-sixth of the world's population uses *Ayurveda* as its primary form of medical care.

Although *Ayurveda* treats diseases, in its purest original form it is a comprehensive system of *preventative* medicine. It masterfully teaches people how to become and stay healthy. I think of *Ayurveda* as the cosmic download of all the timeless laws of Nature that help guide us to keep our mind/body strong. It describes thousands of laws governing the intricacies of our complex, sophisticated, and infinitely amazing physiology.

You can use these laws of Nature expressed in the principles of *Ayurveda* to help you make intelligent choices that beneficially impact your health. This knowledge can help guide you to choose only those things that are health-supporting and avoid those things that are not. The *Ayurvedic* principles will also give you a context in which to understand each item presented in this book. They give you a broader and deeper understanding of why each item benefits your health and protects you from developing diseases, especially breast cancer.

At the heart of *Ayurveda* is the recognition of a divine, natural healing intelligence that exists in each of us. According to *Ayurveda,* diseases arise from imbalances that occur when this intelligence is subverted by poor choices, such as certain foods and lifestyles. These imbalances block the full expression of this healing intelligence, eventually weakening it to where it can no longer keep you well. In time, the body begins to break down and diseases begin to manifest.

Health is only regained and maintained by enhancing the healing intelligence, keeping it lively and flowing.

In *Waking the Warrior Goddess,* this healing intelligence is personified as a Warrior Goddess. This is not just a creative archetype. When considering the human body and all its extraordinary complex functions, the image that emerges that best represents the managing intelligence is one of a multitasking Warrior Goddess. She is supernatural in strength and power and vastly discriminating in her intellect. Yet, she is delicate and very particular. This metaphor accurately reflects both the mastery and the magnificence of the intelligence that manages the trillions of biochemical reactions simultaneously occurring in our bodies at any given moment. It also provides a new perspective for appreciating the importance of providing attentive care and nurturance for this extraordinary body that each of us has been given. Like a Goddess, this managing intelligence's majesty and splendor depends on respecting its very precise and specific demands. *Waking the Warrior Goddess* teaches a woman about her Warrior Goddess—what weakens her, and what makes her strong and invincible. The symbol of the Warrior Goddess also helps to transform the abstract—but nonetheless phenomenal—physics, chemistry, and biology of the body into an intimate, personal, and powerful friend.

Because every woman's risk of breast cancer is real, I encourage you to begin the thirty-step program immediately. Make it fun. Make it an adventure. Find a girlfriend to join you. Or organize a group of friends, and meet once a week to encourage and support one another and share experiences. Research shows meeting with a group of supportive friends regularly is strong preventive medicine, too. Adopting even some of these simple, but powerful techniques will improve how you feel and lower your risk of breast cancer. Depending on your current state of health, the improvement could be quite dramatic.

My greatest wish, hope, and dream is this: that this knowledge becomes common knowledge; that people use this information and adopt these health-preserving habits; that the incidence of breast cancer radically drops; and that the world is filled with people experiencing perfect health and enlightenment.

Though no one can go back and make a brand new start,
anyone can start from now and make a brand new ending.

—AUTHOR UNKNOWN

Part One

Modern Beast and Ancient Slayer

The Basics of Breast Cancer and *Ayurveda*

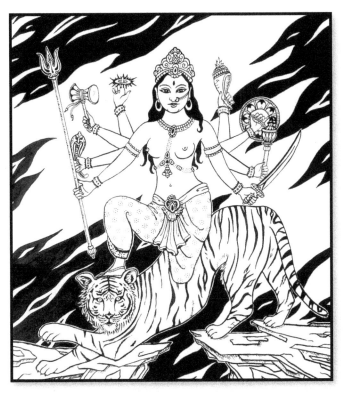

Durga, the Warrior Goddess

Chapter 1

Breast Cancer Epidemic
The Numbers, the Fears,
and the Possibility of Prevention

When solving problems, dig at the roots
instead of just hacking at the leaves.

—ANTHONY J. D'ANGELO, *THE COLLEGE BLUE BOOK*

reast cancer is a killer beast with a voracious appetite. Every year it attacks tens of thousands of women. It isn't attracted to children, but once a woman reaches her mid-twenties, she will catch its attention and it will start to stalk her. Generally, like most hunters, breast cancer prefers a slower easier target, so it particularly likes older women—in fact, the older the better. And the more meat on their bones—actually, the more extra fat—the better. This savage killer finds women particularly delectable if they have just been brought to their knees by a major emotional trauma. It doesn't care about race, religious beliefs, finances, or marital status.

Breast cancer is a womanizer. It finds most women equally desirable, but there are a few things that make a woman absolutely irresistible. If breast cancer were to place an ad for the female of its dreams, it would go something like this:

> SEARCHING FOR AN OVERWEIGHT, older, American or Western European woman to take on a short, extremely emotional ride; someone who loves to stay up all night drinking alcohol and eating red meat, junk food, and sugary desserts—that is, on the nights she's not working the graveyard shift; a woman who thinks organically raised fruit, vegetables, and whole grains aren't foods; a person who loves to burn the candle at both ends, thrives on stress, isn't into exercising, has been a smoker since she was a teenager, and who puts everyone else's needs before her own.

Not the normal type of ad you'd see in a singles column, but for breast cancer, this type of woman is perfect.

Although breast cancer loves all women in general, the good news is, it has preferences. By being aware of them, you can make yourself much less desirable. This book will teach you how to make yourself as *unattractive* to this monster as possible.

First, let's take a look at the breast cancer battlefield. You need to know a few things about the enemy's current position and force: where it is, how far it has advanced, who is on the front lines and at greater risk, and the current casualty and death toll. Then, you'll learn about its strengths and weaknesses, and together, we'll plan a strategy to slay this beast. What you'll learn in this book will cut the enemy's supply lines and raise a wall of protection. Breast cancer can be conquered. Knowledge is power. Together, we can end this epidemic.

YOUR RISK

Breast cancer is the most common cancer among American women and the second-leading cause of cancer deaths. In 2013, the latest statistics available from the American Cancer Society, the Centers for Disease Control and Prevention, and the National Cancer Institute's SEER (Surveillance Epidemiology and End Results) Cancer Statistics Review were from data collected through 2009. At some point in their lives, 12.4% of American women will be diagnosed with this deadly disease. The older a woman is, the higher her risk. At age thirty, her risk is 1 in 227. At forty, her risk climbs to 1 in 68. A woman at age fifty has a 1 in 42 chance, and at age sixty the risk elevates to 1 in 28. If she lives to be more than eighty, her risk is 1 in 8. Conversely in a more optimistic view, the chance that an American woman will never develop breast cancer is 87.6 percent or about 7 in 8. The 1 in 8 risk of an American woman developing breast cancer you hear most commonly quoted, actually refers to a woman's *lifetime risk*—in other words, what a woman's risk is if she lives to the average life expectancy of seventy-five years or older.

It is also important to remember that these statistics are based on averages for the whole population. A woman's individual risk may be higher or lower depending on many different factors. The good news is that most of those factors are within your control and when you finish reading this book, you'll have all the tools you need to lower your risk as much possible.

The American Cancer Society (ACS) estimates that in 2011, 230,480 women were diagnosed with invasive breast cancer (versus 211,731 in 2009), and nearly 39,520 died because of it. An additional 57,650 women were diagnosed with in situ carcinoma, which is considered a tumor marker—meaning, those who have it are at a much higher risk of developing invasive breast cancer in the future. However, most women who are diagnosed with carcinoma in situ will never develop the invasive disease.

Men can develop breast cancer, but the incidence is rare. Ninety–nine percent of all breast cancers arise in women and only 1 percent occurs in men. In 2011, about 2,140 men were diagnosed with breast cancer and 450 died from this disease. The National Cancer Institute (NCI) estimates that in 2011 in the United States, 2.6 million women were alive who have had a history of breast cancer.

Between the years of 1990 and 1998 the incidence of breast cancer rose approximately 1.7 percent per year. Starting in 1998, for the first time the rate began to fall. From 1998 through 2002, it dropped approximately 1 percent per year. A study that was conducted at MD Anderson Cancer Center in Houston and presented at a breast cancer symposium in San Antonia, Texas, on December 14, 2006 found that 14,000 fewer women were diagnosed with breast cancer in 2003 than in 2002—a 7 percent drop in the rate of breast cancer in just one year. The incidence of estrogen-sensitive tumors in women ages fifty to sixty-nine in 2003 fell even more: 12 percent. Although it will take years of data analysis to determine exactly why the rate suddenly dropped, many researchers theorize that the significant decrease in prescribing hormone replacement therapy (HRT) after it was found to increase the risk of breast cancer, as well as several of other serious health conditions, may be the primary reason. However other researchers, such as Samuel Shapiro's group at the University of Cape Town in South Africa, point out that a causal relationship cannot be concluded from the HRT/breast cancer studies and that declines in breast cancer incidence should have continued if that were true. But, breast cancer rates have remained relatively stable in women since 2003. The reasons for the decline may be impossible to determine.

The incidence of advanced breast cancer in American women younger than forty years old, however, is on the rise according to an analysis that was published in February 2013 in the *Journal of the American Medical Association*. Data collected from 1976 to 2009 found that the incidence for women between the ages of twenty-five and thirty-nine, who were initially diagnosed with breast cancer that had spread to other areas of the body, almost doubled during that time. The reason for this rise is impossible to know for sure, but researchers suspect it may have something to do with environmental causes, including rising obesity rates, stress, poor diets, and endocrine-disrupting chemicals commonly found in our food, water, and environment.

Even with the numbers staying relatively stable in the last decade, these statistics are alarming and most women are terrified of getting breast cancer. Being diagnosed with breast cancer, even at early stages is bad enough, but worse yet,

RISK AND BRCA GENES

On May 14, 2013, the world woke to the shocking news that Angelina Jolie, a young actress and humanitarian graced with exceptional beauty and fame, and a mother of six, had undergone a double mastectomy and breast reconstruction. A blood test revealed that she had the BRCA1 gene mutation. Her doctors told her that her risk of developing breast cancer was 87 percent. Angelina said that the reason she decided to let the public know about her health situation was to raise awareness about this genetic condition and to help other women not to be afraid to take action. Surgery may have been the best course of action for Ms. Jolie, but it may not be for many other women with the BRCA gene mutations.

What BRCA Genes Do

The BRCA1 and BRCA2 genes are classified as tumor-suppression genes. The acronyms come from the full names of the genes: breast cancer susceptibility gene 1 and breast cancer susceptibility gene 2. They give instructions for proteins to suppress tumor growth and to help repair damaged DNA. Your DNA is a frequent target for assaults from a variety sources, especially from oxygen free radicals and toxins. Because injuries are common, your body keeps a repair crew on call to fix the damage. But, if the crew lacks the right tools to repair the DNA—as it does with BRCA gene mutations—misinformation can be passed on that may lead to cancer.

Specific types of mutations of the BRCA1 and BRCA2 genes are associated with a significantly higher risk of breast and ovarian cancer. These abnormal genes also increase the risk of other cancers including cancers of the cervix, uterus, pancreas, colon, stomach, gallbladder, and skin (melanoma). Men can also have a BRCA1 mutation and they are at a higher risk for developing prostate cancer at a younger age.

Most women do not carry the BRCA mutations. In fact, over 99 percent of us do not. Only about 5 to 7 percent of women diagnosed with breast cancer have this defect. This means that for the vast majority of women, the major risk factors for developing breast cancer are not genetic, but rather come from influences under our control, such as diet and lifestyle. These same diet and lifestyle factors also impact the risk of breast cancer in women with malfunctions in their BRCA genes.

Should You Be Tested for BRCA1 and 2?

Because problems in the BRCA genes are uncommon, testing is not routinely recommended. Women with a strong family history of breast and ovarian cancer, especially diagnosed at younger ages, may want to seek genetic counseling. There are many controversial issues regarding genetic testing that you should fully explore with your doctor before you consent to the test. If you do decide to be tested for the BRCA genes, make sure you educate yourself as much as possible about all of your options.

How to Dodge the BRCA Bullet

The most important point for you to know is this: Not everyone who has a BRCA gene mutation develops breast cancer. Estimates currently are about 80 percent of women with this defect will develop breast cancer if they live to be eighty years of age—20 percent will not. When the family lineages for those who carry the BRCA gene mutations have been traced back in time, the risk of developing breast cancer in the past was found to be much lower. A study published in 2008 found that women who were born before 1930 with mutations of the BRCA genes, had an 8 percent chance of developing breast cancer before age forty, whereas those born after 1940 have a 22 percent risk. In other words, the risk of breast cancer is three times higher now than it used to be.

With this news, two important questions may have popped up for you: Why do some women with the gene mutations avoid cancer? And why was the risk much lower in the past? No doubt the answers are linked to diet and lifestyle choices—just as they are for women who do not have this genetic defect.

There are few published studies that focus on the influence that diet and lifestyle have on the risk of breast cancer in women with BRCA mutations. However, the studies that are available do show that consuming certain foods and dietary supplements reduces the risk—substantially. The foods and supplements include:

❏ **Caffeinated coffee** (Chapter 11, page 127): Drinking several cups of joe a day can drop the risk for those with the BRCA1 gene mutation by as much as 70 percent!

❏ **Selenium** (Chapter 13, page 144): This essential mineral has several anticancer properties, including helping to repair oxidative DNA

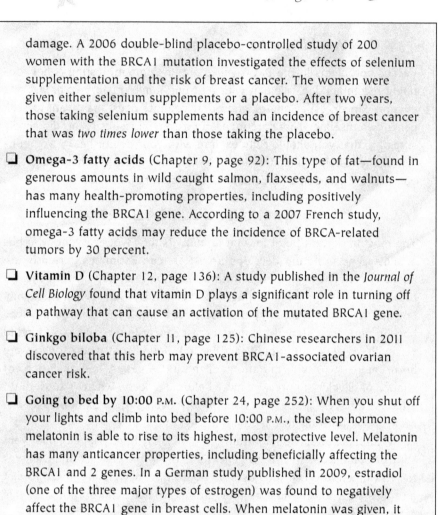

damage. A 2006 double-blind placebo-controlled study of 200 women with the BRCA1 mutation investigated the effects of selenium supplementation and the risk of breast cancer. The women were given either selenium supplements or a placebo. After two years, those taking selenium supplements had an incidence of breast cancer that was *two times lower* than those taking the placebo.

❑ **Omega-3 fatty acids** (Chapter 9, page 92): This type of fat—found in generous amounts in wild caught salmon, flaxseeds, and walnuts—has many health-promoting properties, including positively influencing the BRCA1 gene. According to a 2007 French study, omega-3 fatty acids may reduce the incidence of BRCA-related tumors by 30 percent.

❑ **Vitamin D** (Chapter 12, page 136): A study published in the *Journal of Cell Biology* found that vitamin D plays a significant role in turning off a pathway that can cause an activation of the mutated BRCA1 gene.

❑ **Ginkgo biloba** (Chapter 11, page 125): Chinese researchers in 2011 discovered that this herb may prevent BRCA1-associated ovarian cancer risk.

❑ **Going to bed by 10:00 P.M.** (Chapter 24, page 252): When you shut off your lights and climb into bed before 10:00 P.M., the sleep hormone melatonin is able to rise to its highest, most protective level. Melatonin has many anticancer properties, including beneficially affecting the BRCA1 and 2 genes. In a German study published in 2009, estradiol (one of the three major types of estrogen) was found to negatively affect the BRCA1 gene in breast cells. When melatonin was given, it almost completely counteracted the bad effects of estradiol.

BRCAs on-the-Blink Means Choices

If you are diagnosed with a BRCA gene mutation, surgery may be a good choice to cut your risk, but don't think it's your only choice. Research supports that adopting as many healthy diet and lifestyle habits presented in this book as possible will dramatically reduce your odds. There are many safe and very effective technologies, such as thermography and ultrasound (discussed in the next section) that can be used to monitor the health of your breasts and ovaries. With regular screenings, potential problems can be caught in their earliest stage—before they become a serious or life-threatening problem. The radiation from mammograms or other imaging devices for women with the BRCA gene mutations can cause a significant jump in breast cancer risk, especially for women under thirty. So I recommend that you avoid these tests and instead choose those that do not use radiation.

Keep in mind that if you carry the BRCA gene mutations, there are many options to lower your risk. Numerous considerations go in to determining what course of action may be best for each individual. Surgery may be the superior approach in certain situations. However for most women, effective safe alternatives to surgery may be a wiser. As a former surgeon, I recommend you consider them first. Your circumstances are unique, so make sure you educate yourself as much as possible to determine which path is right for you.

can be the treatments of this disease. Although they may be effective for many women, the treatments can be horrendous: potentially mutilating surgery, damaging radiation, and injections of severely toxic chemical poisons. As Dr. Susan Love, author of *Dr. Susan Love's Breast Book* and *Dr. Susan Love's Hormone Book*, says, the treatment of breast cancer is "slash, burn, and poison." No wonder women are terrified.

Examination Isn't Prevention

Doctors aren't taught much about prevention because Western medicine does not make prevention a priority. The priority is to treat a disease you already have, not prevent you from getting it in the first place.

When I was trained as a surgeon and as a spokesperson for the American Cancer Society, I was taught that there was no known cause and no known cure for breast cancer. The belief was, the only thing you can do is to try to catch the disease "early" using mammograms and breast exams. But catching a cancer in a "treatable stage" isn't what you really want, either. Anyone who has been diagnosed with breast cancer (or is close to someone who has) knows that the diagnosis of breast cancer is devastating—no matter when it is detected. Who wants to be slashed, burned, and poisoned? And, after going through all these treatments, there's no guarantee that your cancer is gone. These treatments don't always work, even for cancers that are caught "early." For instance, my mother never missed an annual mammogram and regularly examined her own breasts.

Her cancer was caught "early" by Western standards. The tumor was less than 1 cm in diameter and had not spread to her lymph nodes. Statistically, she shouldn't have died from breast cancer—but she did, five years later in 1994.

Although the Western medical community's intentions are good, this approach to mammograms and breast exams is *not* prevention. It only exposes the disease once you have it. Given these facts, it wouldn't be surprising if you believed that there isn't much you can do to decrease your chances of getting breast cancer. You may believe it's all due to bad luck or bad genes.

If you believe that, you're mistaken.

Mammograms and Other Technologies

There's no question that mammograms are a useful screening tool. They have helped us find cancers at earlier, more treatable stages and have helped save lives. However, mammograms aren't perfect. This test uses potentially dangerous radiation, can be painful, can't see through "dense" breast tissue (found typically in most women younger than forty which is why mammography is not recommended for that age group), and doesn't work well for women with breast implants. At its best, a mammogram can only "see" breast cancers that produce calcium or significant masses—about 70 to 80 percent of all breast cancers. Regardless of their size, 20 to 30 percent of breast cancers won't show up on a mammogram. So, women with these "invisible" tumors feel falsely reassured by normal mammograms, and diagnosis of their cancers may be dangerously delayed. In addition, *80 percent* of the findings on a mammogram that are "suspicious" enough to lead to a breast biopsy are *not* cancers. In other words, mammograms wrongly suspect the presence of breast cancer *80 percent of the time*! In a study published in the *Archives of Internal Medicine* in May 2004, obese women were found to have a 20 percent increased risk of having false-positive mammography results.

The financial and emotional costs of the "false-positive" readings from mammography are enormous. More than 1 million breast biopsies are performed in the United States every year. That means approximately 800,000 women undergo expensive, physically traumatizing, and emotionally devastating surgical breast biopsies *unnecessarily* every year. False-positive mammograms don't just cause immediate emotional distress; they also cause long-lasting psychological problems, according to an article published in the *Annals of Family Medicine* in March 2013. Psychological testing showed that women who were given a false-positive diagnosis on their mammogram remained as upset six months later as those women who were diagnosed with breast cancer. Three years later, women with false-positive mammograms still exhibited psychological disturbances.

The most concerning problem with mammography comes from the fact that this technology requires potentially health-damaging radiation. In the past, the risk of radiation associated with mammography was hypothetical. But now, there are numerous studies documenting that mammograms increase the risk of the very disease from which they are supposed to save lives! For certain groups of women, the risk is not small. A European study published in 2012 found that when those who have the genetic predisposition for breast cancer (BRCA1 or BRCA2 gene mutation) are exposed to any diagnostic radiation before age thirty, their risk of breast cancer increases by 90 percent. The study also found that a history of mammography before age thirty raised the risk by 43 percent. In fact, even one mammogram before the age of thirty for those with the BRCA1 gene mutation was associated with an increased risk.

Because of the well-recognized shortcomings and potential dangers of mammography, additional tests, such as ultrasounds and magnetic resonance imaging (MRI) scans, are frequently employed. An ultrasound uses sound waves to show images of the tissues in the body. It is safe, noninvasive, and painless. But the conventional B-mode ultrasounds don't give enough information to be valuable as a screening or diagnostic tool for breast cancer. This type of ultrasound can only be used to determine whether a breast mass is cystic or solid (solid masses are of more concern). Recently, a more sophisticated type of ultrasound called a "3-D ultrasound" has been shown to be particularly helpful for screening women with dense breasts. A 2012 study found that it was able to detect three times the number of breast cancers compared to mammography alone in women with greater than 50 percent breast density.

Another type of ultrasound was developed in the United States in the 1990s and became commercially available in the 2000s that has an additional software technology called "elastography." Based on the fact that cancerous tissue is generally stiff compared to benign tissue, this ultrasound uses a color mode that shows the elastic or flexible properties of tissues. Firm tissue associated with cancer will show up as a different color than benign processes and softer background tissue. A study published in the 2007 *Journal of Ultrasound Medicine* compared ultrasound elastography, mammography, and conventional sonography in the diagnosis of a solid breast tumor. The researchers found that ultrasound elastography was superior to conventional sonography, and equal to, or superior to mammography in differentiating benign from malignant lesions in the breast. A combination of sonography with elastography ultrasound had the very best results in detecting cancer. This study, as well as many others published since then, conclude that elastography ultrasound may be very helpful for detecting cancers without using harmful radiation and for reducing the number of unnecessary biopsies from false-positive mammography readings.

MRI scans use a magnetic field instead of radiation to generate images of the interior structures of the body. These scans are safe for most people, painless, and noninvasive. They are very good at revealing the minute structural changes associated with breast tumors, including those that mammograms might miss. But like mammograms, MRI scans aren't very specific; they frequently show areas that are "suspicious" for breast cancer, but that are actually benign. So MRI scans also lead to excessive numbers of unnecessary biopsies. Another downside of MRI scans is that they are very expensive. The average cost for a breast MRI in 2013 was $2,850—a price too high to make it practical as a primary screening tool.

We need a highly accurate, inexpensive, noninvasive, painless, safe test that can show abnormalities at very early stages. Recent research shows that there is a reemerging technology with all these qualities that shows tremendous potential as a screening tool for breast cancer. It's called "thermography."

Thermography uses infrared technology to detect heat. It was first developed by the military in the early 1950s as a way to see enemy forces at night—by sensing their heat and movement. In the early 1960s, thermography was introduced in a very rudimentary form for medical use. It was approved by the FDA in 1982, but unfortunately, this promising technology fell out of favor when it was prematurely, hastily, and haphazardly included in the Breast Cancer Detection Demonstration Project, a large national study of mammography. Poor training, quality controls, and equipment led to misinterpretations and the false conclusion that thermography wasn't a valuable screening tool for breast cancer. But a few individuals, believing in its potential, persevered.

Since then, thermography equipment has vastly improved. The digital cameras and computer-software systems that are now available are so sophisticated that their high-resolution images and precise heat-variation calculations generate extremely valuable information. Research shows that, unlike mammograms, when thermography suspects something is wrong, it usually is. A study published in the *American Journal of Radiology* in January 2003 concluded that this technology could help prevent most unnecessary breast biopsies: "Infrared imaging (thermography) offers a safe noninvasive procedure that would be valuable as an adjunct to mammography in determining whether a lesion is benign or malignant."

A breast thermogram is a digital infrared picture that reveals the heat and vascular patterns of the breast tissue. These patterns change when a breast tumor starts to grow. Breast cancer cells require new blood vessels to feed them nutrients and oxygen. These new blood vessels don't grow like normal blood vessels. Instead, they grow in characteristically abnormal patterns, and they generate increased heat that is detectable by thermography.

Thermography can detect breast cancers much earlier than any other available technology. Because blood vessels ordinarily start to grow *before* any other significant changes and tumor growth, a thermogram can "see" these abnormal physiological processes as early as five to ten years *before* a cancer can be seen by a mammogram, MRI, or ultrasound or felt by a physical exam. What is most exciting is that when these abnormal processes are caught this early, they are *reversible*. The warning patterns seen by thermography have been found to resolve and return to normal after only a few short months of the healthy diet and lifestyle changes presented in this book. Simply taking certain dietary supplements can also cause dramatic improvements in a few weeks. Thermographers have reported consistent striking improvements in thermograms in just eight to twelve weeks in women who took *Protective Breast Formula*—a tablet which contains a combination of seven dietary supplements, including turmeric, green tea, maitake mushrooms, vitamin D_3, grape seed extract, and two plant chemicals found in cruciferous vegetables: diindolylmethane (DIM) and calcium D-glucarate. You can read more about it on my website: www.drchristinehorner.com.

A very simple way to understand thermography is to think of it as a thermometer. Long before a tumor forms, your breasts will usually become inflamed and run a fever. A thermogram shows you a picture of the temperature of your breasts. If one or both of your breasts are running a fever—a thermogram will show you. For a fever, aspirin usually helps bring it down. Similarly, if you take dietary supplements that have strong anti-inflammatory, antioxidant, and other health-promoting properties, your breast fever will improve.

Thus, thermography is the first tool we have that shows promise at being able to pick up changes in the breast that are so early—at a stage that involves only precancerous physiological changes—that women can reverse these changes and avoid getting breast cancer by making a few simple diet and lifestyle modifications.

The potential of this technology is electrifying. In the near future, thermography may play a dominant role in the screening and prevention of breast cancer. But before that can happen, many well-designed studies must be conducted to understand what the full potential of thermography really is: its precise capabilities and limitations, how it can best be used, where it fits in with other technologies, and how to properly evaluate and interpret the information it generates.

How to Lower Your Risk

Research shows that there are many natural, nonpharmaceutical, nonsurgical approaches that can substantially lower your risk of developing breast cancer. The medical literature is full of studies that have found strong anticancer effects in many foods, spices, herbs, and dietary supplements. There are also techniques that fit under the umbrella of complementary and alternative medicine that have been shown to be effective. For example, simple regular aerobic exercise can lower your risk of breast cancer by as much as 30 to 50 percent.

The amount of risk reduction associated with each of these items is not small. Many of them lower your risk by as much as 50 percent or more. And their protective effects multiply when you do more than one. For instance, later in this book, you'll learn that the spice turmeric greatly enhances the breast cancer–blocking qualities of soy. And when turmeric is consumed in the same meal with green tea, each makes the other's anticancer properties more powerful: Turmeric makes green tea eight times more effective, and green tea, in turn, makes turmeric three times more effective.

If you have breast cancer, this information can help you, too. Studies show that many of the items that lower your risk also help to improve your outcome and chances of survival if you have the disease. For example, many spices, herbs, supplements, or techniques can help prevent metastasis (the spread of the tumor), decrease the risk of the tumor's coming back, and stop new tumors from growing. Best of all, everything that lowers your risk of breast cancer also decreases your risk of developing a multitude of other diseases. This collection of risk-reducing habits not only lowers your chances of developing breast cancer, but also helps you to achieve an excellent robust state of health.

You're Not to Blame

Don't use the information in this book to beat yourself up. It's not designed for that. It's designed to empower you. It's not your fault that you didn't know this information before. No good comes from blaming yourself or feeling guilty. The most powerful and productive thing you can do is to start taking action now. Accept whatever situation you find yourself in today as simply "what is" with no judgment. It's called the power of living in the "now." You have no power over the past. Your real power exists in the present moment. This belief has been taught by wisdom traditions throughout the centuries. For a clear picture of this empowering way of living, I recommend reading *The Power of Now*, an excellent book by Eckhart Tolle. Then, start the "thirty-step" program (see Chapter 29) and celebrate every step you take.

> *The secret of health for both mind and body is not to mourn*
> *for the past, worry about the future, or anticipate troubles,*
> *but to live in the present moment wisely and earnestly.*
>
> —BUDDHA

Your Doctor's Not to Blame

Don't blame your doctor for not telling you all the facts on breast cancer prevention. Most doctors don't know them; they know only the basics of prevention: don't smoke; don't drink too much alcohol; exercise; and eat more fruits and vegetables instead of hamburgers, French fries, and doughnuts. That's about it. Although it's good advice, this list barely touches upon what you need to know to stay healthy. Medical education concentrates on the surgical and pharmaceutical treatment of diseases—*after* you have them. Most doctors know very little about prevention because it's not a focus in Western medical school training. Topics on natural prevention are rarely, if ever, included in traditional continuing-medical-education conferences, either. One reason for this is that most of the money for research comes from the pharmaceutical industry. Doctors would have to attend "holistic" medical conferences, usually sponsored outside their traditional medical society, to learn about natural prevention. The only other option doctors have is to research the medical literature, as I have done. And that takes a lot of time—time most doctors don't have.

It's the system of medicine that's broken. Our current approach to "healthcare" is actually one of "disease care." Except for acute care, such as trauma, this system doesn't work very well. If you have a broken bone or a gunshot wound, there's none better, but Western medicine doesn't know much about the prevention or treatment of chronic disorders. The "root causes" of a disease are not part of its vocabulary. The best that you can hope for, for most chronic disorders, is to suppress the symptoms without creating side effects that are worse than the disease itself.

A Quantum Leap

The paradigm of Western medicine and how it views the human body needs a radical shift. In the first half of the twentieth century, physicists discovered that the structure of our universe and how it operates are fundamentally very different from what we had previously thought. The concepts and laws of Newtonian physics were replaced with those of the radically different quantum physics. But surprisingly, Western medicine hasn't caught up with this scientific revolution. It still treats the body as if it were a machine of unrelated parts. It doesn't see the unified field of intelligence described by quantum physics that underlies and coordinates body, mind, and consciousness. It doesn't understand that everything affects the complex balance of your physiology in one way or another for good or ill: everything you eat, everything you do, every thought you think, the company you keep, the music you listen to—everything. Western medicine doesn't understand that all diseases come from imbalances or that correcting those imbalances causes most chronic illnesses to improve and, sometimes, to be cured. It doesn't understand that imbalances caught and corrected early will prevent chronic disorders from manifesting. Worse, it has no technology or diagnostic technique to catch a disease "early." Rather, its tests can only detect diseases at late stages, once they have caused structural changes in the body.

What if I were to tell you that there's a system of medicine that contains very detailed and sophisticated knowledge about how to stay healthy and prevent diseases, such as breast cancer, arthritis, asthma, and heart disease? Even better, what if I were to tell you that this system's in-depth understanding of human health, physiology, and consciousness is so profound that if you follow its advice, you can achieve a state of extraordinary and vibrant health beyond what you thought possible—a state of perfect health? Would you believe me? And what if I told you that this system of medicine has been around for a very long time, that the human race has held the secrets to extraordinary health for thousands of years—in fact, 5,000 years? You'd probably find it very hard to believe, but it's true!

This astounding ancient system of holistic medicine is called *Ayurveda*. The next chapter will tell you about a few basic principles and techniques of this wonderful and profound system of medicine.

Chapter 2

Rediscovering Ancient Healing

Ayurveda: A Comprehensive Holistic Preventative System of Health

*W*hen I went to medical school in the early 1980s, I was taught how to try to fix existing medical problems, but I wasn't taught how to prevent disease or how to achieve and maintain health. Twenty years after I left medical school, I went back to my alma mater—the University of Cincinnati—to lecture to the students. I can tell you that not much changed in those twenty years. Still today, almost nothing is taught in medical school about prevention or nutrition, or about attaining and preserving good health, because Western medicine doesn't know much about these subjects. But *Ayurveda* does.

When I was first introduced to *Ayurveda* and began to study it in 1996, I'm embarrassed to say that I had previously never heard of it, even though over 1 billion people—one-sixth of the world's population—use it as their primary form of healthcare. During the past two decades, I have dedicated myself, in large part, to the study of this miraculous system of healthcare, and I have never lost my awe at its power to create perfect health. In fact, my awe simply increases with each passing year.

Ayur means life, and *veda* means knowledge, so *Ayurveda* literally means "the knowledge of life." I'm sure you can get the sense just from its name that the approach of this system of health and its reservoir of knowledge are very different from those of Western medicine.

Ayurveda teaches how to live life to its fullest potential. It's the science of how to live a long, perfectly healthy life by achieving and maintaining a fine state of balance in your physiology. All the techniques and recommendations of *Ayurveda* are designed to bring you into balance and keep you there. *Ayurveda* underscores this core truth: *Perfect balance is the foundation and key to perfect health.*

A HOLISTIC APPROACH

Ayurveda is a holistic system of health. It holds that there is no separation between mind, body, spirit, and consciousness or anything seemingly outside you in the universe. Quantum physics has shown that this is true. Everything inside you and everything outside you, at the most finite level, is intimately connected. So, everything affects everything. In other words, any technique—be it mental, physical, or spiritual—has profound effects on your entire physiology. Naturally, it follows that everything in your environment affects your health, as well.

Ayurveda emphasizes the experience of higher states of consciousness, which are characterized by an expanded awareness that brings profound balance to the mind/body. Research shows that people who practice techniques that enliven higher, more expanded states of consciousness regularly enjoy so much balance that they are dramatically healthier than the average American. Studies show that these individuals use the healthcare system, overall, 50 percent less often and have 87 percent fewer hospital admissions for cardiovascular diseases!

But the ultimate intention of *Ayurveda* goes far beyond preventing disease. Its goal is to produce robust perfect health for the mind/body and the consciousness. This level of health is of paramount importance because it helps us to achieve higher states of consciousness—and ultimately, enlightenment. Enlightenment is the highest state of human awareness; it is the ability to see and know the reality of all things and to enjoy mastery over the physical state of being.

Clearly, the goals and objectives of *Ayurveda* are very different from the Western model of healthcare. I like to put it this way: Western medicine is about suppressing the symptoms of disease; *Ayurveda* is about creating profound health. Because we have grown up with a "disease-care" system of medicine (as opposed to "healthcare" system), most Americans have no idea how to create extraordinary health—or even that it's possible. Fortunately, *Ayurveda* can teach us that.

The History of *Ayurveda*

Ayurveda dates back at least 5,000 years and is thought to be the oldest comprehensive system of medicine still practiced. The *Vedic* culture, a visionary society that lived in an area of the world that is now India, is credited with being the original source of this knowledge. Initially, all the wisdom held in *Ayurveda* was passed down through oral tradition. Then about 2,500 years ago, it was written down in two texts: the *Charaka Samhita* and the *Sushruta Samhita*. Both of these astoundingly broad repositories of ancient knowledge are still used by students of *Ayurveda* today.

Although *Ayurveda* is thousands of years old, it is an extremely sophisticated system of medicine that has many specialty divisions—branches of medicine—that have lasted through time. In fact, they make up the fundamental structure of our medical system today: internal medicine, ENT (ear, nose, and throat), ophthalmology, obstetrics and gynecology, pediatrics, and surgery. As a plastic surgeon, I was fascinated to learn that the preferred surgical technique for reconstructing the nose after trauma or cancer that was taught to me during residency was first described in *Ayurvedic* texts thousands of years ago.

Ayurveda went through some rocky times when the British invaded India. All the *Ayurvedic* medical schools were closed, and practicing *Ayurveda* was declared illegal. After India gained its independence in 1947, attempts were made to reestablish *Ayurveda*. Not surprisingly, much of the ancient knowledge had become fragmented and some of it had been lost. The practice of *Ayurveda* had degenerated essentially into an herbalized form of Western medicine. Prevention and techniques of consciousness were no longer at the forefront of the medical field.

Then, in the early 1980s, Maharishi Mahesh Yogi, the person who introduced Transcendental Meditation (TM) to the West, recognized that the world was in desperate need of *Ayurveda*—the original comprehensive *Ayurveda*. He brought the top *Ayurvedic* doctors (called *vaidyas*) together to reconstruct the lost knowledge. They were given the task to carefully read the original *Ayurvedic* texts and then select the most effective techniques that would best suit our culture now. This form of *Ayurveda* is distinguished by being called Maharishi *Ayurveda* or Maharishi *Vedic* Approach to Health (MVAH).

Navigating Alternative Medicine

If you've ever looked into using complementary and alternative medicine (CAM), I'd be surprised if you haven't become confused and overwhelmed. On the surface, it appears to be a smorgasbord of hundreds of different health practices with no apparent link. Without expert guidance, the average person can't select the right combination of techniques or approaches to most effectively meet his or her individual needs.

Most of the techniques used in CAM today have their roots in *Ayurveda*, including such diverse treatments as yoga, massage, meditation, music therapy, sound therapy, aromatherapy, herbs, breathing techniques, special diets, and detoxification, to name just a few. *Ayurveda* also teaches a group of simple but profound principles that provide a broad, yet fundamental understanding of all the different techniques included in CAM. Its basic principles form a framework for understanding these techniques and how they fit together into a comprehensive model of healthcare.

These timeless truths are actually laws of Nature that govern health. They reveal how and why certain techniques work to improve health. Throughout *Waking the Warrior Goddess*, *Ayurvedic* principles are presented to help give you the "big picture"—a deeper and clearer understanding of each element of the program. If all the methods to lower your risk of breast cancer were presented without teaching you about their underlying *Ayurvedic* principles, they would seem like a long list of unrelated items that you could easily forget. But when you understand them in relationship to the fundamental laws of Nature, you understand them on a much deeper level. They make sense, and they stay with you.

To give you an idea of what I'm talking about, let's look at an example. One *Ayurvedic* principle is: *Food is medicine.* We don't usually think of food as medicine in our culture. For the most part, we are unfamiliar with the medicinal qualities of foods, because Western doctors don't prescribe foods; they prescribe pharmaceutical medications. That's why we're all very familiar with how to approach common, uncomplicated health problems using medications, such as aspirin or Pepto-Bismol. But very few of us know the names of the spices, herbs, and foods that may be just as effective.

Ayurvedic physicians, on the other hand, prescribe food as one of the first lines of treatment. Instead of reaching for aspirin for a painful swollen joint, their patients would most likely seek relief by turning to the cooking spices turmeric and ginger, and the vegetables asparagus and spinach. For acid indigestion, instead of a couple of tablespoons of a bright-pink liquid, they would eat rice, *mung dal* (lentil soup), pumpkin, squash, pomegranate, fennel, cumin, coriander, or turmeric.

Thousands of years ago, the intelligence contained in food was well recognized for its ability to induce balance and increase the healing intelligence of our bodies. Modern science is now confirming what ancient physicians knew: The right food *is powerful medicine.* Part Two of this book reveals the medicinal foods that modern research shows can substantially lower your risk of breast cancer. But protecting against breast cancer isn't the only thing they do. They also lower your risk of most chronic disorders and can dramatically improve your overall health.

> *Sickness is the vengeance of nature*
> *for violation of her laws.*
>
> —CHARLES SIMMONS

Two Underlying Principles of *Ayurveda*

All the techniques and principles in *Ayurveda* boil down to two grand underlying principles. The first and foremost one is this:

Perfect balance brings perfect health.

Ayurveda emphasizes that everything you do or eat—every day—either brings you into balance or throws you out of balance. The trick is to know the difference. If you choose only those foods and activities that bring balance, you can create perfect health.

The second most important principle is:

Perfect health is achieved through enlivening your inner healing intelligence.

In other words, all health-promoting foods, activities, herbs, and so on work by making your body *stronger* and *smarter* at repairing itself and resisting disease. At their most fundamental level, all the seemingly unrelated techniques presented in this book lower your risk of breast cancer by enlivening your body's inner healing intelligence and inducing balance.

It's equally important to recognize not only what brings you into balance, but also what throws you out of balance—what to avoid. These are the activities you do or the foods that you eat that weaken you because they violate the natural laws governing your mind/body. Knowing these laws of Nature in advance helps to keep you from making the mistakes or creating the habits that obstruct your inner healing intelligence.

The principles of *Ayurveda* are the keys to understanding all the rules that govern your health. When you know the rules and follow them, you thrive abundantly, avoid catastrophes, and pave the path to the immense pleasure of extraordinary balance and health.

Without a doubt, the medicine of the future will reincorporate these ancient truths. It's already happening. An integrated system of medicine—one that combines the best technologies of Western medicine with those of ancient holistic systems of medicine—will serve us best. Imagine a system of medicine that uses all of the best knowledge and techniques of health from every culture in the world, where rapidly advancing sophisticated technology is built on a base that includes everything we have learned about our bodies and health over thousands of years since the beginning of recorded time.

Chapter 3

The Birth
of the Beast

How Breast Cancer Grows

*I*nside the human body, there is a fascinating universe of spectacular intelligence. In a healthy body, every structure and every cell work together in perfect coordination and harmony. It's important to understand a few basic facts about the anatomy and physiology of the human body because it will enhance your grasp of each subject presented in this book. This fundamental knowledge will help you to comprehend more fully how and why each one influences your risk of breast cancer.

The human body is composed of cells, each of which functions like its own city. The boundary of every cell is defined by a cell membrane—like a protective bubble surrounding the city. Within each cell city, there are many different structures, all with special functions. There are power plants that make energy, construction crews that build new structures and repair damaged ones, and demolition crews that tear down faulty or decaying sections so that new better functioning ones can be built in their place.

In the center of every cell (except red blood cells) is a very important structure called the nucleus. It contains the DNA. A simple way to understand DNA is to think of it as the source code for every structure and function in the body. In other words, it supplies the information that tells every cell and every molecule in the body what to do, when to do it, and how to do it. It's like a set of blueprints. DNA comes in strands that form a double helix. Our DNA is not packaged in just one long strand; instead, it is divided up into separate chunks called chromosomes. There are twenty-three pairs of chromosomes or forty-six individual chromosomes in every cell. A chromosome is made up of various amounts of defined sequences of DNA called genes. The largest chromosome is called chromosome 1 and contains about 2,000 genes. Human DNA contains a total of about 25,000 genes—much less than originally thought.

New cells are constantly being created to replace old, damaged, or worn-out cells through a process called cell division. When your cells divide to form new cells, the DNA in the cell must make an exact copy of itself. Sometimes, DNA becomes damaged due to environmental toxins, pesticides, radiation, viruses, inflammation, or any of a variety of other factors. When a cell containing damaged DNA divides, a copy of the DNA with damaged genetic information is passed on to the new cell, so some part of the information passed on to the new cell will be wrong.

Depending on where the mistake occurs, it might be the spark that ignites a deadly disease such as cancer, or it might not create any problems. For instance, let's assume that the part of your DNA that contains the instructions telling the construction workers when to *stop* building becomes damaged. They will start to erect a structure and finish it, but because they receive no instruction telling them to stop, they continue building—*forever*. That's exactly how cancer can form. In a healthy balanced body, DNA controls cell division. However, if the gene that governs cell division becomes damaged, cells may start to divide wildly, initiating the growth of a cancer. Cell division out of control is cancer.

ESTROGEN'S ROLE

Estrogen is the hormone that causes female characteristics to develop. It influences the shape of the body, hair distribution, voice, emotions, skin texture, and a myriad of other effects. It also makes breast tissue grow by increasing the rate at which breast cells divide. Too much estrogen causes breast cells to divide too rapidly and to keep on dividing. With every cell division, there's a chance for a mistake to occur that could lead to cancer. So, the faster breast cells divide, the higher the risk of breast cancer.

Scientists have found that it's not uncommon for cancer cells to form as a result of damaged DNA. This is largely because DNA must replicate itself each time a cell divides. This is a complicated process with a high probability of error. Mathematically speaking, the chances of a mistake occurring during DNA replication are extremely high. There are tens of thousands of opportunities for a mistake to occur in each cell in your body *every* time a cell divides. And you have *trillions* of cells that are continuously dividing.

With those odds, it should come as no surprise that your body constantly produces cancer cells. Fortunately, you were created with this fact in mind. The extraordinary internal healing intelligence inside you organizes many layers of protection against this normal, but potentially disastrous occurrence. Using the construction analogy again, you have quality-control teams that detect damaged DNA and send in repair crews. If the repair crews are overwhelmed with work, they can't keep up with all the mistakes, and cancer cells may start to grow. Fortunately, there are other workers who back up these repair crews. They flag the newly formed cancer cells and instantly call in another crew to come and destroy them. A tumor only forms when mistakes happen so rapidly and cancer cells form so quickly that the detection and repair crews can't keep up.

The Risk with Estrogen

Breast cancer is considered a hormonal disease because a hormone initiates and fuels it by causing cells to grow and divide. In breast cancer, that hormone is estrogen. The more estrogen you're exposed to, the higher your risk of breast cancer is.

Contrary to a common misconception, the term "estrogen" includes many different types of molecular compounds, not just one. There are three major types of estrogen naturally made by the body: estradiol, estrone, and estriol. Estradiol is the most abundant and the most potent of the three. It's the type of estrogen that contributes the most to increasing your risk of breast cancer. The more estradiol your body makes in your lifetime, the higher your risk of cancer.

When you have a menstrual period, your body produces more estradiol. So the more periods you have during your life, the higher your risk of breast cancer. That's why your risk goes up if you start menstruating at an early age or go through menopause at a later age. For instance, if you were younger than age fourteen when you started having periods, your risk of breast cancer is 30 percent higher than if you started when you were sixteen. If you were ten when your periods started, your risk of breast cancer is 50 percent greater than if you had started at age sixteen. If you go through menopause late—at age fifty-five—your risk is 50 percent higher than it would be if you went through it at age forty-five.

The shorter your menstrual cycles are, the more of them you will have in your lifetime, and the higher your risk of breast cancer will be. You might think that the length of your menstrual cycle is completely controlled by genetics, the phases of the moon, or some other factor beyond your control, but it's not. There are certain foods you can eat to naturally lengthen your menstrual cycles and lower your risk; these foods will be discussed in Part Two.

Pregnancy also influences your risk of breast cancer. If you never had a child or had your first child after age thirty, your risk is higher than if you had a child before you were thirty. The reason, again, has to do with estrogen. When you're pregnant, you don't have menstrual periods, so you don't make much of the strong kind of estrogen (estradiol) that increases your risk of breast cancer.

But, you say, this doesn't sound right. You may remember from high school biology that your body produces high amounts of estrogen when you are pregnant. So, why does pregnancy cause your risk to go down? When you are pregnant, estradiol doesn't go up; a different kind of estrogen—estriol—does. Estriol is the weakest of the three natural estrogens. It is only $\frac{1}{1000}$ the strength of estradiol. That means that for every 1,000 cells that divide in response to estradiol, estriol will cause only one cell to divide. When there's more estriol and less estradiol, breast-cell division is thousands of times slower. The slower breast cells divide, the lower your risk of breast cancer. That's why high estriol levels during pregnancy can significantly lower your risk of breast cancer.

The protective effect of estriol can be substantial. Research shows that when compared to women who have given birth, women who have never had a child have a 20 to 70 percent increased risk of breast cancer by the time they are forty-five. You can lower your risk even more by breastfeeding your baby. Most women don't ovulate or have menstrual cycles during the first few months of breastfeeding.

Your risk of breast cancer goes up as you age. The older you are, the greater the amount of estrogen your body has made, and the higher the accumulation of damage from toxins and bad habits. At age twenty, your risk is about 1 in 1,681; at age forty, it is estimated to be 1 in 68. Approximately 77 percent of all breast cancer cases occur in women over fifty years of age. By the time you are eighty, your risk is about 1 in 8.

The Estrogen Pathway

Understanding how estrogen is produced, used, broken down, and eliminated from your body—the estrogen pathway—is important. It adds to your understanding of how and why the factors discussed in this book have an impact on your risk of breast cancer. It's a complicated process. Estrogen is produced primarily by your ovaries before you go through menopause. Other tissues make estrogen too. After menopause, estrogen is primarily made by fat cells and by the adrenal glands, which sit on top of the kidneys. A tiny amount is also made by your muscles.

To understand the estrogen pathway better, let's use the analogy of a car ride. Your trip begins in the ovaries where estrogen is made and then is released into the blood. The blood vessels are like highways, and estrogen flows through these blood-vessel highways to get to its target destinations. When estrogen travels in the blood, it either travels alone or is attached to a substance called a "protein binder"—the difference between driving alone in your car and carpooling. When you carpool in certain cities, you can use a special high-speed lane, usually on the far left. In this lane, you can't exit from the highway. If you're driving alone, you can't use these high-speed lanes. You must travel in lanes that have access to the exit lanes. Like the person driving alone, only the estrogen that travels alone—without a protein binder—can exit from the blood-vessel highway. In this case, we are concerned about the off-ramp for only one destination: the breast tissue.

When estrogen reaches the breast, it looks for a place to "park." Parking spaces represent the "estrogen receptors," which estrogen binds to on the breast-cell membranes. There are estrogen receptors all over your body, but the highest concentrations are found in the uterus and breast. Men also have a high concentration of estrogen receptors in their prostate gland. Because of the relatively large number of estrogen receptors in these tissues, they respond more to estrogen than the other tissues in the body do.

When estrogen binds to an estrogen receptor, it "turns it on." A turned-on receptor causes cells to start dividing. Estrogen receptors don't turn on like a simple on/off switch. Instead, they turn on like a rheostat, a light switch with a dimmer.

The rate at which cells divide in response to estrogen is affected by many factors. First, the rate depends on the strength of the estrogen. There are strong and weak estrogens. Strong estrogens speed up cell division and, therefore, increase the risk of cancer. Weak estrogens slow down cell division, decreasing the risk of cancer. You can think of it like this: The driver of the estrogen car, say, estriol or estradiol, starts blowing bubbles, which represent the new cells formed by cell division in response to estrogen. If the driver is strong (estradiol), he or she can blow a lot of bubbles very quickly, creating a big soapy mess in the car (aka cancer). If the driver is very weak (estriol), he or she can hardly blow any bubbles. One or two bubbles doesn't cause any harm.

Parking at an estrogen receptor causes a lot of wear and tear on the estrogen. After a while, it needs to go in for service. So, the estrogen leaves the estrogen receptor and heads for the liver (service station). The liver is the great detoxifier of the body. It breaks down toxins and other natural substances to prepare them for elimination.

Estrogen is broken down in the liver, and is influenced by the presence of certain chemicals. It is either broken down into a "good" kind of estrogen or a "bad" kind of estrogen. For instance, substances in cruciferous vegetables and flaxseeds create more of the good kind while environmental toxins create more of the bad. The difference between good and bad estrogen is that good estrogen causes breast cells to divide very slowly, whereas bad estrogen causes them to divide rapidly. Bad estrogen can also cause mutations or mistakes in how the cells grow that increase your risk of cancer even more.

The good estrogen causes no damage and drives immediately to the colon or to the bladder where it leaves the body. The bad estrogen backfires, gets stuck in reverse, and speeds back to the breast where it wreaks havoc (see Figure 3.1 on page 42). If this bad estrogen finds a parking spot on a breast cell, it will rapidly speed up cell division. If you have a lot of bad estrogen in your body, your risk of breast cancer goes up significantly.

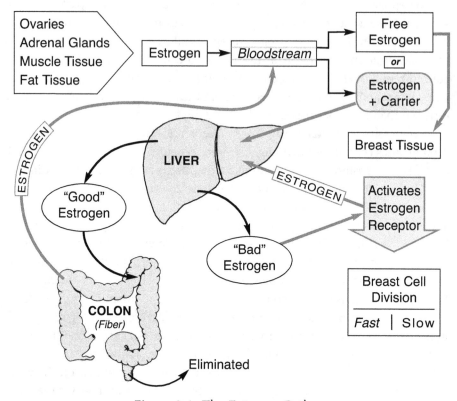

Figure 3.1. The Estrogen Pathway

In the colon, estrogen is either eliminated or absorbed back into the blood. If it is absorbed back into the blood, it adds to the total amount of estrogen in your body, and therefore, adds to your risk. There's a simple solution: Eat more fiber. Fiber binds to estrogen in your colon and eliminates it. (See Chapter 7 for more on fiber.)

Now that you understand the fundamental process that links estrogen to breast cancer, we are ready to move on to learning about all the natural ways that you can protect against and fight breast cancer.

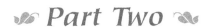

Part Two

A Banquet
Fit for a Goddess

Foods That Heal

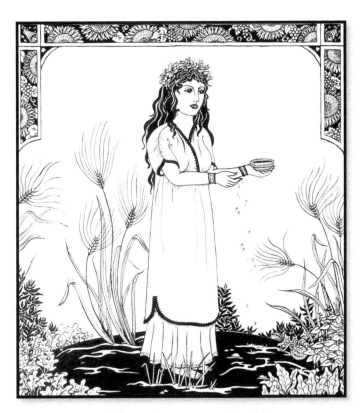

Goddess of Harvest and Fields

Chapter 4

Let Food Be Your Medicine
Rediscovering a Forgotten Ayurvedic Pillar of Health

*A*t the heart of *Ayurveda* is your relationship to your inner healing intelligence. It teaches that you can achieve a perfect state of health by enlivening that intelligence with specific foods and behavioral choices. If you make poor choices that sabotage your inherent capacity to heal, imbalances arise that further block the full expression of your healing intelligence. Eventually, poor choices will weaken it to where it can no longer keep you well. In time, your body will begin to break down, and diseases will start to manifest. Health is only regained and maintained by enhancing this healing intelligence and keeping it lively and flowing.

The divine, natural healing intelligence inside you manages trillions of biochemical reactions simultaneously at every moment of your life. The image that emerges for me when I think of this intelligence is one of an extraordinary multitasking Warrior Goddess—supernatural in strength and power and vastly discriminating in her intellect. Yet, she is delicate and very particular.

Like a Goddess, the magnificence of this managing intelligence depends on respecting her very precise and specific demands. When you think of the phenomenal biology, physics, and chemistry that keep you alive and well, embrace them as your Warrior Goddess: an intimate, personal, profoundly intelligent, and powerful friend.

Having the knowledge of what empowers your Warrior Goddess and what drains her strength endows you with the power of choice—the choice about how you treat her and, thus, the direction of your health. But, if you aren't aware of her likes and dislikes, you're like a ship lost at sea, unable to find the course that leads to achieving and maintaining good health. You won't be able to choose the best direction to excellent health—no matter how much you want to—because you lack the skills and equipment for the task. Chances are, sooner or later, you'll crash on the rocks, get stuck on a sandbar, or suddenly find yourself in a hostile foreign land filled with life-threatening diseases. However, if you choose to honor and empower your Warrior Goddess, she will steer you to a land of perfect health—an enchanting place filled with the treasures of clarity, abundance, fulfillment, peace, wisdom, and beauty.

Never does Nature say one thing and wisdom another.

—Juvenal, *Satires*

FOOD FOR A GODDESS

All ancient systems of medicine recognize that one of the most important determinants of your health is what you choose to put in your mouth. The right foods bring balance and greatly increase the healing intelligence of your body. The wrong foods can act as poisons—junk foods, for example. They contain health-damaging chemical additives and preservatives, and most of their nutrients have been destroyed during processing. Processed foods, canned foods, frozen foods, and leftover food all have lower nutritional values. They have qualities that aren't good for your mind/body, and should be avoided.

Your stomach shouldn't be your wastebasket.

—Author unknown

Some foods are filled with so many health-promoting and anticancer properties that they can be thought of as medicines. As mentioned earlier, this is an important *Ayurvedic* principle: [*The right*] *food is medicine*. Most medicinal foods come from the plant world. Physicians trained in *Ayurveda* possess an extremely sophisticated knowledge of the medicinal qualities of plants. Because of this, they prescribe fruits, vegetables, grains, seeds, spices, and herbs as the initial approach for the prevention or treatment of any health condition. Not only do they know the medicines contained within each plant, but they also know the ideal harvesting, processing, and mixing procedures to maximize the plant's healing potential.

The most health-promoting foods you can eat are fresh, organically grown fruits, vegetables, nuts, seeds, and whole grains—especially if they are locally grown. Research shows that eating these foods can have a dramatic effect on lowering your risk of breast cancer. Since these foods also enhance your inner healing intelligence, try to favor them. Think of it this way: Make every meal a banquet fit for a Goddess. When you feed your Goddess what she needs, you arm her with powerful weapons. Her ability to keep you well is amazing. When you give her the right raw materials, she can create a multitude of masterful protective devices. This is why *Ayurveda* places great importance on diet and digestion. In fact, there may be nothing that has more influence on your health.

Together, diet and digestion comprise one of the three pillars of *Ayurvedic* health. The other two are proper lifestyle and rest. According to *Ayurveda*, about 80 percent of all illnesses arise from improper diet and digestion.

What you eat is important, *Ayurveda* says, but *how* you eat is just as important. If you don't digest your food properly, it doesn't matter if you have the best diet in the world; it won't do you any good. You have to digest your food well in order to absorb the nutrients. It's the only way you can be nourished by the food you eat.

The Top 12 Aids to Digestion

Ayurveda recommends twelve ways to help you digest your food properly.

1. Eat your main meal at noon.
2. Don't eat again until your previous meal has been digested (about three hours).
3. Keep regular mealtimes.
4. Don't overeat. Eat to fill three-quarters of your stomach's capacity.
5. Eat in a settled atmosphere.
6. Don't eat when you are upset.
7. Always sit down to eat.
8. Don't talk while chewing.
9. Favor lightly cooked foods over raw foods.
10. Avoid cold drinks.
11. Favor fresh wholesome foods, such as organic fruits, vegetables, and whole grains.
12. Put your full attention on your food.

Most of these recommendations are self-explanatory, but a few of them need further clarification. *Ayurveda* recommends that you *eat your main meal at noon* because your "digestive fires" are at their peak from 10:00 A.M. to 2:00 P.M. In other words, your body's metabolism is revved up during these hours, and you can digest your food better than you can early in the morning or later at night. If you eat a big meal late at night, it won't digest well, and your sleep will be disturbed. I'm sure you've had this unpleasant experience at least once or twice. However, the times you've *eaten light in the evening and gone to bed early,* you more than likely woke up feeling great. Most of the principles and recommendations of *Ayurveda* are as simple as this one, but don't let their simplicity fool you. Their effects can be very profound.

Cold drinks should be avoided, especially during a meal, because according to *Ayurveda,* a cool drink cools down and dilutes the digestive fires. In Western scientific terms, cool drinks slow down the action of your stomach's digestive enzymes, which work best at body temperature or a little above. At the temperature of an iced drink, the effectiveness of your digestive enzymes is cut almost in half. If you want to drink something with your meals, *Ayurveda* recommends that you have sips of hot water only. Don't drink too much water with your meal, either, because water will dilute the enzymes in the stomach, making them less effective.

The *Ayurvedic* recommendation to *favor fresh wholesome foods* is a key principle of diet, and it plays a big role in lowering the risk of breast cancer. The 2,500-year-old text of *Ayurveda,* called the *Charaka Samhita,* proclaims the importance of a wholesome diet: "The distinction between health and disease arises as the result of the difference between wholesome and unwholesome diet." Wholesome foods are considered to be primarily fresh organic fruits, vegetables, and whole grains.

According to *Ayurveda,* when foods are lightly cooked they are easier to digest and, therefore, more nutrients are absorbed. Overcooking foods or cooking foods at high temperatures should be avoided because it destroys nutrients and creates harmful substances.

Finally, when you eat a meal, it is ideal to *put your full attention on your food.* Don't watch TV or read the newspaper. When your full attention is on your meal, you're more likely to chew your food well, eat smaller portions, and digest your food better.

If you eat highly nutritious foods and follow these simple recommendations, you can provide your body with the best materials and the most competent and proficient team of builders to design, construct, and maintain the foundation of your health. If you choose poor materials and unskilled workers, your foundation will be weak, and no matter what else you do to support your health, it will crumble. With a strong foundation, you can build a structure so solid that it becomes impenetrable against even the most aggressive and ruthless enemy—breast cancer.

Chapter 5

An Organic Pharmacy
"Chemotherapy" from Organic Fruits and Vegetables

ruits and vegetables are virtual anticancer pharmacies. Thousands of studies have shown that a diet high in fresh fruits and vegetables is associated with a lower risk of many different types of cancers and chronic diseases. Scientists have found that these plants contain a wide variety of natural chemicals that are extremely powerful at protecting against cancer and help to fight it once it has formed.

The remarkable natural "chemotherapy" found in fresh fruits and vegetables is safe and free of side effects, and it expresses an intelligence of such brilliance that pharmaceutical companies study these plants to learn how to create pharmaceutical chemotherapy—in fact, approximately 60 percent of chemotherapy drugs are estimated to be based on plant medicine. *Ayurveda* explains that the reason these plants are so protective is that they contain high amounts of "intelligence." They transfer this intelligence to your body, increasing its natural healing intelligence, its ability to keep you healthy, and its power to ward off disease. Animal-based products, especially those high in saturated fat, tend to have the opposite effect. In other words, they decrease or block the healing intelligence of your body. The result is an increased risk of cancer and other chronic disorders.

Scientists have studied many of these plants to determine what causes them to be so protective. Most fruits and vegetables have several common beneficial properties that are associated with a lower risk of cancer. These beneficial properties are:

1. They are low in fat and high in fiber. (See Chapters 7 and 8.)

2. They are high in antioxidants and vitamins. (See Chapters 12 and 13.)

3. They have fewer calories than animal foods, high-fat foods, and simple carbohydrates, so the people who eat a lot of them on a regular basis generally have less body fat than those who don't.

THE INTELLIGENCE OF PLANTS

Plants contain specific cancer-fighting and disease-battling substances called "phytochemicals," or plant chemicals. Each plant contains anywhere from dozens to hundreds of different plant chemicals. Scientists think that plants developed these phytochemicals to protect themselves against predators, such as insects, bacteria, and fungi. Phytochemicals aren't nutrients and don't provide calories. Rather, they function as medicines—natural medicines with an extraordinary array of healing benefits.

Research has shown that phytochemicals can protect you from cancer in several different ways. Many of them are powerful antioxidants that protect your cells and DNA from damage caused by oxygen free radicals—damage that can lead to cancer. Some plant chemicals inactivate carcinogens and other substances that can damage your DNA and lead to cancer. Others can block one or more of the steps required for a cancer to grow.

Carotenoids

One of the most powerful cancer-fighting groups of phytochemicals is carotenoids. All carotenoids are potent antioxidants, but they each have unique healing properties. For instance, one class of carotenoids might significantly reduce one type of cancer by blocking steps in its growth, but it might have little effect on another kind of cancer. For example, the carotenoid lycopene is very protective against breast and prostate cancer, but it doesn't do much to protect against leukemia.

Carotenoids give a plant its color and contribute to its flavor. For instance, lycopene gives tomatoes their red color, and beta-carotene gives carrots their orange color. But you can't always tell which carotenoids are present by the color of the plant. Sometimes, you can't see the color of a carotenoid, even though it's present in large amounts, because another color is covering it up. For example, lutein has a yellow color and some very important health-promoting qualities; it is found in high quantities in leafy green vegetables, such as kale. You don't normally see the yellow color of lutein in kale, however, because it is camouflaged by the green chlorophyll. When kale starts to age, it loses some of its green chlorophyll, and then you can see the yellow of the lutein. This is exactly what happens to the leaves of deciduous trees in the fall. Tree leaves change their color when they lose enough green chlorophyll to expose the color beneath it.

Carotenoids also help to protect against many other disorders besides breast cancer. For instance, lutein helps to prevent macular degeneration, the most common cause of adult blindness.

Flavonoids

Also called bioflavonoids, these phytochemicals contribute to the color and flavor of a plant. Flavonoids are antioxidants and have other powerful anticancer properties, too.

In a study published in 2003 in the *British Journal of Cancer,* one group of flavonoids in particular, flavones (commonly found in leafy green vegetables and herbs), was found to dramatically lower the risk of breast cancer. Just 0.5 milligram (mg) a day of flavones, about what one-eighth of a green pepper contains, decreased the risk of breast cancer by 15 percent. For every additional 0.5 mg of flavones that a woman ate each day, her risk dropped another 15 percent.

Indole-3 Carbinol

Another group of plant chemicals that's particularly helpful in reducing the risk of breast cancer is known as indole-3-carbinol (I3C), which is found in all "cruciferous" vegetables. The cruciferous family includes the following:

- Bitter cress
- Bok choy
- Broccoli
- Brussels sprouts
- Cabbage
- Cauliflower
- Collards
- Horseradish
- Kale
- Kohlrabi
- Mustard seeds
- Radishes
- Rutabaga
- Turnip
- Watercress

Researchers have found that indole-3-carbinol attacks breast cancer with a diversity of weapons. It's like a superhero's Swiss army knife, fighting the deadly disease in many different ways. Here are some of them:

1. Indole-3-carbinol stops breast cancer cells from growing by shutting off a key enzyme (cyclin-dependent kinase) necessary for the cells to grow.

2. It interferes in the relationship between estrogen and the estrogen receptors in breast cells. Normally, their interaction ignites the rapid reproduction of cells. Indole-3-carbinol dampens that flame to a mere flicker. In other words, when estrogen binds to the estrogen receptor with indole-3-carbinol present, breast cells don't divide as fast as they usually do.

3. It forces estrogen to break down into a "good" (protective, non-cancer-promoting) type of estrogen. As you saw in Figure 3.1 on page 42, indole-3-carbinol is involved in breaking down estrogen in the liver. The liver converts estrogen into either "good" estrogen or "bad" estrogen. Indole-3-carbinol ensures that more estrogen is transformed into the "good" type.

4. It beneficially influences DNA and the instructions that DNA passes on. For

example, it activates a "tumor-suppression" gene, which contains the commands for several internal tactics that stop tumor growth. Not all your genetic material is read or turned on at any one time. Only part of the information in your genes is expressed. Certain substances—indole-3-carbinol, for one—can turn genes on, meaning they give the command for a specific gene's information to be read and the instructions carried out. Certain other agents, such as enzymes, proteins, or other chemical substances, can also turn genes on and off.

Indole-3-carbinol turns on the gene that contains the DNA message to slow down tumor growth. In addition, this tumor-suppression gene sends messages that prevent tumor cells from invading bodily tissues, spreading to other areas of the body, and from adhering together. (Adhesion, which is the ability of cells to stick to one another and other tissues, is necessary for a tumor to grow and spread successfully.) A 2011 Canadian study found two other genes involved in cancer growth that a derivative of I3C, called diindolylmethane, quiets: transcription factor Sp1 and fatty acid synthase.

5. It blocks the estrogen receptor, preventing strong natural or chemical estrogens from attaching to it and turning it on.

6. It encourages the production of something called p21 which stops cell growth in both estrogen and progesterone positive and negative tumors.

7. It prevents the initiation of tumor growth by stimulating immune function in many different ways, including increasing a substance in the immune system called interferon; upping the production of immune cells in the spleen; and improving the function of a cell in the immune system called a macrophage, which gobbles up foreign invaders including cancer cells.

8. It dissuades the growth of new blood vessels into tumors by as much as 76 percent.

9. It stops some of the cancer-promoting effects of the COX-2 enzyme, which is also involved in inflammation.

Of all of these effects, scientists think that indole-3-carbinol's ability to influence the liver to make more of the "good" kind of estrogen and less of the "bad" may play the biggest role in lowering the risk of breast cancer. Researchers have found that "bad" estrogen is a significant instigator of breast cancer. In one study, the amounts of "good" estrogen and "bad" estrogen were measured in two different groups of women. One group was composed of healthy women and the other group was composed of women who had breast cancer. Those with breast cancer had almost twice as much "bad" estrogen as the healthy women.

If you have breast cancer, indole-3-carbinol's influence on a tumor-suppression gene may be extraordinarily beneficial in improving your chances of survival.

When indole-3-carbinol is ingested, it is converted by stomach acid to diindolylmethane, or DIM. DIM is simply two molecules of indole-3-carbinol joined together, and has a stronger effect on the body than I3C. For example, DIM appears to be much more powerful at blocking the estrogen receptors compared to I3C. According to a study published in the *Journal of Nutritional Biochemistry* in 2006, DIM was twenty times stronger.

If you have a particularly aggressive form of breast cancer which over-expresses a gene called HER2/neu, a study published in the May 15, 2006 *Journal of Surgery Research* found that DIM may improve your chances of survival by enhancing the anticancer drug Paclitaxel's ability to stop tumor cell growth and kill tumor cells. A 2011 study from Wayne State University in Detroit confirmed these findings, and in 2013 this same group of researchers found that DIM enhanced the effectiveness of another chemotherapeutic drug used specifically for HER2/neu cancers called Herceptin.

Sulforaphane

Another anticancer phytochemical in cruciferous vegetables—particularly broccoli sprouts which contain twenty to fifty times more than a mature broccoli head—is worth noting. It's called sulforaphane, and it helps to stop cancer before it even begins. Sulforaphane increases the activity of the liver enzyme responsible for deactivating or destroying carcinogens and getting them out of your body. It also causes cancer cell death called apoptosis, decreases several different growth factors including epidermal growth factor, stamps out breast cancer stem cells, and impedes the spread of a tumor. Sulforaphane has been shown to hinder the growth of a variety of different types of cancer, including cancers of the breast, prostate, colon, lung, cervix, and stomach.

D-Glucaric Acid

Cruciferous vegetables, as well as fruits (such as oranges, apples, and grapefruit) also have a high concentration of another phytochemical that's effective in protecting against cancer, especially breast cancer—D-glucaric acid.

The liver manufactures a substance called *glucuronic acid,* which binds to toxins (including the "bad" estrogen) in the liver and deactivates them. But the enzyme beta-glucuronidase can interfere with this effort. It splits the toxins off glucuronic acid and reactivates them (see Figure 5.1 on page 54). Researchers have found that people with a high amount of beta-glucuronidase in the blood have an increased risk of various cancers, particularly the hormone-dependent ones, such as breast, prostate, and colon cancers.

Here is where the phytochemical D-glucaric acid comes to the rescue: It stops the activity of beta-glucuronidase, keeping the harmful estrogens and other toxins bound to glucuronic acid (see Figure 5.2 below) and deactivated.

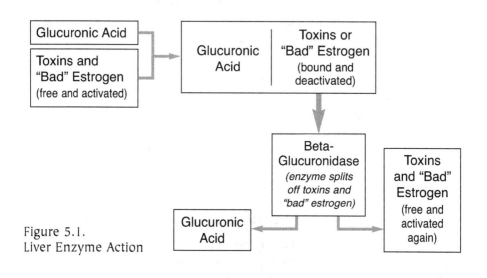

Figure 5.1.
Liver Enzyme Action

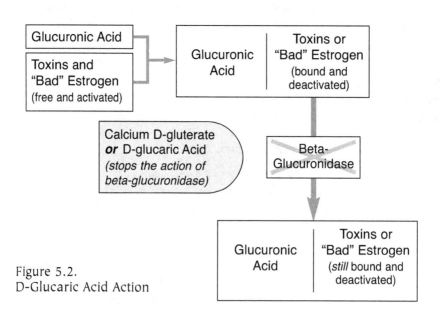

Figure 5.2.
D-Glucaric Acid Action

Simply put, D-glucaric acid strengthens the body's natural defenses against toxins. The liver makes a small amount of D-glucaric acid, but not enough for you to reap the greatest benefits. You can significantly increase the level of this protective substance in your body by eating plenty of cruciferous vegetables and certain fruits or by taking a supplement that comes in the form of a calcium salt called calcium D-gluterate or calcium D-glucarate. Research shows that this supplement is just as effective as natural D-glucaric acid. Taking supplemental calcium D-gluterate may give some added protection against breast cancer, but long-term studies still need to be done.

Eat Your Broccoli!

The results of consuming all the cancer-fighting phytochemicals in cruciferous vegetables are impressive. Researchers have found that women who eat the most cruciferous vegetables have as much as a 40 percent lower risk of breast cancer than women who eat few, if any, of these vegetables. A Chinese study published in 2012 tracked 5,000 women who had been diagnosed with breast cancer for five years. Those who ate the most cruciferous vegetables—about 150 grams per day or just one cooked cup—reduced their overall risk of dying of breast cancer by 62 percent compared to the women who ate the least amount of these vegetables. The women who ate the most cruciferous vegetables were also 35 percent less likely to have their breast cancer recur or come back. Breast cancer isn't the only type of cancer that cruciferous vegetables deter. They also appear to lower risk of cancers of the prostate, colon, stomach, lung, brain (glioma), and possibly cervix.

Chapter 6

Mother Nature Knows Best

Growing Foods to Enhance Their Healing Intelligence

If you're going to America, bring your own food.

—FRAN LEBOWITZ, JOURNALIST

The *way* your food is grown can have a powerful influence on the quality of its healing intelligence and, therefore, a significant impact on your risk of breast cancer. Think of it this way: When you eat plants that have been grown with techniques that maximize their quality and vitality, they supply your Warrior Goddess with the highest level of healing intelligence and the most sophisticated weaponry possible to defend against disease.

Conventionally grown foods may look and smell wholesome, but lurking on and under the surface is often a toxic mix of poisons that includes the residues of chemical fertilizers, pesticides, herbicides, hormones, and toxic additives. Organically grown foods, on the other hand, are carefully cultivated to avoid these chemicals. The reasons you don't want your foods grown with synthetic chemicals are simple: They are usually damaging to your health and the environment. Some of these chemicals have been found to increase your risk of breast cancer—and other cancers, as well. Many agricultural and additive chemicals can also disrupt your immune, nervous, endocrine, and reproductive systems.

There is another important health issue concerning conventionally grown food: Some seed producers change the characteristics of a plant by modifying its DNA. This process is known as "genetic modification." The intent is to increase crop production or commercial viability by adding so-called "beneficial" traits to a plant's DNA. For instance, companies add genes to plants to make them grow bigger, to be more resistant to pests, or to increase their shelf life. The problem is that scientists don't know what the long-term effects of eating these types of foods will be on human health—or on the environment. No human studies were done to evaluate their safety before they were put on the market. In other words, you and your family are Guinea pigs in one of the largest nonconsensual human experiments in history! This "experiment" *will* find out what happens to humans when they eat these foods over a long period of time—and *we* are the ones who will most likely suffer for it—we and our children and future generations!

Problems are already showing up in several short-term studies of genetically modified organisms (GMOs). In a study conducted at the University of Cincinnati by I. L. Bernstein and published in 1999 in *Environmental Health Perspectives*, allergic reactions were found among farm workers using *Bacillus thuringiensis*, a pesticide that's genetically spliced into corn. There have been many case reports of allergic reactions ranging from mild to severe. Even more alarming, a researcher in England found significant organ damage in rats that were fed genetically engineered potatoes.

The only way to reduce your health risk from GMOs is to buy only organically grown foods. Unfortunately, you can only decrease your risk of consuming GMOs because accidents happen. Genetically altered foods have accidentally been mixed with biologically normal foods. For instance, in 2000, genetically altered corn called StarLink, which had not been approved for human consumption, was found in Kraft taco shells. The problem was traced to a silo in Iowa where StarLink corn had accidentally been mixed with non-GMO corn.

A front-page story in *The New York Times* on June 10, 2001, reported that genetically altered DNA had been found in organic foods. Reporter David Barboza said that the reason was, "More than 100 million acres of the world's most fertile farmland were planted with genetically modified crops last year ([in] 2000) . . . Wind-blown pollen, commingled seeds, and black-market plantings have . . . extended these products of biotechnology into the far corners of the global food supply—perhaps irreversibly." In other words, organically grown plants can become contaminated with genetic modifications. For the most part, however, certified organic foods are free from GMOs and are the only way to reduce your risk of consuming genetically altered foods.

There is an excellent book by Jeffrey Smith entitled *Genetic Roulette: The Documented Health Risks of Genetically Engineered Foods*, and an award-winning documentary based on it called *Genetic Roulette: The Gambles of Our Lives*, which I highly recommend if you are interested in learning more.

High-tech tomatoes! Mysterious milk! Supersquash!
Are we supposed to eat this stuff? Or is it going to eat us?

—ANNITA MANNING

WEED KILLER COULD KILL YOU

Conventionally grown foods are sprayed with chemical pesticides, herbicides, fungicides, and fertilizers. These chemicals are popular because they are effective, but most of them are also highly toxic. They can damage your health in a variety of ways, causing everything from cancer to nervous, endocrine, and reproductive system damage. Chemicals that damage your nervous system are classified as neurotoxins. They impair IQ, memory, coordination, and the ability to concentrate. Other chemicals, known as endocrine disrupters, disturb the delicate balance of the hormones that regulate your body's functions, including reproductive functions. Most samples of conventionally grown fruits and vegetables contain the residues of several of these dangerous chemicals.

Let's take a close look at one chemical, the pesticide dichlorodiphenyl-trichloroethane (DDT). First developed in 1873, DDT wasn't recognized as a pesticide until 1939 when a Swiss citizen, Paul Meuller, discovered this functional use and was awarded the Nobel Prize in 1948 for his discovery. Initially, DDT was thought to be safe and the answer to the world's pest problems. But then wildlife, especially birds, began to die by the thousands. Certain populations of birds, such as the American bald eagle, dropped almost to extinction. The reason why this happened is because DDT softens the birds' eggshells so much that they can't support a developing embryo.

DDT was sprayed on fruits and vegetables grown in the United States from the early 1950s to the late 1960s. It was found to be harmful to humans by increasing their risk of certain cancers. Because of the serious environmental damage and human-health issues linked to this pesticide, it was banned in the United States in 1972. Unfortunately, DDT is persistent. It doesn't break down quickly and lasts for decades in our soil, water, and bodies. Animals pick up DDT from the environment through the plants, water, and animals they consume. When an animal or a fish ingests DDT from another creature or from the environment, this pesticide concentrates and stores in its fat, and stays there. The level of DDT in an animal's fat is about 700 times greater than the level in its blood.

Each time a bigger animal or fish eats a smaller one, it eats all the stored and concentrated DDT in that animal. So, huge amounts of DDT can accumulate in larger animals after a lifetime of eating smaller ones. This process is called "bio-concentration." Ultimately, when you eat an animal or fish, you ingest all the DDT (not to mention many other concentrated toxins) from all the smaller animals and fish that *that* creature ever ate. That is why the biggest sources of pesticides in your diet are fish, poultry, pork, beef, and other animal products.

You might think that DDT doesn't pose much of a health threat anymore because it was banned so long ago. Unfortunately, that's not true. Despite the ban on using it in the United States, American companies still manufacture DDT and sell it to other countries, such as Mexico, where it's legal. Mexican farmers spray DDT on their fruits and vegetables, and then—you guessed it—they export that produce right back to us. Our government checks only about 1 percent of imported produce, so fruits and vegetables sprayed with DDT, as well as other banned pesticides, come into the United States essentially without restriction. This toxic chemical–boomerang effect is called the "circle of poison." Recent research has found that the levels of many banned pesticides, including DDT, are rising in Americans.

One of the reasons DDT poses such a big threat to breast health is that it mimics estrogen. It acts just like the human estrogen molecule in your body, but with one big difference: This man-made chemical is much more powerful than natural estrogen. DDT significantly increases the rate at which cells divide in the breast—so much so that it dramatically increases your risk of breast cancer. It also steps up the production of natural estrogen in the body by stimulating aromatase—a key enzyme involved in the process.

DDT breaks down in the body into dichlorodiphenyldichloroethylene (DDE). Some studies show that women with the highest DDE levels have a 400 percent higher risk of breast cancer, but other studies don't show any increase at all. A significant percentage of the studies that showed no effect, however, were sponsored by the very chemical companies that make DDT. Because of their vested interest, companies have been known to skew the data or design of a study to make their chemicals look safe when they really aren't.

A study published in 2000 of more than 400 women in Denmark found that those with breast cancer had significantly higher levels of DDE than those who were healthy. Those with the highest levels of DDE were found to have a 300 percent higher risk of breast cancer. A prospective study conducted by the Public Health Institute in Berkeley, California, and published in 2007, found that girls who were under fourteen years of age and exposed to high levels of DDT around 1945, had a fivefold increase of breast cancer compared to girls who were older than fourteen at that time. The researchers emphasized from this finding that the age a person is at the time of exposure to toxins, such as DDT, can significantly influence the amount of damage these chemicals may cause. Hundreds of other pesticides have been manufactured, and many currently in use are far more toxic than DDT. For instance, benzene hexachloride (BHC) is nineteen times more powerful as a carcinogen than DDT. To play it safe, avoid chemical estrogens by eating only organically grown fruits, vegetables, and other foods.

The Poison Cocktail

We humans aren't exposed to just one pesticide or harmful chemical at a time. We're exposed to a "soup" of toxins every day. These toxins come from our food, the air we breathe, and the chemicals that outgas in our homes, in the buildings where we work and shop, and in our cars. They also come from dry-cleaned clothes, home-cleaning supplies, and beauty and personal-care products. In addition, some toxins stay in our bodies for decades, creating an ever more complex, chemical cocktail.

The big question is: What happens when these chemicals mix together? Do they interact in some way and become even more toxic? Because most of these chemicals haven't been studied, we don't know; however, the few studies that have been done suggest that this may be *exactly* what happens. A study conducted at Tulane and Xavier Universities in New Orleans found that when two pesticides, endosulfan and dieldrin, were combined together, the estrogenic effect of endosulfan increased 160 times and that of dieldrin increased 1,600 times. When the researchers combined endosulfan with chlordane (a pesticide banned in the United States but still used in third-world countries and sold back to us on the food we import), the endosulfan's estrogenic activity increased 100 times. There have been many other similar studies testing the effects of mixing together various endocrine-disrupting chemicals, and all show that the toxic effects are amplified.

ORGANIC: IT'S WORTH IT

Concern over harmful chemicals is probably the biggest reason why organically grown crops and organic products are the fastest growing sector of the agriculture economy, averaging 20 percent growth per year for more than a decade. Another reason may be that organic foods taste better. That's why many chefs at finer restaurants prefer to use them. In addition, most studies comparing the nutritional quality and content of organic foods to conventionally grown foods have found that organic foods fare much better. For instance, a study conducted at the University of California, Davis, found that corn grown without pesticides had 58 percent more antioxidants when compared to conventionally grown corn. Researchers also found that organically grown Marion berries (a type of blackberry) had 50 percent more antioxidants and organically grown strawberries had 19 percent more antioxidants than the same fruits grown conventionally.

There have been about thirty studies comparing the nutritional qualities of conventional (chemically grown) foods to organically grown foods. Drawing accurate conclusions from comparisons can sometimes be difficult, because in any crop—organic or nonorganic—nutrient content can vary. Sunlight, temperature, soil quality, and rainfall all affect the nutrient content of a plant. In addition, fruits and vegetables that are vine-ripened have more nutrients than those picked before they are ripe and held in storage for weeks. Despite these variations, researchers were able to calculate statistically significant differences between organic and conventionally grown crops using more than 300 different comparisons. Organically grown crops were found to have a higher nutritional value 40 percent of the time, whereas conventionally grown crops had a higher nutritional value only 15 percent of the time. Organic crops had an equal or higher nutrient content than conventionally grown foods 85 percent of the time. Three nutrients stood out as being consistently better in organic crops: On average, they have about 20 percent more vitamin C, better protein quality, and about 20 percent fewer carcinogenic nitrates than conventional crops.

Nutrients don't tell the whole story of a plant, however. The best test is to observe what happens to human beings and animals when they eat organically grown crops compared to what happens when they eat chemically grown crops. Are there any differences in their health? Animal experiments have been done with the intent to find the answer to that question. A review of these studies was published in the journal *Alternative Therapies* in 1998. Most of the studies included in the review found a significant difference. The animals that were fed organic foods were healthier. The biggest differences were seen in animals that were sick or very young: The organically fed animals tended to have a higher reproductive capacity, better survival of the young, less illness, and better recovery from illness. Across generations, there was a decline in reproductive ability in the animals fed chemically grown foods: Sperm motility decreased, and ovum production went down.

Organically grown foods are somewhat more expensive than conventional crops, but their superior power as natural medicines makes them well worth the difference. Think of it as a commitment to your health. It's a small price to pay for food that delivers the most nutritional value, tastes better, is free of (or has *very* low amounts of) dangerous carcinogenic chemicals, and is grown in a way that doesn't damage the environment. Remember, too: Buying organic foods saves you money in the long run because cancer, or any chronic disease, costs you time and drains you physically, emotionally, and financially.

Organic Isn't Just About Food

Foods aren't the only products grown with chemicals. Farmers put huge amounts of pesticides on cotton plants grown for fabric. In fact, more pesticides are used on cotton than on any other plant. Every year, one-fourth to one-third of all the pesticides used in the world is used on cotton. Pesticides contaminate the cotton plant and the environment, get into the food chain, and then set up residence in *you* (more on this in Chapter 21). Other dangerous chemicals are used, or created, in the processing of the cotton, too. For instance, when cotton is bleached white, dioxins are created as byproducts of the bleach, and dioxins are the most powerful carcinogen known. Buying organic cotton clothes, towels, and linens will help to stop this unhealthy practice.

Government Organic Standards

The U.S. Department of Agriculture (USDA) approved strict, nationwide organic standards in 2002. The purpose was to guarantee to consumers that all foods labeled as "certified organic" were grown according to uniform standards. Prior to this date, several state agencies, each with different guidelines, certified organic foods. Because it was difficult for most consumers to know exactly what "certified organic" meant, the federal government stepped in.

All USDA certified-organic foods are now grown according to the same standards (see the website for the Environmental Protection Agency [EPA] at www.epa.gov). You can identify certified-organic foods by a simple green and white "USDA organic" label stamped on the front (see the figure at right).

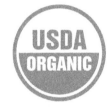

VEDIC ORGANIC AGRICULTURE

"Why do we eat in the first place? We eat to gain a blissful state of life, maximum coherence, health, and vitality." This simple statement by the monk Maharishi Mahesh Yogi expresses why *Ayurveda* considers high-quality food so important to your health. Your body and mind are literally created from the food you eat. Your food *becomes* you. On the horizon is the revival and reestablishment of an ancient agricultural technology that takes certified-organic foods to the next level, creating maximum quality and vitality in food. It's called Maharishi *Vedic* Organic Agriculture (MVOA).

Ayurveda is based on the quantum laws of the Universe, which modern physics has only recently begun to explore. For instance, *Ayurveda* acknowledges that everything in life is intimately connected, expertly managed, and based on the laws of the Universe. So, that which is fundamentally good for human health is also good for all forms of life, including animals and plants.

MVOA uses the same *Ayurvedic* principles and techniques that govern human health to help plants grow to their highest potential. For example, *Ayurveda* teaches that following the natural rhythms of Nature will enhance your health and ignoring them will damage it. If you sleep at the proper times at night, you are working with the rhythms of Nature and your physiology responds by gaining balance and strength. On the other hand, if you work against the rhythms of Nature by sleeping during the day and staying awake all night, your physiology becomes unbalanced, weak, and prone to disease. Similarly, the health of a plant depends on how well the farmer works with the rhythms of Nature.

Jyotish and the Rhythms of Nature

Farmers are extremely aware of the rhythms and cycles of Nature. To produce successful crops, they must work within these laws. For instance, crops are planted in the spring and harvested in the fall. Crops planted in the fall in Northern climates are doomed to failure. Everyone knows this because the cycles of the seasons are so obvious. However, there are cycles and rhythms to Nature that are far more subtle and specific that can also have a significant impact on the growth and quality of plants. MVOA uses a special, ancient mathematical system, called *Jyotish,* to map out these more subtle cycles.

The *Jyotish* calculations help the farmer to determine when to begin certain activities, such as planting and harvesting, with much more precision. Having a deeper knowledge of the more subtle cycles creates a higher probability of success for the crops. For instance, a farmer may know from experience that a crop should ideally be planted by the second week in May. *Jyotish* calculations are much more specific. They can tell the farmer the exact day and the precise time on that day—down to the minute—to begin planting.

The importance of identifying the best day and time to plant and harvest crops is not a strange or foreign concept. One of early America's most influential figures, Benjamin Franklin, recognized the importance of working with the rhythms of Nature to produce the best crops. To help farmers do just that, he published *Poor Richard's Almanack* [sic].

Jyotish calculations go deeper, however. They are based on the influence and movements of the planets and stars. Because all things in the Universe are connected on the quantum level, *everything influences everything.* That's why the planets have a significant effect on us. The influences of the sun and moon are very familiar. The daily cycles of the sun establish the rhythm for every life form on this planet. The moon creates daily and monthly influences. It causes tides to rise, regulates a woman's monthly menstrual cycle, affects moods, and influences the incidence of crime. Some people have a harder time believing that the more distant planets affect us, too, but quantum physics tells us that they do.

Ayurveda uses *Jyotish* to predict the planetary impact on the present and the future. The constantly changing configurations of the planets are mathematically measured, and detailed information can be determined about every aspect of your life, from the probability and timing of potential health problems or accidents, to the best time to begin a new project, such as constructing a new house or getting married. If you know about potential problems *before* they happen, you can do something to try to prevent them and protect yourself. *Jyotish* is said to help you "avert the dangers not yet come." For example, if you know you have a day when the probability of accidents is extremely high, you might choose to not drive on that day. If the *Jyotish* calculations say that there's a strong probability of your developing a particular illness, you might pay closer attention to your diet, rest, and take preventative herbs. In short, *Jyotish* helps you to work with precision with the rhythms of Nature, instead of leaving things up to chance.

Musical Medicine

MVOA uses music and sounds to enhance the growth of plants. Decades of research have determined that certain *sounds and music can induce balance and promote health*—not just in humans, but also in plants. This fundamental principle of health was recognized in *Ayurveda* thousands of years ago, and not surprisingly, this system of medicine contains detailed, sophisticated knowledge about using sounds for health.

The fact that music can affect the growth of plants should come as no surprise. More than thirty years ago, modern scientists rediscovered the powerful effects of music on plants. In the 1970s, classical music was observed to cause plants to grow faster and stronger, whereas hard rock-and-roll caused them to droop and wilt.

Instead of classical music, *Ayurveda* prescribes specific sounds, called primordial sounds, and music, called *Gandharva Veda*. There are many types of *Gandharva Veda* music, and each one is designed to be used during different hours of the day. Precise types of music are also prescribed for various health conditions. MVOA uses these same primordial sounds and music for the benefit of crops. Research has shown that playing primordial sounds, called *Sama Veda,* and the music, *Gandharva Veda,* at prescribed times helps to bring balance and coherence to plants and causes them to grow to their full potential.

In addition to *Sama Veda* and *Gandharva Veda,* there is a wide variety of *Ayurvedic* tools that can be used to help prevent disease, promote growth, and enhance the healing qualities of plants. They include techniques of consciousness, medicinal smoke pots, aromatherapy, herbal medicines, and specially timed and prescribed performances of traditional ancient vibrational chants, called *yagyas.*

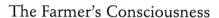

The Farmer's Consciousness

Vedic agriculture recognizes that the consciousness of the farmer and those who work on the farm also has a significant influence on the health and nutritive value of a plant. Science shows that people create "field effects," that is, they generate measurable influences on the environment. People are influenced by other people's states of consciousness, too. For instance, if you are in an extreme state of bliss or if you are in a horrible rage, you create a field around you that influences the people and the environment around you.

Research also shows that when people collectively experience higher states of consciousness—particularly during group meditation—the field effect of each individual merges with the others, intensifies, and creates specific and measurable benefits. For instance, when groups of individuals practice a form of meditation called Transcendental Meditation (TM) and an advanced meditation technique called the TM *Sidhi* program, the surrounding geographical area is beneficially affected by a calming influence. In a study published in 1988 in the *Journal of Conflict Resolution,* groups of meditators during the Lebanon war were found to produce an influence that resulted in a significant reduction in war deaths and casualties, when compared to those that occurred on days when no meditators were present. In the summer of 1985, an assembly of thousands of meditators convened in Washington, D.C. During their stay, crime rates went down and the incidence of violence and accidents dropped by 25 percent.

How does the field effect of consciousness work? It works at the quantum level (see Quantum Physics and Consciousness on page 289). Quantum physics says that everything in the universe, when reduced to its finest level—the quantum level—is interconnected and composed of the same material. In other words, if you look beyond the atom, beyond the subatomic parts, you find a nonchanging field of quantum forces/particles that physicists have called the "unified field." This field holds all the laws of Nature. Scientists say that what lies beyond this physical unified field is a unified field of consciousness. The practice of TM strengthens your connection to this unified field of consciousness. When the unified field is directly experienced during the practice of TM, it is enlivened. Because this field holds the laws of Nature, enlivening this field enlivens natural law. The result is that the health of your mind/body is automatically supported and nourished.

Since everything is connected on the quantum level, it's easy to understand how the farmer's consciousness can create a nourishing field of influence on his or her crops. Experiencing the unified field through the regular practice of TM enlivens the laws of Nature, creating a powerful beneficial influence on the plants. You can think of *Vedic* agriculture as quantum-mechanical farming.

Sthapatya Veda Architecture

Because *Vedic* agriculture as a quantum-mechanical science recognizes that all things are interconnected and influence one another, it gives serious thought to the influence caused by the characteristics of the land, its slope, orientation, and other special features, as well as all the buildings on the farm. To optimize a nourishing influence on the growth of the plants, the fields and buildings should be designed according to an ancient form of architecture called *Sthapatya Veda*. Its structures are known to have an extraordinary influence on plant growth. For example, a tree next to a temple in India that was built according to this design blooms twelve months out of the year.

You may be familiar with a similar, but different, form of Chinese architectural design called *feng shui*. Historians believe *feng shui* may have developed from *Sthapatya Veda*. Both systems of architecture are based on the recognition that the structures you live and work in, as well as the characteristics of the land, have powerful effects on your mind/body. The direction in which a building faces, the dimensions and layout of its rooms, the thickness of its walls, the materials used for its construction—all have a predictable influence. *Sthapatya Veda* buildings are designed to create optimal harmony between the individual and all things in Nature, enhancing human physiology and everything in the surrounding area.

On the Vine

A final important step in *Vedic* agriculture is to allow fruits and vegetables to ripen on the vine before picking them. The maximum nutritional benefits of a plant can be achieved only by allowing its produce to vine-ripen. Those of you who have a garden know that there are no words to adequately describe what happens when you bite into freshly picked, vine-ripened food. The explosion of flavor is so incredible compared to "store-bought" foods, it's startling. That's because the taste of vine-ripened food reflects its nutritional qualities.

All the techniques of *Vedic* agriculture are designed to create foods with the highest possible potential for medicines and life-giving nutrients, which then thoroughly metabolize and integrate into your body. As Maharishi Mahesh Yogi so eloquently said, "Conventionally grown foods poison you; organically grown foods won't hurt you; and MVOA foods produce a blissful state of life, maximum coherence, health, and vitality." (See Resources under Maharishi *Vedic* Organic Agriculture.)

Chapter 7

Fields of Gold

How Whole Grains
and Fiber Protect You

*P*icture rolling hills covered with amber fields of whole grains danc-ing in the wind. Their majestic beauty hints at their special power. The rustling sound they make as they gently brush against one another whispers the suggestion that Nature has bestowed upon us another plant food that contains powerful medicine. These fields of gold are teeming with plant medicines—medicines so potent and varied that they protect against breast cancer and other diseases in a multitude of ways. For your War-rior Goddess, they are mighty shafts of intense potential—fundamental instru-ments of focused plant intelligence that can fortify you against even the fiercest of foes.

Whole grains have been a primary food staple in the diet of many cultures for thousands of years, and for good reasons. They are rich in antioxidants, vita-mins, trace minerals, fiber, and lignans, all of which promote health and protect against diseases, especially cancer, cardiovascular disease, diabetes, and obesity. Not surprisingly, researchers have found that people who consume diets high in fresh organic fruits, vegetables, and whole grains have the lowest risk of chron-ic disorders. For example, women who regularly eat these foods cut their risk of breast cancer by more than 50 percent.

A FEAST OF FIBER

Most plant foods are rich in fiber, particularly whole grains. Fiber is much more than an effective laxative. It has many medicinal qualities that make it extreme-ly adept at preventing and combating breast cancer. Research shows that women who eat a high-fiber diet have up to a 54 percent lower risk of breast cancer. For women who have had breast cancer, many studies have found that high dietary fiber improves their survival and significantly lowers overall mortality. For instance, the Health, Eating, Activity, and Lifestyle (HEAL) study in 2011 found an inverse relationship between dietary fiber intake and breast cancer mortality.

There are two major types of fiber: soluble and insoluble. Each is important for good health, and each has special anticancer properties.

Soluble fiber is found in fruits, vegetables, and certain grains, such as oats. This type of fiber is processed by intestinal bacteria and converted into a powerful deactivator of carcinogens in the colon. Think of it like a bomb squad deactivating bombs. This is one of the reasons why high-fiber vegetarian diets are associated with a much lower risk of colon cancer.

Soluble fiber doesn't add much bulk to your stool, but *insoluble* fiber does. It, therefore, assists in regularity. When there's a lot of bulk to your stool, the time it takes to pass through your colon is much shorter. The faster carcinogens in your stool get out of your colon, the less likely they are to cause damage.

Insoluble fiber is found in large amounts in wheat bran and corn bran. This type of fiber also absorbs and retains water like a sponge—an important characteristic when it comes to protecting against cancer. Insoluble fiber absorbs so much water that it dilutes carcinogens, making them less dangerous. But this is no ordinary sponge; it's a special weapon against breast cancer, absorbing and binding all kinds of potential enemies.

Take, for example, the fact that insoluble fiber binds to estrogen in the colon and eliminates it. If you review Figure 3.1 on page 42, you'll see that estrogen is broken down by your liver, and then sent to the colon to be eliminated. If there is insoluble fiber in your colon, it will bind to the estrogen and facilitate its removal from your body. As a result, the total amount of estrogen in your body will be reduced. Experimental animals fed high-fiber diets (containing both soluble and insoluble fiber) were found to excrete twice as much estrogen in their feces as animals fed low-fiber diets.

Fiber has the same beneficial estrogen-lowering effects in humans, too. In a study of women who ate wheat bran, researchers found that the more wheat bran a woman consumed, the lower her estrogen levels were.

There are several other ways that fiber helps to lower the risk of breast cancer as well. Insoluble fiber takes away much of the threat of certain adversaries, such as simple carbohydrates (including refined sugars) and harmful fats, by slowing down their absorption. But its cancer-fighting abilities don't stop there. Insoluble fiber regulates insulin and glucose, two high-threat opponents that can significantly elevate the risk of breast cancer. Glucose is the principal form of sugar that your cells use for energy. High glucose and insulin levels are one of the biggest risk factors for breast cancer (see Chapter 16).

High-fiber diets also lower the risk of obesity by promoting weight loss. Obesity is thought to be a major contributor to at least 40 percent of all breast cancers diagnosed after menopause. In addition, fiber cuts your risk of obesity and breast cancer by decreasing the amount of fat you absorb from your food, thereby lowering blood-fat levels. High amounts of saturated fats and certain other types of unhealthy fats are also associated with a higher risk of breast cancer.

Whole grains and bran are also rich in antioxidants, vitamins, and trace minerals, all of which support the exceptional ability of your internal healing intelligence to keep you healthy and ward off disease. In addition, whole grains are endowed with generous amounts of a substance called "lignans." Lignans are what give stiffness to the structure of a plant. They are extremely medicinal and can have a big impact on lowering your risk of breast cancer. Scientists have mapped out at least a dozen different ways that lignans help to reduce your risk. The cancer-fighting properties of lignans are discussed in detail in Chapter 9.

Chapter 8

Fats: The Good and the Bad

Fats That Poison and Fats That Protect

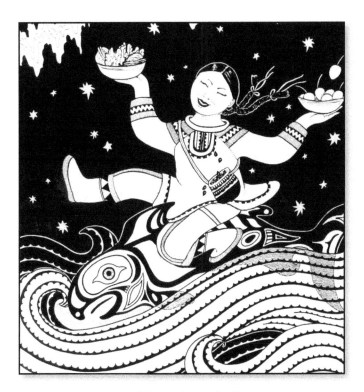

Goddess of Good Oils

Intellectuals solve problems; geniuses prevent them.

—Albert Einstein

*F*ats aren't ambivalent when it comes to breast cancer. They're either miraculous in their power to protect or terrible in their power to destroy, accelerating the initiation and growth of breast cancer. Contrary to a common misconception, *not all* fats are bad for you. In fact, certain fats are life-sustaining and absolutely essential to enable your body to function properly. Your Warrior Goddess finds a multitude of uses for these fundamental substances of life. When she is given proper amounts, her energy is boundless, her movements are as agile and lyrical as a dancer's, and her complexion is luxuriant and glows like the full moon. She exudes these qualities because you have provided her with the resources she needs to stay strong and supple. You have also given her the material she needs to craft her many sly and slippery modes of defense against disease. In order to more fully understand how she does this, it is important to first discuss basics about nutrition.

The food you eat each day is composed of nutrients. These nutrients supply your body with fuel for energy production, with building blocks for tissue repair and construction, and with all the substances your body needs to initiate chemical reactions and carry out body functions. The nutrients you consume influence your risk of breast cancer. Depending on what you eat, they can increase your risk, decrease your risk, or have no effect on it whatsoever.

There are two broad categories of nutrients: macronutrients and micronutrients. Macronutrients are the nutrients that we need in relatively large amounts. They are carbohydrates, fats, and proteins. All packaged-food labels list the amounts of these three macronutrients. Because we also need water in large amounts each day, some nutritionists consider water a macronutrient, too. Micronutrients—vitamins and minerals—are discussed in Chapter 12.

Your body is constantly rebuilding itself, and carbohydrates, fats, and proteins supply the fuel and building materials. Most of the cells in your body have preprogrammed deaths. That means they are designed to live for a certain amount of time and die. New cells then replace these worn-out cells. This process is called "cell turnover."

Cell turnover plays an important part in your risk of cancer. Certain cells in your body turn over at a faster rate than other cells. For example, the lining of the intestines and breast and prostate cells turn over fairly frequently. The faster the cells turn over, the higher the risk is of a cancer developing. That's why cancers of the breast, prostate, and colon are so much more common than cancers in other parts of your body, where cells turn over slowly or, perhaps, not at all, like the heart.

There are different kinds of proteins, carbohydrates, and fats, and each of them has a different effect on your body and on your risk of breast cancer. Later in the book we will look at certain proteins and carbohydrates and how they affect your risk of breast cancer. Meanwhile, let's take a closer look at fat.

FATS AREN'T ALL BAD

Fat has gotten a bad rap. It's a substance that we have been taught to avoid, but the truth is certain fats are vital to life. For instance, every cell in your body has a membrane that is composed primarily of fat. Without proper amounts of fat in your diet, your cells can't function well. All your nerve cells, including those in your brain, are coated with fat. And this fatty sheath is what enables electrical impulses to travel through them. If there's a problem with this fatty sheath, as there is in multiple sclerosis, the ability of nerve impulses to move along these pathways is severely impaired and, as a result, so is your ability to move and think. Fat also serves as your body's main storage unit of fuel. It provides insulation, assists in wound healing, is used to make hormones, and protects you from trauma.

Fats make up the fundamental structure of every cell membrane. You've heard the cliché "You are what you eat." This statement is absolutely true. Your body can only use the materials you supply to rebuild itself. That means the type of fat structuring your cell membranes can *only* be the type of fat you have eaten. The specific type of fat that predominantly makes up your cell membranes determines how well those membranes will function. It also affects how well your whole body functions. If your cell membranes are composed primarily of health-promoting fats, they will be able to carry out their duties with perfect competence and ease. If health-destroying fats have the upper hand, the ability of your cell membranes to perform their tasks will be severely impaired.

Here's a good analogy: Your car needs certain fats—oil—to run properly. If you don't put oil in the engine, you're headed for big trouble. The engine will soon suffer irreversible damage. If you put the wrong kind of oil in the engine, it won't run very well or very efficiently, either. Over time, this misguided choice of oil will clog the engine. However, if you put the ideal high-quality oil in your car, the engine will run extremely well. And if you keep using top-grade oil in the right amounts, your car's engine will continue to run well for a long time.

Balance Is Everything

Although you need fats for your body to run well, too much of a good thing can be bad. This concept is expressed through the *Ayurvedic* principle: *The right things in the right amounts at the right times will bring balance.* Remember, perfect balance means perfect health. If you eat the wrong things in the wrong amounts at the wrong times, you cause imbalances, and all diseases start as imbalances.

Eating excessive amounts of fat, especially certain types of "bad" fats, significantly increases your risk of several types of cancer, including breast cancer, as well as other serious diseases. High-fat diets increase your chances of developing breast cancer because they amplify the production of estrogen in your body. Remember, the more estrogen your body makes, the higher your risk is. Researchers have found that diets high in saturated animal fats may boost your risk of postmenopausal breast cancer by 50 percent or more. If you have breast cancer, eating a diet high in fat may decrease your chances of survival. Out of fourteen studies looking at women with breast cancer and their intake of dietary fat, eight showed that the women who ate a high-fat diet had a higher death rate than those who ate diets that were lower in fat.

The good news is, if you reduce the amount of fat in your diet, you can substantially lower your risk of breast cancer. A study published in the *British Journal of Cancer* confirmed this fact. The women in the study were put on a low-fat diet. Their daily intake of calories from fat normally made up about 30 to 40 percent of their total calories. They were given a diet in which fat supplied only 15 percent of their daily calories. The amount of estradiol (the most common and most potent type of natural estrogen in your body and the one that correlates to your risk of breast cancer) in their blood was measured before they went on the low-fat diet. It was measured again after they had followed the low-fat diet for two years. Researchers found that the level of estradiol in these women dropped by 20 percent over the two years. That means that their risk of breast cancer dropped substantially *more* than 20 percent, because small changes in estradiol translate into big changes in your risk.

Another study investigated the influence of a low-fat diet on total estrogen levels (all three types of natural estrogens—estradiol, estrone, and estriol) after a much shorter period of time. The women in this study had a 20 percent drop in their estrogen levels after an average of only five to six months on a low-fat diet.

BAD FATS

Certain types of fat are very bad for your body. They damage your overall health and significantly increase your risk of breast cancer as well as many other types of cancer and serious diseases, such as heart disease. The worst types of fats are saturated fats—especially animal fats—and fats that have been chemically altered, called trans fats or hydrogenated fats.

Saturated Animal Fats

Eating a diet high in saturated animal fats, like those found in red meat and high-fat dairy products, notably increases your risk of breast cancer. A study published in the *Journal of the National Cancer Institute* in 2003 interviewed 90,655 women and found that premenopausal women between the ages of twenty-six and forty-six who consumed the highest amounts of red meat and high-fat dairy had a higher risk of breast cancer than those who ate only a small amount of these fats.

What's interesting, according to the study's principal researcher, Eunyong Cho, is that this study "found that earlier [dietary habits] have a stronger impact on later breast cancer risk. In other words, women had an increased risk if, as young adults, they had a higher intake of animal fat, mainly from meat and dairy fat." But don't think that this means there's nothing you can do now to reverse the damage. You can. Remember, other studies show that decreasing your saturated-fat intake lowers your estrogen levels and significantly reduces your danger of developing breast cancer.

When you eat saturated animal fats, they make the cells throughout your body more insulin resistant and consequently increase the level of insulin in your blood. This seemingly innocent, normal response actually brings on a flood of increased risk; high insulin levels are one of the biggest risk factors and promoters of breast cancer. Women with abnormally elevated insulin levels have a 283 percent higher risk of breast cancer than those with normal insulin levels (see Chapter 16).

Saturated animal fats are a storehouse for concentrated toxic chemicals such as pesticides. Some of these chemicals mimic estrogen and make cell division in the breast speed up rapidly. As you now know, the faster cells divide in your breast, the higher your risk of breast cancer. If the animals and animal products you eat were not organically raised, the level of toxic chemicals in them can be quite high. In addition, these animals are commonly given hormones and growth factors that, when you ingest them, speed up breast-cell division. These hormones are also very dangerous for women with breast cancer, because they cause breast tumors to grow more rapidly.

Organic, but Not Toxin-Free

By law, organically raised animals must be fed only organically grown foods. They cannot be given any antibiotics, hormones, or growth factors. Despite this, organically raised animals aren't always completely toxin-free. Some of them may have small amounts of toxic chemicals concentrated in their fat. Why are there toxins in organic animals? Primarily because, instead up being confined in stalls, they graze in pastures. Although being outdoors is a good thing, our environment is contaminated with hundreds, if not thousands, of toxins. Rainwater may, and often does, contain poisonous chemicals. When it rains, these dangerous compounds fall onto the pasture and into the ponds where organic animals eat and drink.

There's another reason why organically raised animals may contain toxins. Harmful chemicals are generally very persistent in our environment. That means that they don't break down easily. For a farm to become certified organic, no synthetic or potentially unsafe chemicals may have been used on the land for at least three years. But some of these toxins persist in the soil for much longer than three years. In fact, it's not unusual for them to last twenty years or more.

IGF-1: A Top Breast Health Enemy

The body naturally produces insulin-like growth factors (IGFs). In normal concentrations, they play a necessary role in the manufacture of body tissue. However, an elevated level of insulin-like growth factor-1 (IGF-1) is a huge promoter of breast cancer, as well as prostate and colon cancers. In fact, a few studies have found that there's nothing we know of that stimulates breast cancer or prostate cancer more than IGF-1! Promoting excessive amounts of this growth factor is like throwing rocket fuel onto the flames of cancer.

You can avoid inundating your body with excessive amounts of IGF-1 by steering clear of conventional dairy products. In the United States, cows are routinely injected with the genetically engineered growth hormone recombinant bovine growth hormone (rBGH). When rBGH is injected into a cow, it causes the natural growth factor IGF-1 to be released into the body of the cow. Cows injected with rBGH have been found to have unusually high levels of IGF-1 in their fat and milk. When you consume IGF-1 in animal products, it normally breaks down in your stomach and causes no harm. But when IGF-1 is consumed in milk, it doesn't break down. The protein in milk, called casein, prevents IGF-1 from breaking down, so it's all absorbed into your body.

A study published in the British journal *The Lancet* in 1998 documented the enormous risk associated with high levels of IGF-1. The risk of breast cancer among premenopausal women younger than fifty-one who had the highest levels of IGF-1 in their blood was found to be 700 percent higher than the average.

Other studies also show a significant increased risk of breast cancer associated with high IGF-1 levels. For instance, a study published in the July 29, 2006 issue of the *International Journal of Oncology* found that women who had the highest ranges of IGF-1 and the IGF-1 binding protein (IGFBP)-3 in their blood had 3 times the incidence of estrogen and progesterone receptor-positive tumors compared to those with the lowest ranges, and a 2.4 times higher incidence of estrogen and progesterone-negative tumors. In this same study, the hormone testosterone was also found to increase the risk of breast cancer. Women with the highest range of testosterone levels were found to have a 4 times higher incidence of breast cancer overall and a 5.8 times higher incidence of estrogen and progesterone receptor-positive tumors. Those women who had both high IGF-1 and testosterone levels had a risk of breast cancer that was up to 26.4 times higher!

The reason that the IGF-1's bite is so venomous is because there are IGF-1 receptors on breast cells, just as there are estrogen receptors. Research has found that IGF-1 and estrogen interact. According to a study from Georgetown University published in 2002, estradiol and IGF-1, through a complex "cross-talk" mechanism, stimulate normal breast cells to start dividing.

In summary, when you eat the nonorganic saturated animal fats found in meat and dairy products, your risk of breast cancer escalates from a triple threat:

1. High insulin levels (as a response to the saturated fats),

2. High IGF-1 levels (from rBGH-injected cows), and

3. Toxic estrogenic hormones and chemicals (either injected into or fed to the cows).

This is why you should avoid nonorganic red meats and dairy as much as possible. If you simply must have dairy products, you can minimize your risk by eating only those that have been organically produced and are low in fat.

Trans Fats: Another Top Enemy of Breast Health

Of all the fats you can eat, trans fats are the most dangerous. Trans fats are manmade. They are natural fats that have been chemically altered by adding extra hydrogen atoms. That's why they are also called "hydrogenated" or "partially hydrogenated" fats. Chemical engineers created these fats in an effort to make processed foods taste better and to increase their shelf life. They were successful. Hydrogenated fats make foods such as potato chips crispier, and they increase the shelf life of processed foods such as crackers, chips, cookies, and baked goods. But what the engineers didn't know was that the fats they created would also promote serious diseases, including heart disease and cancer.

Michael Jacobson, executive director of the Center for Science in the Public Interest, states that trans fats cause about 50,000 premature deaths each year. New York City became the first city to ban trans fats in its restaurants when city health officials mandated that trans fats be banned from food served at the city's 20,000 restaurants by July 1, 2007. Many companies have stopped using trans fats. McDonald's announced on January 30, 2007, that it had settled on a new formula for its frying oil and would begin using this trans-fat-free oil sometime in 2007 or 2008.

The reason trans fats are so bad for you is because they promote oxygen free radicals—molecules that cause damage to your cells and DNA, damage that can lead to cancer. (For more about oxygen free radicals, see Chapter 13.) Trans fats also encourage inflammation, which, in turn, creates more oxygen free radicals. Chronic inflammation has been identified as a key factor in the initiation and progression of breast cancer.

All these ill effects add up to a high probability of developing not only breast cancer, but also cancers of the prostate and colon. Research has found that women with the highest amounts of trans fats in their bodies, documented by serum blood samples, have a 40 to 75 percent increased risk of breast cancer. A 2011 study from the Fred Hutchinson Cancer Research Center in Seattle, Washington, found that women diagnosed with breast cancer had a 40 percent higher risk of dying from any cause if they consumed a high amount of saturated animal fats in their diet. If they consumed a high amount of trans fats, their risk of dying was 78 percent higher! And if that isn't bad enough, cancer isn't the only disease provoked by chronic inflammation. It's thought to play a large role in many degenerative diseases, including heart disease, the number-one killer of American men and women.

Omega-6 Fatty Acids

Fats are made up of smaller units of molecules called fatty acids. Omega-6 fatty acids are needed by your body to function properly. They are important for normal brain function, and growth and development. But if you eat too much of them they can have detrimental effects, especially by increasing inflammation. Researchers believe this may be one of the main reasons why excess omega-6 consumption has been found to increase your risk of breast cancer. Studies have found that women with the highest amounts of omega-6 fatty acids in their bodies have a 69 percent increased risk of breast cancer. If you have breast cancer, eating large amounts of omega-6 fatty acids can make your prognosis—and your chance of survival—worse. A high intake of these fatty acids increases the likelihood that your cancer will metastasize, spreading to other parts of your body. The following is a partial list of the foods and oils that are high in omega-6 fatty acids.

- Commercial salad dressings
- Margarine
- Safflower oil
- Corn oil
- Mayonnaise
- Sesame oil
- Cottonseed oil
- Peanut oil
- Soybean oil
- Grape seed oil

Omega-6 fatty acids are essential for your body to function properly, so don't eliminate all omega-6 fatty acids from your diet. In the following section "Omega-3 Fatty Acids," there's more information on the best amounts to consume. Also, see the section Conjugated Linoleic Acids (CLAs) on page 87 for a discussion of this health-promoting type of omega-6 fatty acid.

GOOD FATS

As the ancient Chinese described, there is a yin (dark) and yang (light) side to all things; fats are no exception. The devastation caused by destructive fats is inversely proportional to the powerful shielding force of protective fats. Certain types of fats have extraordinary healing benefits. These "good" fats help your body to function properly and noticeably reduce your risk of such diseases as heart disease and cancer.

Omega-3 Fatty Acids

The most health-promoting type of fat you can eat is composed of omega-3 fatty acids. They reduce your risk of breast cancer considerably in three major ways. First, omega-3 fatty acids decrease the power of estrogen in the breast, so that cells won't divide as quickly in response to estrogen. Second, they act to subdue inflammation and all the ill effects of an enzyme involved in inflammation called the COX-2 enzyme. In fact, a study published in 2012 from the University of San Diego found that omega-3s had the most powerful anti-inflammatory effects of any substance tested because they block *all* of the inflammatory pathways! Third, omega-3s mop up oxygen free radicals.

Omega-3 fatty acids also help to fight breast cancer if you already have it, and they do so very impressively. Research has found that they cause breast tumors to shrink in size and prevent them from metastasizing. In fact, omega-3 fatty acids are so powerful in subverting the spread of tumors in the body that women with the highest levels of omega-3s in their bodies have only one-fifth the incidence of metastasis that occurs in women with the lowest levels.

Ten of the specific ways that omega-3s subdue tumor growth are as follows:

1. Omega-3s disrupt key enzymes necessary for breast cancer to grow (protein kinase A and the PKC-alpha isozyme of protein kinase C).

2. Omega-3s stop tumor cells from sticking together.

3. Omega-3s prevent tumor cells from migrating or spreading to other areas of the body.

4. Omega-3s cause cell death by apoptosis.

5. Omega-3s influence syndecan-1 (a protein on the cell membrane that regulates many biological processes, including growth factor signaling and cell to cell adhesion).

6. Omega-3s stop new blood vessels from growing into tumors.

7. Omega-3s work synergistically to enhance the effectiveness of several chemotherapeutic agents, including tamoxifen, doxorubicin, and a drug used to treat women with breast cancers that express the HER2/neu gene called Herceptin. Omega-3s also directly and dramatically suppress the HER2/neu gene.

8. Omega-3s reduce the receptors for epidermal growth factor—a tumor promoter.

9. Omega-3s decrease breast density.

10. Omega-3s lower insulin resistance.

For those who are treated with the chemotherapeutic drug Taxol (paclitaxel), omega-3s are protective against one of its most debilitating side effects—peripheral neuropathy, or nerve damage, which causes numbness and tingling of the hands and feet.

Omega-3s benefit many other common conditions affecting women. In a study published in 2004 in the journal *Obstetrical and Gynecological Survey,* Swedish researchers stated that omega-3 fatty acids improve menstrual and fertility problems by increasing blood flow to the uterus; decrease the risk of premature births; increase the length of pregnancy; increase birth weight; improve placental blood flow; and help to prevent preeclampsia, postpartum depression, postmenopausal osteoporosis, and cardiovascular disease. Nursing mothers may also enhance their baby's brain development by consuming omega-3s.

The health benefits of omega-3s are so great and so broad, that experts recommend that everyone supplement their diets—every day—with omega-3s.

Here is a list of some of the major health conditions improved with omega-3s:

- Asthma
- Cancers of the breast, prostate, and colon
- Diabetes
- Heart arrhythmias
- Heart disease
- High blood pressure
- High cholesterol
- Inflammatory bowel disease (IBD)
- Macular degeneration
- Osteoporosis
- Parkinson's disease

- Periodontitis or gum disease
- Rheumatoid arthritis
- Mental disorders: Depression, bipolar disorder, schizophrenia, attention deficit/hyperactivity disorder (ADHD), Alzheimer's disease, and cognitive decline

- Skin disorders
- Systemic lupus erythematosus (SLE)

The best plant source of omega-3 fatty acids is flaxseeds. Flaxseeds contain considerably more omega-3s than any other known edible plant. When it comes to combating breast cancer, flaxseeds exhibit superhero power. But an abundant supply of omega-3s is only one of the reasons flaxseeds are so beneficial. For more information about flaxseeds, see Chapter 9.

Omega-3 fatty acids can also be found in notable amounts in other foods— for example, chia seeds, algae, walnuts, and certain fish such as wild-caught salmon, herring, and krill. But—and this is a *big but*—*fish is now one of the most toxic foods you can eat* because we've polluted our lakes, rivers, and oceans so badly. In fact, fish contain more concentrated amounts of dangerous chemicals than any other food source.

If you think eating farm-raised fish is safer, think again. An article published in *The New York Times* on July 30, 2003, reported findings by the Environmental Working Group, a nonprofit environmental research and advocacy group, on ten samples of farmed salmon bought at markets on the East and West coasts. (Farmed salmon accounts for 66 percent of all salmon eaten in the United States.) All the fish samples were contaminated with polychlorinated biphenyls (PCBs) at levels far higher than any other protein source, including all other types of seafood. (See Chapter 21 and the inset "What Are PCBs?" on page 84.) For this reason, I don't recommend eating fish to get your omega-3s. (Instead, choose flaxseeds and other good omega-3 sources such as walnuts, pumpkin seeds, hemp seeds, soybeans, some dark green leafy vegetables, winter squash, and ground oregano.)

When it comes to omega-3 and omega-6 fatty acids, it's the ratio that you consume of them that makes all the difference—how much you eat of one compared to the other. The body functions best when you eat a 4:1 ratio of omega-6s to omega-3s. The typical American diet has a dangerous ratio of about 20:1. As you now know, consuming excessive amounts of omega-6 fatty acids is extremely dangerous.

Omega-9 Fatty Acids

Those who follow a Mediterranean-style diet have only half the breast cancer risk of those who follow the standard American diet. Researchers think there are two main reasons for this. First, the Mediterranean diet is high in fruits and vegetables, and second, it includes a lot of olive oil, which is high in omega-9 fatty acids. Omega-9s contain properties that are health promoting in general, as well as specific against breast cancer.

A population-based case-control study conducted in the Canary Islands and published in February 2006 in the journal *Public Health and Nutrition* confirmed the protective effect that olive oil has against breast cancer. They found that women who consumed the most olive oil in their diets (greater than or equal to 8.8 grams per day) had about a 50 percent lower prevalence of breast cancer. In an Italian review of twenty-five studies published in 2011, women who consumed the most olive oil compared to those who consumed the most butter had a five times lower risk of breast cancer!

Olive oil has many different ways that it improves cancer risk and survival. Those who enjoy olive oil frequently and develop breast cancer usually have cancers that are found at earlier stages and have a favorable hormone-receptor

What Are PCBs?

PCBs are a group of 209 different compounds. They were first brought to the market by the Monsanto Corporation in 1929. (Monsanto is also the company principally responsible for creating genetically altered foods.) PCBs were used in electrical transformers, adhesives, fluorescent lighting, flame retardants, and paints. Their primary use, however, was as a dielectric fluid in electrical equipment. Because of their stability and resistance to thermal breakdown, as well as their insulating properties, they were the fluid of choice for transformers and capacitors. As a matter of fact, they were required by some fire codes due to their exceptional fire resistance.

But after a few decades of use, it was discovered that PCBs caused an alarming number of serious health problems, so corporations were forced to stop manufacturing them in the late 1970s and early 1980s. These health problems include suppression of the immune system, headaches, depression, numbness, abnormal heart rhythm, impaired long-term memory, loss of coordination, liver failure, disruption of the endocrine system, and cancer. Pregnant women with high PCB counts are more likely to have children with physical, behavioral, and cognitive problems.

Even though PCBs are no longer made, an estimated two-thirds of all the PCBs manufactured between 1930 and 1970 are still in use or are in waste dumps, slowly leeching into our water supply. PCBs are extremely resistant to status. In other words, olive oil lovers who are diagnosed with breast cancer have a much higher incidence of estrogen receptor-positive (ER+) and progesterone receptor-positive (PR+) tumors than average. Omega-9s also exert positive effects on the structure and function of the cell membranes, cell communication channels, and gene expression. If you have breast cancer, olive oil has many properties that have been shown to help your body fight it. For example, it helps to stop tumor growth, directly kills tumor cells, and prevents tumors from spreading to other areas of the body and invading into surrounding tissues.

What Makes Olive Oil So Protective

Many researchers have been analyzing olive oil for decades to find out why it is so effective at warding off cancer. In a study published in 2000 in the *European Journal of Cancer,* German researchers identified an abundance of antioxidants in extra-virgin olive oil (polyphenols such as oleuropein, aldehydic secoiridoids,

---

degradation. So, scientists say that the remaining one-third are still somewhere in our environment. Disturbingly, experts expect that they will persist for hundreds of years.

PCBs are a huge problem in the Great Lakes. They are thought to have entered the lake water from contaminated landfills, leaking tankers, rainwater, and birds. The levels of PCBs in lake water measured between 5 and 60 parts per thousand (ppt) at its worst in the early 1970s. Although the level has dropped considerably since then, it is still considered unsafe. PCBs, like other toxins, become concentrated in animal flesh, and it is this "bioconcentration" phenomenon that poses significant danger to us.

Here's how it works: Medium-sized fish eat hundreds of small fish, each with concentrated toxins stored in their flesh. The toxins from these hundreds of small fish then concentrate into the medium-sized fish's flesh. Then, a bigger fish eats hundreds of these medium-sized fish and concentrates all of their toxins into its flesh, and so on. This is why fish that are large enough for human consumption usually have perilous amounts of toxins. For example, commercial-sized fish from the Great Lakes are found to have PCB levels as high as 4.83 parts per million (ppm). According to the EPA (www.epa.gov), levels greater than 2ppm pose health risks. Women who eat the most fish from the Great Lakes give birth to children with a multitude of problems, especially attention deficit hyperactivity disorder (ADHD), learning disabilities, and reproductive disorders.

flavonoids, and lignans). Antioxidants neutralize oxygen free radicals—tiny unstable molecules of oxygen formed in our bodies as a natural byproduct of metabolism. When there is an excess of oxygen free radicals in our body (stress, pollution, and toxins are common causes) they can damage our cells and DNA and contribute to the initiation and acceleration of a variety of chronic disorders, including cancer.

Spanish researchers, J. A. Menendez and R. Colomer working in conjunction with Northwestern University in Chicago, published three studies between 2005 and 2006 which illuminate some of the very specific ways that olive oil protects against breast cancer. Their findings are a bit technical for a layperson to understand, but worth describing. Olive oil also known as oleic acid, "suppresses the overexpression of HER2 (HER2/neu, erbB-2), a well characterized oncogene playing a key role in the etiology, progression, and response to chemotherapy and endocrine therapy in approximately 20 percent of breast carcinomas." In other words, there are genes in our DNA called "oncogenes" that when activated, promote the growth of cancer. One of those genes is called HER2. About 20 percent of breast cancers are HER2 positive, meaning that this gene is involved in the growth of the tumor. Olive oil suppresses this gene in at least three different ways. Women with HER2-positive tumors are usually given a chemotherapy drug, called Herceptin, to help combat their tumors. Olive oil actually works in a similar manner as Herceptin and is therefore very effective for women with this type of tumor. In fact, a study published in the *Annals of Oncology* in 2005 found that olive oil acts synergistically with Herceptin, enhancing the cancer cell-killing and growth-stopping effects of this drug by 70 percent. These same researchers in 2007 discovered the polyphenol in olive oil with the most potent action against breast cancer—oleuropein aglycone—caused a fiftyfold increase in the efficiency of Herceptin! The HER2 gene also plays a role in ovarian and stomach cancer, so olive oil is protective against these tumors too.

Another way that olive oil lowers the risk of breast cancer is by decreasing the "mammographic density" of the breast. High mammographic breast density has been identified as a significant risk factor for breast cancer. There are many things that effect mammographic breast density, for example, obesity, number of children, and breast feeding. What we consume in our diet can affect it, too. Flax oil, flax lignans, and olive oil all lower breast density.

Many Other Health Benefits of Olive Oil

In addition to its anticancer properties, olive oil also has many other health-promoting effects. When it comes to your heart health, olive oil helps to protect it because it lowers the bad type of cholesterol (LDL, or low-density lipoprotein) and raises the good type, HDL (high-density lipoprotein). It also lowers triglycerides, especially in diabetics, which is important not only to your cardiovascular system, but also to your risk of both breast and colorectal cancers. Olive oil suppresses inflammation and autoimmune diseases. That's why it is beneficial for conditions such as rheumatoid arthritis. It is helpful for your digestion too because it enhances emptying of the gallbladder, and decreases the response that your pancreas and stomach has to food. Finally, it promotes healing of gastric ulcers and makes the stomach lining more resistant to damage by non-steroidal anti-inflammatory drugs.

When you purchase olive oil, *always* remember to buy certified organic. If your local grocery store doesn't carry it, ask the manager to order it. (See the Resources section under "Organic Foods.")

Conjugated Linoleic Acids (CLAs)

Conjugated linoleic acids (CLAs) are a mixture of unique omega-6 fatty acids that have a slightly different molecular structure from the omega-6s associated with an increased risk of breast cancer. CLAs have the opposite effect of normal omega-6 fatty acids; they lower the risk of breast cancer. CLAs occur naturally in certain foods, but not in sufficient quantities. Therefore, to benefit from their anticancer properties, you must take a daily supplement.

Research shows that CLAs work in many different ways to inhibit the growth of breast cancer. For example, CLAs help to prevent the initiation of breast cancer by toxic chemicals. CLAs also cause structural changes in breast tissue that make it more resistant to damage by oxygen free radicals and toxins that are known to initiate breast cancer. According to a study conducted in Finland, these protective effects are profound: Women with the highest amounts of CLAs in their blood had the lowest incidence of breast cancer.

If you have breast cancer, CLAs are beneficial for you, too. They encourage cancer cells to stop growing and deter the tumor from spreading to other parts of your body through a variety of mechanisms. For example, a study published in *Breast Cancer Research and Treatment* in 2013 found that CLAs reduce proliferation, or the speed at which tumors grow, by decreasing the production of fatty acids—a substance required for the growth of tumors (a detailed explanation is given in the next section on Gamma-Linolenic Acid). A French study from 2012 documented several genes that were activated by CLAs, which cause tumor growth to slow down, prevent tumors from spreading to other areas of the body, and kill tumor cells by a process called apoptosis.

CLAs discourage the growth of breast cancer through estrogen and nonestrogen pathways and, therefore, are effective for both estrogen receptor-positive and estrogen receptor-negative tumors. When combined with certain chemotherapeutic drugs such as gemcitabine, CLAs make their antitumor activity much stronger.

Another way that CLAs may help to lower the risk of breast cancer is by promoting higher lean-muscle mass and lower body fat. That's why bodybuilders use CLAs as a supplement. Remember, fat cells make estrogen, and the more estrogen your body makes, the higher your risk of breast cancer. So, reducing body fat is one effective way to lower your risk of this terrible disease. (By the way, when figuring your 4:1 ratio of omega-6 to omega-3, you do not need to take your supplemental CLA into account.)

Gamma-Linolenic Acid

Another special type of omega-6 fatty acid called gamma-linolenic acid (GLA), which is found in high amounts in evening primrose oil, borage oil, and black currant seed oil, appears to mount a powerful defense against breast cancer. GLA contains superb anti-inflammatory and antioxidant properties that help to impede the growth of cancers. It also has many other specific ways it mounts a defense against this deadly disease. For example, laboratory tests conducted at Northwestern University and published in the *Journal of the National Cancer Institute* in November, 2005, found GLA—just like olive oil—inhibits the HER2/neu gene and increases the tumor-cell killing ability of the anticancer drug Herceptin by thirty to forty times! Earlier research at Northwestern University demonstrated that GLA also enhances the effectiveness of several other chemotherapy drugs used for breast cancer, including Taxol, Taxotere, Navelbine, Tamoxifen, and Faslodex.

A study published in the *International Journal of Oncology* in 2004 found another way that GLA helps to combat HER2/neu breast cancer: It inhibits the expression of a critical enzyme involved in the synthesis of fatty acids in mammals called fatty acid synthase (FAS). This enzyme is important for breast cancer because it is found to be over-expressed—meaning that it is produced in excessive quantities, especially in HER2/neu breast cancers. GLA was found to be the most effective of all the oils tested at shutting down the activity of FAS—decreasing it by 75 percent. When FAS levels are low, it causes an accumulation of toxins in the cancer cells and causes them to die.

According to a study published in the *Journal of Nutrition* in November 2003, GLA can also protect against some of the damaging side effects of chemotherapy, especially nerve damage called peripheral neuropathy that manifests as numbness and tingling.

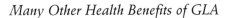

Many Other Health Benefits of GLA

There are many other health benefits of GLA. Here are some of the conditions improved with it:

- **Diabetes.** Patients with diabetes frequently suffer peripheral neuropathy, too. Just like the nerve damage caused by chemotherapy, patients with diabetic neuropathy suffer with numbness and tingling of their extremities. This lack of sensation may lead to unrecognized injuries of the feet and subsequent infections. Several studies, including one that was published in 2003 in the *Journal of the American Board of Family Practice*, show that evening primrose oil significantly improves this condition.

- **Hormonal balance.** Evening primrose oil has been shown to help alleviate hot flashes associated with menopause and has modest benefits for PMS as well. For women who suffer with painful breasts, especially around their menstrual periods—a condition called cyclic mastalgia—evening primrose oil may be extremely helpful. In a study published in the *British Medical Bulletin* in 1991 and another in the prestigious journal the *Lancet*, evening primrose oil improved the symptoms in 77 percent of patients with cyclic mastalgia.

- **Inflammatory skin conditions and autoimmune diseases.** In a meta-analysis (a review of many studies) of randomized placebo-controlled clinical trials of evening primrose oil for atopic eczema, there were clear improvements in itching, crusting, edema, and redness. Evening primrose oil improves a variety of other skin conditions and autoimmune disease including psoriasis, systemic lupus erythematosus (SLE), and multiple sclerosis.

- **Arthritis.** Because evening primrose oil has excellent anti-inflammatory and antioxidant qualities, it should come as no surprise that studies show it helps relieve the severity of the common inflammatory conditions of osteoarthritis and rheumatoid arthritis.

- **Weight control.** GLA may be beneficial for those who are overweight, because according to a study published in *CCL Family Foundations* in 1993, it assists the body in more effectively using fat.

How to Take GLA

The recommended amount of evening primrose oil is 2,600 milligrams (mg) per day. If you are taking it for conditions such as arthritis, asthma, or eczema, up to 4 to 6 grams is recommended. Look for high-quality organically produced evening primrose oil, such as that made by Barlean's Organic Oils. Approximately 280 mg of GLA is contained in the 2,600 mg daily dose. Another excellent product is Barlean's Essential Woman Swirl, which comes in a delicious chocolate-raspberry flavor and tastes like a fruit smoothie. It contains organic evening primrose oil, organic flaxseed oil, and lignans, which are all loaded with powerful anticancer properties.

Chapter 9

A Fortress
of Seeds

Flax—The Medicine Within

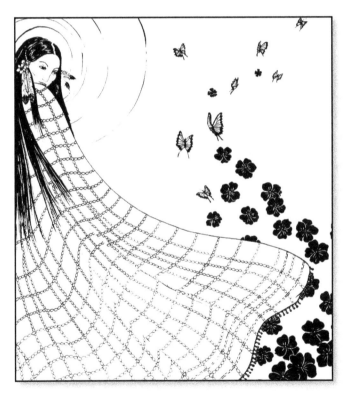

Goddess of Flax

Flowers and fruits are only the beginning.
In the seed lies the life and the future.

—MARION ZIMMER BRADLEY

*H*ippocrates said, "Let food be your medicine and medicine be your food." *Ayurveda* recognized that foods could be a source of medicine thousands of years before Hippocrates and proclaimed, "Food should be the first medicine you take, because without a proper diet, no medicine will work; with a proper diet, no medicine is necessary." The ancient Chinese agreed, stating, "He who takes medicine and neglects diet wastes the skill of the physician."

If you were given only one choice of a food to take as medicine, your best choice would be the tiny seeds from the flax plant. Flaxseeds have more potent medicinal qualities—especially those that fight breast cancer—than any known edible plant. This small seed provides a fortress of protection against this killer.

1. OMEGA-3 FATTY ACIDS

The intelligence contained in flax is so spectacular that it coordinates a sensational offense against breast cancer. Flax has three notable distinctions. First, it's the richest plant source of omega-3 fatty acids. Research has found that women who eat the highest amounts of omega-3s have the lowest risk of breast cancer.

Omega-3 fatty acids help to lower the risk of breast cancer by quieting inflammation and by decreasing the rate at which breast cells divide in response to estrogen. Inflammation is a key factor in the initiation and progression of a variety of diseases including heart disease, rheumatoid arthritis, skin diseases, and cancers (such as breast cancer). If you have breast cancer, omega-3s have been found to help shrink breast tumors and prevent them from spreading to other parts of the body.

2. LIGNANS

The second exceptional quality of flax has to do with lignans. Lignans are natural plant compounds that help to give plants their stiff structure. They also possess extraordinary anticancer properties, with an astonishing ability to help protect against and fight breast cancer. Lignans are found abundantly in certain fruits, vegetables, beans, seeds, and legumes—including garlic, carrots, broccoli, asparagus, dried apricots, and prunes. But the amount of lignans in these plants is miniscule compared to that in flaxseeds. Flaxseeds contain at least 100 times more lignans than any other known edible plant!

Lignans deter and arrest the growth of breast cancer in a multitude of ways. First, they act as a weak estrogen (similar to how genistein acts in soy; see Chapter 10). Second, lignans change the structure of the breast, making it more resistant to the toxins that induce cancer. Third, if you have breast cancer, lignans can stop the tumor cells from growing and help to prevent the metastasis of your tumor. They do this by decreasing two growth factors that fuel the fires of breast cancer: insulin-like growth factor-1 (IGF-1) and epidermal growth factor. As you may recall, IGF-1 is thought to be one of the most dangerous and potent risk factors for breast and prostate cancer.

There is another cancer-enhancing growth factor that lignans thwart, called "vascular endothelial growth factor" (VEGF). VEGF aids in the growth of cancer cells by stimulating new blood vessels to grow. How can new blood vessels affect the rate of growth of cancer cells? Here's how: In order for a tumor to grow larger, it needs more nutrients and oxygen, which can be delivered only by new blood vessels. So, the more blood vessels that grow into a tumor, the more food and oxygen that are delivered to it, the faster it will grow. In fact, without new blood vessels, tumors can't grow larger. Cancer specialists discovered that this anticancer tactic used by lignans—blocking VEGF—is so powerful at stopping tumor growth that they have created anticancer drugs that work this same way. The first VEGF-blocking drug, called Avastin (bevacizumab), was released on the market in 2004. Avastin is currently approved only for the treatment of metastatic colon cancer and must be given in combination with another chemotherapeutic drug called 5-FU. The Food and Drug Administration (FDA) revoked the approval of Avastin for breast cancer treatment in 2011 after it did not show any improvement and caused serious side effects, including high blood pressure and bleeding.

Lignans have several additional ways that they reduce the risk of breast cancer. They create more of the "good" kind of estrogen (similar to how indole-3-carbinol works), and reduce the production of estrogen by fat cells. According to a 1993 study from the University of Rochester, flaxseeds high in lignans also lengthen the menstrual cycle. For example, if a woman has a menstrual period every twenty-eight days and then starts consuming flaxseeds, her cycles may lengthen to every thirty-two days. The longer your menstrual cycles are, the fewer the number of cycles you will have over your lifetime, and the less estradiol you will produce. Simply put, the longer your menstrual cycles are, the lower your risk of breast cancer is.

Lignans also lower the production of estrogen by blocking the aromatase enzyme (similar to the anti-cancer drug Arimidex), block the estrogen receptor (similar to the anti-cancer drug Tamoxifen), improve blood glucose and insulin resistance, decrease breast density, and show excellent antioxidant and anti-inflammatory properties. If you must take Tamoxifen you'll be interested in knowing that a 2003 study conducted by researchers at the University of Toronto showed that the lignans found in flaxseeds enhance the effectiveness of Tamoxifen.

All of the very effective schemes that lignans use to combat breast cancer add up to lots of protection. Research shows that women with the highest amounts of lignans in their urine—a reflection of how much they consume in their diet—have the lowest risk of breast cancer. Women who consume high amounts of lignans and develop breast cancer are far less likely to be diagnosed with invasive, aggressive and/or triple-negative tumors, and their survival is better.

In the fall of 2003, a supplement made of isolated, purified, and concentrated lignans from flaxseeds, called Brevail, was released on the market. The dose in one daily capsule was strategically designed to create levels of lignans in the body that are in the same range as those found in women with the lowest risk of breast cancer. There are two major benefits to taking supplemental lignans. First, the amount of lignans in flax can vary from crop to crop by as much as 300 percent, whereas those in the supplement are standardized so you always get the optimal amount. Second, studies show that the lignans in Brevail are absorbed eighteen times more effectively than they are from ground flaxseeds. So, taking lignans in this supplemental form guarantees that you get the healthiest dose of lignans every day. Brevail is not recommended for women who are pregnant or currently breastfeeding, not because it isn't safe, but because no studies have been conducted yet on this special group of women to analyze the effects and proper dose.

Taking Brevail with other cancer drugs is also not recommended because this product hasn't been studied in women currently undergoing cancer treatment. However, that may change in the near future. A study published in the journal *Breast Cancer Research and Treatment* in July 2003 found that lignans enhance the effectiveness of the common cancer medication Tamoxifen. Researchers J. Chen and Lillian Thompson found that lignans and Tamoxifen, alone and—better yet—in combination, reduce the ability of estrogen receptor-negative tumor cells to stick together, invade, and migrate—all important properties in cancer's metastasis. More research is needed to determine the exact role this supplement may play in cancer treatment.

Brevail is standardized to one type of lignan found in flax, "secoisolariciresinol diglycoside" (SDG). Of all the lignans found in flax, SDG is the one found in the highest amounts and is possibly the most potent. If you decide to take Brevail, I think it's a good idea to eat flaxseed, too. In addition to the advantages of lignans, flax has many other anticancer properties that you wouldn't want to miss out on.

I recommend eating at least 3 tablespoons of *ground* flaxseeds a day. The hard seeds can't be digested, so grind them in a coffee grinder until they become a fine nutty powder. Add the ground seeds to just about anything you like: vegetable dishes, salads, smoothies, baked goods such as muffins, and cereal.

Many Health Benefits of Lignans

Supports breast health

❏ Decreases production of estrogen

❏ Blocks environmental estrogens from attaching to estrogen receptors

❏ Creates more of a "good" protective type of estrogen

❏ Causes breast tissue to be more resistant to environmental toxins

❏ Decreases three different growth factors that speed up the growth of breast cancer:

   • VEGF

   • Epithelial growth factor

   • IGF-1

❏ Kills tumor cells

❏ Prevents the spread of tumors

❏ Increases protein hormone binders in the blood

❏ Lengthens the time between menstrual cycles

❏ Blocks the aromatase enzyme (just like the anticancer drug Arimidex)

❏ Decreases tumor growth and invasion

❏ Reduces the risk of other cancers, including cancers of the prostate and colon

Helps hormonal balance

❏ Improves PMS and perimenopausal symptoms including hot flashes, mood swings and cognitive function

❏ Supports bone-mineral density

Other health benefits

❏ Cardiovascular:

   • Lowers blood pressure

   • Decreases total cholesterol and LDL while raising HDL

   • Prevents blockages in arteries

❏ Diabetes:

   • Improves blood glucose and insulin resistance

   • Has strong anti-inflammatory and antioxidant properties

3. FIBER

The third property of flax that lowers your risk of breast cancer is its abundant fiber. High-fiber diets are associated with a 54 percent lower risk of breast cancer. One way that fiber helps to lower your risk is by decreasing the amount of estrogen in your body by binding to it in your intestines and then expelling it from your body. You can review the many other ways that fiber helps to lower your risk in Chapter 7.

A MAGNIFICENT CAPE

To put the power of flaxseeds into perspective, consider this: If your Warrior Goddess were to create a majestic cloak of divine protection for herself, she would require a fabric made of the finest natural substance possessing a multitude of miraculous powers. She would search the world until she found the most magnificent fiber she could to create her cape of supernatural strength. Her expedition would end the moment she encountered the flaxseed. Her refined intuition would instantly tell her that this tiny seed was no ordinary seed. Rather, flax is the source of a rare and astonishing intelligence, the perfect material for creating a barrier against breast cancer.

Chapter 10

Asian Defense
Soy Foods

Never be afraid to try something new.
Remember, amateurs built the ark;
professionals built the Titanic.

—AUTHOR UNKNOWN

he East is known for its martial arts: elegant beautiful forms of movement that can be used to induce balance and healing or to deliver deadly blows to ward off formidable foes. Several foods in the traditional
Asian diet, especially soy foods, strengthen the physiology, and attack and
defend against breast cancer with the skill of a *Ninja* warrior. These foods are
some of your Warrior Goddess's favorite weapons against this enemy—eating
these foods is like arming her with *samurai* swords, *nunchucks*, and *shurikens*
(throwing stars).

Soy—a superstar in your arsenal against breast cancer—has been a food staple in the Asian diet for thousands of years. Asia has far lower rates of cancer
than the United States does, and researchers think that eating a lot of soy may
be one of the reasons. Japanese men and women eat about ten times more soy
than American men and women. According to many studies, if you eat an adequate amount of soy often enough, your risk of breast cancer will drop by 30 to
50 percent. For instance, a study published in the *Journal of the National Cancer
Institute* in June 2003 found that women who ate three bowls of miso soup (a
soup made with soybean paste) a day had a 40 percent lower risk of breast cancer. Those who ate two bowls of miso soup a day cut their risk by 26 percent.

GENISTEIN—SOY'S MOST IMPORTANT PHYTOCHEMICAL

There are several substances in soy that are active against breast cancer. A particular type of phytochemical called genistein appears to be one of the most

important. Genistein is classified as a phytoestrogen, or plant estrogen, because it has a weak estrogenic effect. Two other major phytoestrogens in soy are daidzein and glycitein. However, genistein is the most abundant and well researched of the three and is usually the only one that is listed on the label of soy products.

Research shows that genistein is extraordinarily effective at reducing the risk of breast cancer. It has been shown to stop tumor growth, prevent metastasis, and shut off new blood vessels in growing tumors. According to a 2006 study published in *Medical Hypothesis,* genistein attaches to a "beta" type of estrogen receptor (ERbeta), which has an antiproliferative effect as opposed to the "alpha" type of estrogen receptor that stimulates cells to grow and divide. It also blocks the cancer-promoting estrogens from attaching to the alpha estrogen receptors on breast cells.

Let's review how this beast grows. Breast cancer is a hormonal disease. That means that a hormone causes the cancer to develop by inciting cells to grow and divide. For breast cancer, that hormone is estrogen. The more estrogen you are exposed to, the higher your risk of breast cancer is.

Estrogens come in different strengths and behave differently. Strong estrogens increase your risk of cancer because they tell cells to grow and divide rapidly. Phytoestrogens and other weak estrogens decrease your risk of cancer because they slow down cell division. Genistein acts like a weak estrogen in the body. It blocks the effects of strong estrogens and slows down cell division. Genistein is very weak—in fact, less than $1/100$ of the strength of estradiol (the most potent type of natural estrogen). So, if genistein attaches to an estrogen receptor, the rate of cell division is only $1/100$ of the speed that it is if estradiol attaches to the receptor. The more genistein there is to compete with estradiol, the slower the rate of cell division and the lower your risk of breast cancer.

This is an extremely simplistic look at a very complicated process. Remember, soy is composed of hundreds of components all interacting together. Genistein doesn't act alone. If it's extracted from whole soy foods and then isolated and consumed without the other soy ingredients, it can actually have detrimental effects (see The Soy Controversy on page 103). Other substances in soy, for instance, phytoalexins glyceollins I, II, III, have been found to suppress tumor growth, to reduce the risk of developing breast cancer by protecting cells from toxins, and to inhibit BRCA1 mutant tumor growth through activation of DNA damage checkpoints, cell cycle arrest, and mitotic catastrophe (meaning that when cells try to divide and grow, they die during the process instead).

Understanding Phytoestrogens

There is currently a lot of confusion and misinformation about phytoestrogens. It is important to understand that plant estrogens are not the same as the estrogens our bodies make or the synthetic estrogens found in hormone replacement therapy (HRT) or birth control pills. They are very different. Most act more like selective estrogen modulators (SERMs), such as the cancer medication Tamoxifen, and as inhibitors of the enzyme aromatase (which is used in the production of estrogen), like the anticancer drug Arimidex. In other words, phytoestrogens act more like estrogen blockers than like estrogen. They have also been shown to lower the production of estrogen by hindering the aromatase enzyme, prevent new blood vessels from growing into tumors, and enhance the anticancer effects of vitamin D_3. Phytoestrogens act in so many complex ways that we may never fully understand them all.

SOY CONSUMPTION IN PREPUBESCENT GIRLS

Many studies show that young girls who eat soy products before they go through puberty have a substantially lower risk of breast cancer later in life. One explanation for this finding is that a woman's breast tissue is considered "immature" before she has had her first baby. Immature breast tissue is more sensitive to environmental toxins and other carcinogens. Soy has been found to help mature the breast tissue, making it more resistant to environmental toxins. According to a study published in *Carcinogenesis* in 2004, exposure to soy prior to puberty triggers another protective action—it "up-regulates" the breast cancer 1 (BRCA1) gene, a tumor-suppression gene. In other words, soy turns on a gene that suppresses tumor growth—and keeps it on. A 2012 study found that consuming soy before puberty may also contribute to lowering the risk of breast cancer by delaying puberty.

GENISTEIN, CANCER CELL DEATH
AND CHEMOTHERAPY

Genistein has also been shown to kill breast cancer cells through a process called apoptosis. Researchers at the Arkansas Children's Nutrition Center reported in their study published in *Carcinogenesis* in 2005 that genistein promotes apoptosis by inducing the production of a tumor suppressor protein known as "PTEN."

In a study published in the *Journal of Nutrition* in 2003, genistein was found to work synergistically with indole-3-carbinol in not only blocking the alpha-estrogen receptor, but also in increasing apoptosis of cancer cells. Both genistein and indole-3-carbinol were found to induce the BRCA1 and BRCA2 breast cancer genes that help to inhibit the stimulation of the estrogen receptor by estradiol and increase breast cancer cell death according to researchers at Georgetown University. Japanese researchers found that genistein also works synergistically with omega-3 fatty acids to increase apoptotic tumor cell death in their study published in the *Journal of Cancer Research and Clinical Oncology*. Researchers at the National Institute of Health found that breast cancer tumors that have a mutant BRCA1 (responsible for the genetic type of breast cancer) are more sensitive to the killing effects of genistein compared to other types of cancer cells.

Genistein enhances the killing effects of several chemotherapeutic drugs. Chemotherapeutic agents are known to induce nuclear factor kappaB (NF-kappaB) activity in tumor cells resulting in reduced cell killing and higher drug resistance. In contrast, genistein has been shown to inhibit the activity of NF-kappaB and the growth of various cancers cells without causing toxicity to the body. In a study published in the journal *Cancer Research* in 2005, cells pretreated with genistein exhibited cell growth inhibition and increased apoptosis when given each of the chemotherapeutic drugs cisplatin, docetaxel, or doxorubicin. The NF-kappaB inducing activity of these drugs was completely blocked when the cells were pretreated with genistein. Japanese researchers found that genistein enhanced the cell killing effects of yet another common chemotherapeutic drug used to treat breast cancer: Adriamycin. In their 2003 study, they found the combination of genistein and Adriamycin remarkably inactivated the HER2 gene, which plays a significant role in about 20 percent of breast cancers.

Other ways that research shows that soy may help lower the risk of breast cancer include: protecting against the effects of high estrogen in the postmenopausal breast; decreasing breast density in postmenopausal women; preventing the induction of tumor growth by toxins; decreasing activation of procarcinogens to carcinogens; regulating genes involved in tumor initiation, promotion, and progression; repressing the formation of cancer stem cells; and inactivating the HER2 receptor.

All of these anticancer effects help to explain the results of a meta-analysis published by researchers at John Hopkins University and published in the *Journal of the National Cancer Institute* in 2006. Eighteen epidemiological studies from 1978 to 2004 were analyzed and the researchers concluded that high soy intake is associated with a lower incidence of breast cancer, especially in premenopausal women. Other studies have shown that higher intakes of soy are associated with a greater decrease in the risk of postmenopausal breast cancer. Breast cancer survivors benefit from eating soy as well. Many studies conclude that women who eat higher levels of soy have improved survival and lower recurrence rates.

A meta-analysis of eighteen studies published in 2011 by Chinese researchers suggested that the protective effects of soy at reducing the incidence and recurrences of breast cancer were significant for Asian populations and not Western populations. However, an in-depth analysis of combined cohort studies of U.S. and Chinese women published by Vanderbilt University researchers the following year found that soy benefited both populations. In this large study, women who had been diagnosed with breast cancer and who consumed more than 10 milligrams (mg) of soy isoflavones per day had a decreased risk of recurrence and mortality—regardless of where they lived.

SOME SOYS ARE BETTER THAN OTHERS

There are dozens of different types of soy foods available, but when it comes to nutrients and health-promoting qualities, not all soy products are the same. Some soy foods are far better for you than others. Here are six great ones:

1. **Steamed or boiled soybeans in the pod, also called** *edamame.* Only the beans are eaten; the tough, fibrous pod is discarded.

2. **Dry roasted soybeans.** These make a great snack food. There are several different flavors to choose from, including ranch and, my personal favorite, Cajun.

3. **Tempeh.** This traditional Asian and Indonesian food is growing in popularity, so you can find it in most grocery stores. It's a cultured soy cake that sometimes has other grains or spices added to it. You can cook tempeh a number of ways: Sauté it in olive oil, bake it, crumble it into salads or stews, use it as a sandwich filling, or add it to a stir-fry dish.

4. **Tofu.** Made from soymilk curd, tofu looks a little like cheese. Its own flavor is very mild, but it will pick up the flavor of any dish you add it to. You can use it in at least 101 different ways, so I suggest you get a good tofu cookbook and experiment. (For a list of some tofu cookbooks, see the Recommended Reading section.)

5. **Miso.** Miso (fermented soybean paste) is a salty condiment that can be used to flavor a variety of dishes. Added to boiling water, it makes an excellent soup.

6. **Natto.** This form of soy is made from fermented cooked whole soybeans. It

comes in a variety of flavors and is commonly used in sushi rolls and with rice in Japanese restaurants. It's less popular than other soy products, so you are more likely to find it in an Asian market than at your local grocery store.

How much soy should you consume each day to lower your risk of breast cancer? Experts say about 4–12 ounces of a quality soy product. However, if you want to eat a little less soy than that but still get the same (or even better) cancer-fighting effects, you can add certain traditional Asian spices to your soy dishes. (See the inset "Add a Little Spice to Your Life" on the opposite page.)

THE SOY CONTROVERSY

Some physicians warn their patients not to eat soy foods because they fear that soy may increase the risk of breast cancer instead of decreasing it. Their mistaken fear came initially from a study from the University of California, San Francisco, published in October 1996. In this study, women were given 38 grams of genistein a day for one year. It's important to note that these women were not given genistein as it occurs naturally in whole soy foods. Rather, they were given genistein that had been extracted and isolated from soy foods and prepared as a supplement—a supplement composed *only* of genistein with none of the hundreds of other nutrients in soy.

The researchers were surprised to discover that instead of having a protective effect, the genistein supplement appeared to be harmful. After one year on the genistein supplement, the women had elevated the amounts of estradiol in

---

Add a Little Spice to Your Life

When you cook soy, you can exponentially enhance its anticancer power by simply adding a pinch of turmeric or cumin. Both of these spices defend against and sabotage the growth of breast cancer in many clever ways (see Chapter 11).

A 1997 study from Tufts University in Boston found that when turmeric and genistein are combined, they have a synergistic effect. In other words, each one makes the other more effective. Researchers used certain highly estrogenic pesticides, endosulfan/chlordane/DDT, to start some breast cancer tumors—estradiol for others—growing in the laboratory. Both genistein and curcumin (an active ingredient in turmeric and cumin) prevented the growth of the tumor cells—but not completely. When they were added together, the effect was so strong, all tumor-cell growth stopped.

their blood and their breast cells showed signs of stimulation and increased growth. This unexpected result concerned researchers. Could soy actually *increase* the risk of cancer? Hundreds of other studies show that women who eat the most soy have the lowest risk of breast cancer. So, how could a genistein isolate have the opposite effect? Remember the *Ayurvedic* principle: *Favor fresh whole foods.*

The women in the controversial study didn't eat fresh whole soy foods. They were given an isolate of genistein—something that doesn't naturally occur in Nature. When you isolate a substance from the whole, it often behaves differently. Your body was designed to eat, digest, and metabolize fresh *whole* foods, which contain hundreds, even thousands, of substances all interacting with one another. Those interactions can be critically important. One substance may balance the effect of another, make it more or less effective, take away its toxic effects, increase its absorption, or modify how your body uses it in some important way.

Research shows that when genistein is consumed as part of whole soy foods, it's absorbed very differently from how it is in an isolated supplemental form. Genistein in whole soy is activated by intestinal bacteria during digestion, whereas genistein taken as an isolated supplement is absorbed *before* it reaches the bacteria in the intestines. This may be part of the reason that genistein supplements appear to have an effect different from that of whole soy foods. So, until research shows otherwise, stay away from genistein supplements and eat whole soy foods.

Smelling a Rat: Rodents Aren't Human

Another contributing factor to the confusion about soy's effect on breast tissue comes from the fact that rodents metabolize soy differently than humans do. Researchers from Cincinnati Children's Hospital Medical Center pointed out in their study published in 2011 in the *American Journal of Clinical Nutrition* that the metabolism of soy isoflavones differs markedly in rodents compared to humans. Therefore, caution and doubt should be used when taking conclusions about soy in rodent studies and assuming those results will be also true for humans, especially regarding soy's effect on breast tissue.

Rodents and humans also appear to handle soy differently when it comes to the mineral iodine, which is important for healthy thyroid function. Animal studies raise concern that soy interferes with iodine absorption and may lead to hypothyroidism and goiters. However, there are no human studies that show any detrimental effects to the thyroid. A review of studies involving soy consumption and measures of thyroid function in humans was conducted by researchers at Loma Linda University and published in the journal *Thyroid*. None of the studies reviewed showed any unfavorable influences on the thyroid.

The Problem with Isolated Plant Elements

The isolated "active" ingredients of a plant don't express its full intelligence. Products that contain only certain elements of whole plants can miss out on all the other healing qualities of the plant delivered in the way Nature intended. Worse, sometimes isolates can have undesirable health effects because we are consuming substances in a concentration and form not found in Nature.

A whole plant contains hundreds, if not thousands, of different substances all interacting together. When you disrupt the balance in the plant, it's more than likely that you will disrupt the balance in yourself. Good health is all about balance. You don't want to take something for its medicinal qualities if it's going to throw the rest of you out of balance, sparking the development of another disease that may be worse than the one you're treating or trying to avoid. This is a common problem with pharmaceutical medications. They treat one problem, but often create others.

Ayurveda, on the other hand, contains an extremely sophisticated knowledge of the ideal way to administer herbs so that they *don't* create imbalances. *Ayurvedic* herbal medicines are usually mixtures of several different herbs acting synergistically, one enhancing or balancing the effects of another. So, according to the ancient time-tested principle of *Ayurveda,* isolating the "active ingredient" is a step in the wrong direction, away from trying to create an ideal medicine.

This brings up another important *Ayurvedic* principle: *Never sacrifice health for the sake of a cure.* Treatments should not create imbalances or disease. All the herbs and treatments in *Ayurveda* are formulated and designed to enhance balance and increase the body's healing intelligence. If an herb is used to help suppress a symptom, other herbs are also used to balance its effects or enhance the strength of the whole body. That's why eating a wide variety of whole organic foods is important, too. If you eat the same food every day, you'll miss out on important plant synergies and certain nutrients. There's a good chance that you will develop imbalances and eventually get sick.

When you compare certain pharmaceutical drugs to their herbal or natural counterparts, the reasoning behind the principle of favoring whole foods becomes very clear. Herbs are composed of whole plants or whole parts of a plant, such as the leaves and the roots. Pharmaceutical drugs take the active ingredient out of the plant, synthesize it, and then make it into a pill. Usually, the results are an effective substance, but with a catch— unwanted, potentially toxic, side effects. One-third of all patients admitted to the hospital are there due to iatrogenic causes (that is, health problems inadvertently induced by a physician, healthcare providers such as nurses, aides, and therapists, medical treatment, or diagnostic procedure). Each year, an estimated 250,000 people die from iatrogenic causes and, according to Dr. Gary Null and Dr. Carolyn Dean, that number may be much higher. In a paper they coauthored in 2003, "Death by Medicine," and then in the 2005 book *Death By Modern Medicine* by Carolyn Dean, M.D., N.D., and Trueman Tuck, the total number of annual iatrogenic deaths they calculated (based on medical peer-review journals) may be closer to 784,000. That means that the "American medical system is the leading cause of deaths and injury in the United States!" Approximately 106,000 of those deaths are due to adverse drug reactions and interactions.

Herbs aren't just weak pharmaceuticals. They're completely different. When taken properly, they work in harmony with the body, create an abundance of side *benefits*, and rarely have side effects. If they do have side effects, they are usually mild. Similarly, whole foods work in harmony with the body by increasing its healing intelligence in many ways. Isolated elements of foods aren't foods; they're pharmaceutical preparations of a single, concentrated active ingredient.

ANOTHER SOY CONTROVERSY

Another controversy regarding soy comes from preliminary results published in 2000 of a large prospective study called the Honolulu-Asian Aging Study. This study followed 3,734 elderly Japanese-American men from 1991 to 2012. The early results reported in 2000 found that the men who consumed the most tofu during midlife had up to a 2.4 times increased risk of Alzheimer's disease later in life. There also appeared to be a link between a higher incidence of brain atrophy (shrinkage) in men who ate two or more servings of tofu a week. Experts stress that the conclusions in this study are preliminary and not conclusive. It will take several years after the completion of the study in 2012 before the final results will be ready for publication. The association between soy and dementia has been reviewed by several other studies with mixed results. Some studies show no association, and some show an association with tofu, but the opposite effect—better cognition—with tempeh. I know this all sounds confusing—because it is! As of this date, the link between tofu consumption and brain atrophy continues to be speculative and hasn't been proven.

Some researchers have found substances in soy that may interfere with the absorption of certain minerals and other nutrients. They hypothesize that soy could cause a problem with the brain if it actually does obstruct the absorption of nutrients so much so that their levels become dangerously low. These questionable substances are broken down when soy is fermented. Because of that, some doctors recommend that you should eat only fermented soy products such as miso, tempeh, and natto. If you have healthy intestines, the bacteria in your intestines ferments soy, so nonfermented soy shouldn't interfere with your body's ability to absorb minerals, either. Don't forget that rodents metabolize soy differently than we do and many of these studies were conducted on our furry friends.

My personal opinion is that you should eat a wide variety of whole foods, including organic soy foods. Add spices to your foods to increase the anticancer properties. Don't make your diet all about one food. There are many different foods that fight cancer. Your diet should include as many of them as possible. This concept is expressed in another fundamental *Ayurvedic* principle: *A balanced diet should include a wide variety of fresh wholesome foods.* The greater the diversity of plants that you eat, the broader the spectrum of Nature's healing intelligence that you import into your body.

Chapter 11

Magic Mushrooms and Much More

Specialty Foods with Spectacular Powers

*S*oy isn't the only Asian food that mounts an impressive assault against breast cancer. There is a wonderful array of exotic specialty—many with Asian origins—that have their own magical and spectacular powers against this killer beast. These foods include several fungi, beverages, spices, herbs, and vegetables from the sea.

MEDICINAL MUSHROOMS

Falling in love is like eating mushrooms,
you never know if it's the real thing until it's too late.

—BILL BALANCE

In this kingdom of fungi with over 10,000 species, perhaps no other plant has such a spectrum of diversity. Some are a culinary delight and contain the power to heal, while others possess deadly poisons and the power to kill.

Thousands of years ago, Traditional Chinese Medicine (TCM) doctors discovered many with magical medicinal properties. Today, research confirms that dozens of species hold various compounds that mount an impressive defense against many deadly diseases, including cancer. Let's take a closer look at just a few that are particular potent.

The Maitake Mushroom—Tumor-Cell Assassin

For more than 2,000 years, maitake mushrooms have been part of the pharmacopeia in Japan. Hidden within this enchanting fungus is a powerful army of therapeutic chemical weapons against cancer.

Maitake mushrooms (*Grifola frondosa*) grow in clusters on hardwood trees and are indigenous to the Northern Hemisphere. In Japanese, "maitake mushrooms" means "dancing mushrooms." As legend has it, the name comes from how the ancients danced for joy when they found these extremely valuable mushrooms.

Research shows that the cancer-fighting chemicals in maitake mushrooms arrest the growth of tumors, cause them to shrink, and prevent them from spreading to other areas of the body. Maitake mushrooms also stimulate and boost the immune system by increasing the number and function of two important cells in the immune system—macrophages and T cells.

Three broad categories of cells make up the immune system: two types of lymphocytes, called B cells and T cells, and a third type of cells called macrophages. T cells make up 70 to 80 percent of all the lymphocytes in the blood. They lead the body's resistance force against bacterial infections, viral diseases, and tumors, and help to regulate the immune system. After an initial frontal attack by the immune system's lymphocytes, macrophages (or scavenger cells) strike from the rear to gobble up unwanted invaders in your body, including bacteria and cancer cells.

Most of the medicinal effects of this mushroom are thought to come from a special polysaccharide (a type of sugar). Found in what scientists call the "D fraction" in the maitake mushroom, the polysaccharide contains a substance called "beta-glucans," which, research shows, stimulates the immune system.

Maitake mushrooms' cancer-fighting effects go far beyond just boosting the immune system. This fungus can also kill tumor cells. In a laboratory study from Japan published in the journal *Molecular Biology* in 2002, liquid extracts of maitake mushrooms killed 95 percent of prostate cancer cells within twenty-four hours. In a human study, patients diagnosed as having stage 2, stage 3, or stage 4 breast cancer were given a combination of whole maitake powder and the "D fraction" of maitake mushrooms. Tumors shrank and symptoms improved in 68.8 percent of the patients. Researchers found that the mushrooms helped to shrink cancers of the liver and lung, too.

These amazing mushrooms can also be very beneficial for patients on chemotherapy. Normally, chemotherapeutic drugs dramatically weaken the immune system. But research shows that maitake mushrooms can counteract that effect and keep the immune system strong.

Consuming Maitake

Maitake mushrooms come fresh or dried to be used in cooking. Supplements are also available as powder, capsules, or liquid extracts. The recommended dose of maitake mushrooms is 3–5 grams of the dry powder or capsules each day, or 10–30 drops of the liquid extract three times per day.

Other Cancer-Fighting Mushrooms

Reishi mushrooms (*Ganoderma lucidum*), or the "mushroom of immortality," have been used as a medicine in China, Japan, Korea, and other Asian countries for as long as the maitake. Over 400 different bioactive chemicals have been identified which are responsible for reishi's extraordinary medicinal benefits. Some of those properties include empowering the immune system; dowsing inflammation; relieving pain; promoting sleep; protecting against diabetes and cardiovascular disease; and killing bacteria, viruses, and cancer cells.

Reishi mushrooms pack a particular punch against breast cancer using an arsenal of approaches. For example, they stimulate many cells in the immune system including B lymphocytes, T lymphocytes, dendritic cells, macrophages, and natural killer cells. They also can shut off new blood-vessel growth to tumors, and suppress cell adhesion and migration. These qualities mean that reishi mushrooms not only inhibit the growth of tumors, but they may also reduce the ability of a tumor to invade into both surrounding and distant tissues. Researchers at UCLA found that an alcohol extract of reishi mushroom spores stopped the growth of breast cancer cells in a dose-dependent manner. That means that the higher the concentration of the reishi mushroom extract, the more breast cancer cells it can kill. Therefore, reishi mushrooms may be a valuable dietary supplement for women who already have breast cancer. These mushrooms can also improve the killing effects of chemotherapy and radiation while diminishing many of their side effects.

Researchers at Bastyr University published a study in *Oncology Reports* in February 2006, which found three different mushroom *extracts—Coprinus comatus* (CCE), *Coprinellus sp.* (CME), and *Flammulina velutipes* (FVE)—inhibited the growth and killed through apoptosis, both estrogen receptor-positive and -negative breast cancer cells. When these mushroom extracts were applied to MCF-7 breast cancer cells in a petri dish, CCE and CME reduced cell growth by 60 percent and FVE by 99 percent!

The most commonly eaten mushroom—button mushrooms—mount a good defense against breast cancer, too. In a study published in December 2006 in the journal *Cancer Research*, researchers tested ten different mushroom extracts for their ability to interfere with the aromatase enzyme, which is involved in the manufacturing of estrogen. Half of the mushrooms that were tested—portobello, crimini, shiitake, white button, and baby button—inhibited the aromatase enzyme. Of these five, the common white button mushroom had the strongest effects. White button mushrooms (*Agaricus bisporus*) combat breast cancer in two additional ways: They strengthen the immune system, and directly stop tumor cells from growing and dividing. Researchers recommend 100 grams a day of white button mushrooms to help prevent tumor growth. Shiitake mushrooms (*Lentinus edodes*) are another delicious medicinal mushroom with strong anticancer properties. Research shows that women who eat mushrooms regularly, such as shiitake, have a lower risk of breast cancer.

If you don't like the taste of mushrooms, you'll be glad to know that eating them isn't your only option for enjoying their benefits. In fact, the medicinal powers in supplements and extracts of mushrooms are usually much greater than what you can get by consuming them in your meals. For example, hundreds of studies document that an extract made from the mycelium (roots) of certain shiitake mushrooms, called "active hexose correlated compound" (AHCC), has greatly enhanced medicinal properties. AHCC fights cancer in many different ways, including activating the cells in the immune system that help to destroy cancer cells, stopping tumors from growing and causing them to shrink, decreasing the risk of metastasis and recurrences, enhancing the effectiveness of chemotherapy while protecting against many of its harmful side effects, and improving survival. AHCC has been shown to be beneficial for cancers not only of the breast, but also of the prostate, colon, liver, stomach, thyroid, ovaries, testicles, tongue, kidney, and pancreas. The recommended dose for patients with cancer is 3 grams daily for two weeks, followed by a maintenance dose of a minimum of 1 gram per day.

GREEN TEA—THE #1 ANTICANCER BEVERAGE

More than 4,000 years ago, the Chinese began brewing the leaves of a plant and drinking it as a hot beverage. They called the infusion *cha,* their word for "tea." Now, more tea is consumed around the world every day than any other liquid except water. Research shows that drinking tea, especially green tea, is a wise choice because tea has been found to have many potent health benefits.

Research has shown that green tea is very effective in hampering the growth of at least eleven different types of cancer, including cancers of the esophagus, stomach, colon, bladder, prostate, ovaries, uterus, and breast. Green tea also reduces the risk of lung cancer in smokers, non-Hodgkin's lymphoma, and leukemia. That's why green tea is considered the number-one anticancer beverage. You might think that the impact of a few cups of tea each day on lowering the risk of these cancers would be small, but it's not. Cancers of the digestive tract are as much as 68 percent lower in tea drinkers.

One of the reasons why green tea is so potent against so many cancers is because it contains an exceptional blend of powerful anti-inflammatories and antioxidants. Green tea also has the remarkable ability to amplify the power of the enzymes in your liver that detoxify your body of poisons and carcinogens. It enhances the immune system to make it more effective at finding and destroying cancer cells, and gives the DNA repair team a boost too.

Researchers believe that most of the health benefits of green tea come from substances within it called polyphenols. The three polyphenols considered most important are gallocatechin (GC), epigallocatechin (EGC), and epigallocatechin gallate (EGCG). Of the three, EGCG is the most potent.

Japanese researchers found that among healthy women, those who drank green tea had a lower risk of breast cancer. And those women with breast cancer who drank green tea lived much longer than those who didn't. For instance, women with stage 1 or stage 2 breast cancer, who were green-tea drinkers before they were diagnosed, were found to have a much better prognosis for survival. Also, a 1998 study found that drinking green tea lowered the risk of breast tumors metastasizing and stopped them from recurring after the women had been treated. If you regularly eat medicinal mushrooms while sipping your green tea, according to researchers in Australia, you'll enjoy an exceptional amount of protection.

Several studies show that EGCG inhibits the growth of breast cancer and decreases the incidence of it metastasizing to the lungs. A Japanese study of rats with mammary tumors found that 93.8 percent of the rats given green tea survived, compared to only 33 percent of the rats that weren't given green tea. The rats given green tea also had smaller tumors than those that weren't given it.

Scientists have mapped out many different ways in which green tea combats breast cancer. For one, it increases the number of protein binders in the blood, and the more protein binders there are in the blood, the more estrogen it binds and the less estrogen there is available to attach to estrogen receptors in the breast. Secondly, it turns down the alpha-estrogen receptor so that it doesn't respond as much to estrogen. Green tea also lowers estradiol levels. Postmenopausal women who drink green tea and who are diagnosed with cancer are found to have a higher percentage of tumors that have estrogen- and progesterone-sensitive receptors. This is important, because tumors with receptors sensitive to these hormones respond better to treatment and have a better prognosis.

Green tea provides protection against hormone receptor-negative breast cancers as well. Several studies have documented a number of ways that green tea polyphenols induce cancer cell death, or apoptosis, and prevent invasion, which work through processes that are independent of estrogen or progesterone.

This stellar brew also helps to block the growth of new blood vessels into the tumor—a quality that is technically referred to as antiangiogenic, and subdues several different growth factors, including IGF-1. In 2012, researchers at the University of Tennessee discovered that green tea can reduce the risk of breast cancer caused by chronic exposure to environmental carcinogens. The next year, they found that one way it achieves this is by preventing the transformation of stem cells into cancer cells.

If you are on chemotherapy, green tea can enhance its effectiveness and at the same time protect against many of its dangerous side effects. Japanese researchers T. Sugiyama and Y. Saduka published several studies between 1998 and 2003 showing that green tea and some of its individual components increase the concentration of chemotherapeutic agents, such as doxorubicin (Adriamycin), in tumors by 2.1 to 2.9 times, and decrease the levels of these drugs in normal tissue. It also enhances the effectiveness of Tamoxifen while protecting against the liver damage it may cause. Chinese researchers in 2010 found that EGCG in tea improves the cancer-killing effects of another chemotherapeutic drug paclitaxel (Taxol). Breast cancer cells that are HER2/neu positive are not uncommonly resistant to the drug Herceptin, but according to researchers at Boston University green tea can cause the cells to become more sensitive to this drug. Green tea has also been found to affect the expression of twelve different genes in breast cancer cells that help to reduce their growth.

The results are that when you drink green tea while you're taking these chemotherapeutic drugs, tumors shrink more than they usually do without the green tea. In addition, organs that are commonly damaged by these anticancer drugs, such as the heart and liver, are protected from injury by drinking this potent green brew.

Major Health Benefits

Hundreds of studies show that green tea has many other impressive health benefits, as well. It decreases your risk of heart attacks and strokes by lowering levels of cholesterol and blood pressure, as well as by slowing the development of atherosclerosis ("hardening" of the arteries). Green tea is also superb at killing certain bacteria, especially in the bladder. Its flair for stopping these bladder bugs from propagating is revealed in this statistic: Tea drinkers have a 40 percent lower incidence of urinary tract infections. Green tea also aids digestion by increasing the number of helpful bacteria in your intestines while decreasing the number of harmful ones. In addition, green tea is a thermogenic agent. Thermogenics speed up your metabolism and help you lose weight. And if you're concerned about osteoporosis, drink this healthy brew often. A study published in the *American Journal of Clinical Nutrition* in April 2000 found that women, ages sixty-five to seventy-five, who drank at least one cup of green tea a day had

Cleaning Your Genes with Tea

This may sound like the latest cleaning tip from Martha Stewart, but it's not. Rather, it is an ingenious way that Nature designed to reduce your risk of cancer! In the last several decades we have learned a lot about how the genes in our DNA work. Like a radio, genes are either in the "on" position or the "off" position. When they are turned on, they express themselves and give out all the instructions they have. When they are turned off, they are silenced—so no instructions can be given.

The "off" button for our genes is pushed by something called a methyl group. When a methyl group attaches to our genes, it is called DNA methylation. A number of genes are noted to become abnormally methylated in breast cancer patients. In other words, these genes become stuck in the off position—bound and gagged—by a methyl group. The problem is that the instructions those genes contain are important for preventing the growth of cancer. Without those instructions, our body doesn't have the ability to suppress the growth of tumors very well.

Nature has supplied us with the perfect solution. You can clean your genes of the methyl groups and turn them back on with the magical chemicals contained in certain plants. The plants that possess the most outstanding methyl-plucking talents should come as no surprise. They are many of the top-notch cancer-fighters that we have already discussed, such as green tea, soy, and cruciferous vegetables.

All of the instructions our genes contain, however, aren't good. Some of them give bad cancer-promoting instructions. If these "bad" genes are turned on, they instruct our body to make proteins that can actually help tumors to grow. Obviously, you will want to silence those genes. Once again, Nature can come to the rescue. Certain plants, such as beets, wheat bran, spinach and micronutrients, especially vitamins B and E, zinc, and selenium, contain methyl groups that they can donate to the cause. Methyl groups also have many other important functions, including helping the repair crews in your body.

What to methyl? What to de-methyl? It probably all seems very confusing and complicated to you, but to your body's inner healing intelligence (aka your goddess), it is simple. Just supply her with an array of organically produced fresh plants every day, and she'll handle it for you.

significantly higher bone densities than those who didn't. Finally, green tea may help reduce the risk of diabetes. A 2012 study conducted at Pennsylvania State University reported that animals that were given EGCG before they were fed a high-carbohydrate meal had a 50 percent lower spike in their blood glucose compared to the animals that were not given the green tea polyphenol.

Choosing and Preparing Green Tea

Green tea (*Camellia sinensis*) is processed by steaming the tea leaves at high temperatures. When prepared in this way, the health-promoting polyphenols are preserved. (During the processing of black tea, some of these polyphenols are destroyed, which is probably why green tea has more potent medicinal properties than black tea.)

When you choose a green tea, it's important to buy organically grown tea. An analysis of several nonorganic brands found that they contained traces of the banned estrogenic pesticide, DDT. You don't want to drink something to *reduce* your risk of cancer if it also contains something that may *increase* your risk! Be safe and use organically grown green tea.

To create the best-tasting cup of tea with the highest medicinal qualities, steep your tea bag or tea ball in hot water for three to five minutes. For the maximum protection, drink eight to ten cups of green tea a day. Yes, green tea does contain some caffeine, but there are substances in the tea that seem to modify caffeine's side effects to the point that most of the people who drink it aren't adversely affected. Removing the caffeine from green tea actually *weakens* its anticancer power; the caffeine appears to be an important component of the tea's antitumor effects. If you don't think you can drink this much green tea each day, take a green-tea supplement. Two 250-milligram (mg) tablets a day are recommended.

TURMERIC—A MEDICINAL SPICE OF THE HIGHEST ORDER

From the healing powers of green, we move to the medicinal marvels of blazing yellow-orange. The Indian cooking spice turmeric, responsible for the intense color of curry, is even older and wiser than green tea when it comes to promoting and protecting health. This indigenous plant of Asia and India has been a star of *Ayurvedic* and Traditional Chinese Medicine (TCM) for more than 5,000 years—and for good reason. More than 5,500 studies published in medical journals confirm that this spectacular spice is one of Nature's most intelligent creations. These studies show that of all the known herbs and spices, turmeric possesses more anticancer qualities and healing benefits than any other.

Turmeric (*Curcuma longa*), a plant with beautiful, very large, long lily-like leaves, is indigenous to India and southern Asia. But it's what you don't see—under the ground—that possesses all the magic. The medicinal part of turmeric is its *rhizome* (root); it looks very much like ginger root. That's not surprising because turmeric and ginger are considered cousins. They are members of the same botanical family: *Zingiberaceae*.

The big difference between ginger and turmeric can be seen when you cut open the *rhizome*. Ginger root has a pale, plain white interior, but when you slice into turmeric, what you see is anything but drab. A vibrant, almost iridescent, bright-orange pigment radiates from its interior. Turmeric's visual hue gives a clue to the power of the medicine it holds.

Scientists have confirmed that the substance responsible for the spellbinding color of turmeric—curcumin—has many medicinal benefits. In fact, thousands of studies show that curcumin possesses almost all of turmeric's healing benefits. However, a 1997 study indicates that curcumin may not be the whole story of turmeric. Researchers removed the curcumin from a sample of turmeric, and then tested the curcumin-free turmeric for antitumor effects. They found that the anticancer qualities of curcumin-free turmeric were *more potent* than those of whole turmeric with its curcumin intact.

Like green tea, turmeric stands out from all the other plants in its class in its ability to impede cancer. Research shows that turmeric substantially thwarts dozens of different cancers, including cancers of the breast, prostate, colon, uterus, ovary, lung, mouth, esophagus, liver, kidney, skin (melanoma), head and neck (squamous cell cancers), nervous system, connective tissue (sarcoma), lymph (lymphoma and multiple myeloma), and blood (leukemia). An article published in the *American Association of Pharmaceutical Scientists* journal listed every known way that turmeric has been shown to selectively kill tumor cells. They described over thirty different ways! That's why this amazing spice is considered the number-one anticancer spice.

Here are just a few ways that turmeric impedes the initiation and growth of cancers: Turmeric helps to break down toxins in the liver and prevent carcinogens from forming, possesses dramatic anti-inflammatory properties, has potent antioxidants (300 times the power of vitamin E), and stimulates the immune system. Turmeric also emulsifies fat, so it helps to promote weight loss. Keeping your weight down is important, because obesity raises the risk of many cancers including breast cancer. And if you have cancer, turmeric enhances the effectiveness of chemotherapy against your tumor while it protects your organs from the damage that these drugs often cause.

Turmeric works with your liver in an ingenious way to get rid of the toxins in your body. Your liver has two sets of enzymes, called "phase 1" and "phase 2" enzymes. When a toxin or carcinogen, such as *benzopyrene,* which is found in cigarette smoke and charcoal-broiled meats, comes to the liver, phase 1 enzymes activate it. In other words, the toxin isn't a carcinogen until the phase 1 enzymes in your liver turn it into one. Why would your body want to *create* carcinogens? Because they are easier for phase 2 enzymes in your liver to recognize. Phase 2 enzymes attack carcinogens, break them down, and get rid of them. The problem comes when you overwhelm this system. When too many toxins come into the liver, some of them will escape the mechanisms designed to eliminate them.

Your risk of cancer can be reduced by *blocking* the activity of phase 1 enzymes, reducing the number of carcinogens formed or activated, or by *enhancing* the action of phase 2 enzymes, eliminating more carcinogens. One of the reasons that turmeric is so effective against cancer is because it has the ability to *both* block phase 1 and enhance phase 2 enzymes!

If you think the ability of a spice or an herb to protect your body from toxins isn't very strong, think again. Turmeric has *remarkable* abilities. Here's an example of just how amazing it can be. Mutagens (agents that can cause DNA mutations leading to cancer) are in the food you eat, the air you breathe, and in many things you come in contact with every day. They are activated and broken down in your body. The amount of mutagens in your body can be determined indirectly by measuring the concentration of their metabolites (byproducts of metabolism) in your urine.

The average smoker, not surprisingly, has a lot of carcinogenic metabolites in his or her urine. In a study published in the journal *Mutagenesis* in 1992, researchers measured the mutagen metabolites in the urine of sixteen chronic smokers and sixteen nonsmokers. Then, the smokers were given 1.5 grams of turmeric a day for thirty days. The nonsmokers were *not* given turmeric. At the end of thirty days, the urine of the smokers and nonsmokers were tested for mutagen metabolites. What the researchers found was nothing short of astounding: The level of mutagen metabolites was *lower* in the smokers taking turmeric than it was in the nonsmokers!

Turmeric has many general anticancer effects. It also has a number of amazing properties that specifically prevent and fight breast cancer. One way it lowers the risk of breast cancer is by blocking the toxins that are known to cause it. Some pesticides, such as DDT and chlordane, mimic the estrogen molecule in your body and thereby increase your risk of breast cancer. Turmeric can block the pesticides' estrogenic effects. It also impedes breast cancer tumors from forming in response to estrogen and environmental toxins.

Genistein in whole soy foods stumps the pesticides, too. Researchers at Tufts

University in Boston found that genistein and turmeric work synergistically, meaning that each one makes the other's ability to block estrogen and environmental toxins more effective. When genistein and turmeric were combined together, their ability to hinder estrogenic environmental toxins was extremely impressive. In one laboratory study, the combination of genistein and turmeric inhibited 95 percent of chemically induced breast cancer cell growth. In another study, they stopped 100 percent of the growth—*no* cancer cells grew despite heavy loads of estrogenic environmental toxins!

Turmeric also "down regulates" the estrogen receptor. That means it decreases the sensitivity of the estrogen receptor, reducing its normal response to estrogen. In other words, turmeric affects the estrogen receptor in such a way that when estrogen attaches to it, the rate at which breast cells divide is much slower than normal. However, when it comes to turmeric's ability to combat breast cancer, it could care less whether a tumor is sensitive to estrogen or any other hormone for that matter. This extraordinary anticancer medicine discourages the growth of every type of breast cancer: estrogen/progesterone positive or negative, HER2/neu positive, or even triple negative.

Another one of turmeric's very beneficial attributes is that it inhibits or blocks an enzyme that plays a key role in the initiation and growth of breast cancer, as well as several other types of cancer. It's called the COX-2 enzyme. (There's a lot more about this harmful substance in Chapter 14.) The number of COX-2 enzymes found in breast cancer tumors is frequently much higher than in normal cells. Scientists call it an "overexpression of the COX-2 enzyme."

The COX-2 enzyme is responsible for a long list of dangerous deeds. It encourages tumor cells to divide, prevents the death of tumor cells, stimulates the growth of new blood vessels, makes tumor cells better at invading the surrounding tissues, blocks the important tumor-suppressing effects of the immune system, increases the risk of metastasis, and speeds up the production of mutagens. That's an impressive list of horrific actions, but turmeric can put an end to all of them. It shuts down the COX-2 enzyme and thwarts *all* its harmful actions.

If you have breast cancer, turmeric's anti-COX-2-enzyme abilities can be tremendously helpful. Turmeric prevents tumors from growing, induces apoptosis (cell death), and inhibits cell proliferation. It also stops the growth of new blood vessels that tumors need in order to grow and halts the production of a substance called IL-6 (by your immune system), which makes cancer cells grow faster. Turmeric has anti-invasive effects, too; it helps to prevent tumors from invading surrounding tissues. It dissuades tumors from metastasizing to other areas of the body. And if you're on chemotherapy or receiving radiation, turmeric can increase the effectiveness of both treatments by making your cells more sensitive to their killing effects, while at the same time protecting your normal healthy cells from their damaging effects. A 2013 study showed that turmeric can even make estrogen receptor-negative breast cancer cells sensitive to Tamoxifen—an oral anticancer drug that normally only works against estrogen receptor-positive tumors!

Turmeric and green tea also have a synergistic effect. Green tea causes turmeric's anticancer effects to be three times stronger, and turmeric enhances green tea's anticancer capabilities by a factor of eight.

Turmeric's Other Healing Effects

Turmeric has an impressive array of other health benefits, too. In fact, this miraculous spice—with over 150 distinct beneficial actions that have been identified as of 2012—may help more than 500 health conditions. For example, if you have gallstones, it encourages your gallbladder to expel them. Turmeric aids digestion by increasing stomach secretions and decreasing the amount of gas produced in the intestines. It also protects against stomach ulcers. Turmeric lowers your risk of heart disease by decreasing cholesterol and the formation of plaque in your arteries. It promotes wound healing by decreasing inflammation and stimulating the growth of new blood vessels.

One of the more fascinating features of turmeric is that it clearly expresses its own intelligence. Turmeric *blocks* new blood-vessel growth in cancer to stop further growth of a tumor while it *stimulates* new blood-vessel growth in wounds to help speed healing. The key is that turmeric "knows" when to do each one. It can tell the difference between cancerous tissue and normal tissue and respond appropriately. No doubt, researchers will eventually uncover the elegant mechanisms responsible for this behavior.

In addition, turmeric shields your organs from chemical attack. It minimizes the damage to your brain caused by alcohol, as well as chemical damage to your liver. Elevated liver enzymes are an indication of liver injury. The higher the enzyme level, the more extensive the injury is. When turmeric is ingested, liver enzymes drop, indicating that it effectively helps the liver repair itself. Turmeric also strengthens your connective tissue and prevents the formation of adhesions or scar tissue. And it stimulates muscles to regenerate after trauma.

You can apply turmeric topically to your skin for another whole set of benefits. Turmeric can kill bacteria. If it's exposed to sunlight, its talent for exterminating bacteria improves. It is also effective for treating fungal infections, such as athletes' foot, and skin conditions, such as psoriasis.

There's no other known substance that you can eat or put on your skin that will do all that. All those healing effects from just one miraculous plant? It may sound impossible, but more than 5,500 studies in medical literature prove each and every one of them. When it comes to medicinal plants, turmeric is a super-star. This plant beautifully demonstrates an important *Ayurvedic* principle regarding medicinal plants that is worth remembering: *Plants hold intelligence, and they help us to heal by importing their intelligence into us.*

Taking Turmeric

Turmeric is prepared by soaking and then drying the root. After that, the dried root is ground into a fine powder. Turmeric powder can be found in the spice section of most grocery stores. Remember, organic is always best. *Ayurvedic* physicians recommend adding about one-quarter to one teaspoon to your food near the end of cooking. Turmeric works more in harmony with your body when it is cooked—but not overcooked.

You can also take turmeric as a supplement At least two 500-mg capsules a day is the minimum recommended dose if you are healthy. If you have a condition that turmeric can help to improve, some studies have given up to 4 to 10 grams of curcumin a day without negative side effects. Although there is no established standardized dose for cancer treatment and prevention, most researchers recommend doses over 2 grams a day. In addition, you can consume some of your daily dose of turmeric by sprinkling your foods with a delicious mix of Indian healing spices that includes it called "*churnas.*" *Churnas* are precise recipes of several different spices that can be added to any dish, either during cooking or afterward. *Churnas* usually aren't composed of "hot" spices like chili; rather, they are a delightful mixture of mildly flavorful natural medicines, such as turmeric, cumin, ginger, and fenugreek.

GARLIC—A CANCER NEMESIS EXTRAORDINAIRE

For more than 5,000 years, before even the earliest Chinese dynasties, garlic has been used as a medicine in central Asia. Prized for its health-promoting and health-protecting qualities, it was brought further and further West until it reached Egypt about 4,000 years ago. The earliest surviving written records describing garlic as a medicine are found in the Egyptian Ebers Papyrus written around 1500 B.C.E. Garlic was introduced into Europe in the first century A.D.

With this long history of cultivation, garlic is no longer found in the wild; it is strictly a plant grown by people. Today, it's produced and enjoyed for its excellent taste and diverse medicinal qualities by nearly every culture in the world. One of its distinctive traits is its ability to lower the risk of breast cancer.

An Iowa study of 34,388 postmenopausal women found that those who consumed garlic regularly had a noticeably lower incidence of breast cancer.

Eating just one clove of garlic a week made a significant statistical difference. And a study published in the *American Journal of Clinical Nutrition* in 2006 analyzed case control studies from Italy and Switzerland and found that women who ate the most onion and garlic had up to a 25 percent lower incidence of breast cancer.

There are several ways that garlic helps to protect against and fight breast cancer. Overall, garlic is a good cancer fighter because it has more antioxidants than any other vegetable ever tested. Antioxidants protect your body from the oxygen free-radical damage that can lead to cancer. Garlic usually has abundant amounts of selenium, and this mineral stimulates the production of glutathione, one of the body's natural antioxidants.

Research has found that garlic also boosts the immune system. Specifically, it enhances the activity of natural killer (NK) cells. These immune-system cells are important because, as their name indicates, they naturally kill things you don't want in your body, such as cancer cells, bacteria, and viruses.

Laboratory studies have revealed some of the precise ways that garlic prevents and fights breast cancer. Garlic decreases the formation of carcinogens in breast tissue by as much as 50 to 70 percent. It helps to avert the initiation of breast tumors by preventing toxins from binding to DNA in breast cells. Garlic has also been shown to inhibit or prevent breast tumor cells from growing and dividing, and can directly kill them. It reduces tumor cell adhesion so that cells have a more difficult time sticking together to form a solid tumor, prevents tumors from invading into surrounding tissues, and decreases the ability of a tumor to spread to other areas of the body. If you need chemotherapy, it can help to reduce many of the side effects. In addition, research shows that garlic is very effective at lowering the risk of many other types of cancer, including cancers of the oral cavity, pharynx, esophagus, larynx, stomach, colon, ovary, prostate, and kidney.

Cancer isn't the only disease that garlic helps to prevent. The main problem in AIDS patients is that the HIV virus destroys the immune system. The number and function of NK cells, in particular, drop to very low levels. A 1989 study found that garlic was effective at increasing the activity of NK cells in AIDS patients.

Garlic is especially good for your heart's health. It decreases cholesterol and triglycerides, prevents blood clots, improves circulation, and decreases the risk of atherosclerosis (hardening of the arteries). Garlic also reduces blood pressure. Studies show it can reduce systolic blood pressure (the first or higher number in a blood-pressure reading) by 20–30 millimeters (mm) of mercury (Hg) and diastolic blood pressure (the second or lower number) by 10–20 mm Hg.

Garlic: Nature's Antibiotic

Garlic can kill a whole army of unwanted invaders: bacteria, viruses, fungi, and parasites. In 1858 Louis Pasteur, who developed the "germ theory," discovered that garlic kills bacteria. This was an important revelation, because there were no antibiotics then. For nearly half a century after his discovery, garlic juice was put on wounds to help prevent infections. It was one of the principal antibiotics used during World War I and until the availability of penicillin in 1942.

Many modern-day studies have shown that garlic is effective in killing a wide variety of bacteria including tuberculosis and *Staphylococcus aureus*, a common skin pathogen that frequently causes infections. Studies conducted in the 1980s and 1990s found that garlic is also a good antiviral, antifungal, and antiparasitic medicine.

The Magic Inside

As with any whole plant, it's difficult to describe exactly how garlic works because there are thousands of constituents all interacting together. But a few substances have been identified in garlic that have clear medicinal benefits and specific actions. Something called "alliin" holds many of garlic's health-promoting properties. Alliin is just one of thirty sulfur compounds found in garlic. When garlic is crushed or broken, the enzyme alliinase is released. Alliinase converts alliin to a substance called allicin—the actual active compound. Alliin doesn't have any health-supporting effects until it becomes allicin. So, to gain the full potential of the allicin in garlic, you should crush it and wait at least fifteen minutes before you eat it. Other plentiful health-enhancing compounds found in garlic are selenium and vitamins A, B, C, and E.

Getting Your Garlic

Garlic can be eaten fresh or taken in standardized doses as capsules and tablets. The general recommended daily dose is 600–900 mg, or one or two fresh cloves. Many of the antioxidants in garlic are destroyed if you cook it too much. So, eat it raw, or only lightly sautéed, and add it to foods near the end of cooking. If you are concerned about having "garlic breath," there is an odorless form of garlic available in capsule form.

Side effects have been reported with therapeutic doses of garlic, but they are mild and rare. They include heartburn, flatulence, headaches, muscle soreness, fatigue, dizziness, and allergic reactions. Garlic is *not* recommended if you are on anticoagulants or blood thinners, because it also thins your blood.

SEAWEED—BREAST MEDICINE FROM THE SEA

The last of the Asian secret weapons against breast cancer comes from the sea. A prehistoric plant, seaweed has been gathered from the oceans for centuries and is a prominent vegetable in Japanese cuisine. It is rarely consumed in this country, despite evidence that it is a powerful ally in the fight against breast cancer.

Two types of seaweed—wakame and mekabu—suppress the growth of breast cancer by causing cell death. In other words, these seaweeds kill breast cancer cells—and with quite a bit of might. A study published in 2001 by Japanese researcher H. Funahashi found that mekabu seaweed killed breast cancer cells and stopped the growth of tumors *more effectively* than a common chemotherapeutic drug used for breast cancer. Better yet, this seaweed did not cause normal cells to die as chemotherapeutic drugs often do. Researchers in Malaysia in 2013 reported that another type of seaweed, known as red seaweed (*Eucheuma cottonii L.*), was more effective than Tamoxifen at suppressing tumor growth.

One reason why these seaweeds are so potent against breast cancer is because they are high in iodine. Iodine is toxic to breast cancer cells. It is also involved in the production of antioxidants that protect cells from oxidative damage that can lead to cancer. Researchers have mapped out many different mechanisms through which iodine exerts its anticancer blow. They are too complex to describe—but what's important, is to simply know that iodine works in many ways to protect you from breast cancer. Not surprisingly, low amounts of iodine in the diet are thought to contribute to the risk of breast cancer. Animal and human studies show that molecular iodine ($I_{(2)}$) taken as a supplement suppresses the development and growth of both benign and cancerous tumors. Women with thyroid diseases including hyperthyroidism (overactive thyroid), hypothyroidism (underactive thyroid), thyroiditis (inflammation of the thyroid), and nontoxic goiter have a higher incidence of breast cancer. Many of these thyroid conditions are associated with low dietary iodine, but low iodine doesn't fully explain the association between thyroid disease and breast cancer. At this point, we don't have a clear understanding of why women with thyroid cancer or other thyroid conditions have a higher incidence of breast cancer.

Iodine is a trace element that is normally only taken up by the thyroid gland to make thyroid hormones. Embryologically, the breast and thyroid are derived from similar cells. Breast cells have only a temporary ability to uptake and concentrate iodine during pregnancy and lactation—the purpose being to supply the baby with this important substance through the breast milk. Researchers have found that iodine is also taken up by breast cancer cells, but *not* normal breast cells or any other cells in the body. This fact creates an exciting future possibility for treating breast cancer—using radioactive iodine instead of chemotherapy. Radioactive iodine is a substance used to treat thyroid cancers, and it might also prove to be highly effective against breast cancer. Because iodine is not taken up by any other tissues in the body except the thyroid, radioactive iodine—unlike standard chemotherapy—is harmless to the rest of the body. And the damage caused to the thyroid by radioactive iodine is easily treatable with thyroid hormones.

A study published in 2013 elucidated more details regarding the potential of using radioactive iodine in the treatment of breast cancer. They found that 70 percent of breast cancers have a gene that is overexpressed—or turned on too much—called the human sodium-iodide symporter gene. This gene codes for something called the sodium-iodide symporter (NIS) located in the tumor cell membrane, which has the ability to pump iodine into tumor cells. NIS is not found in normal healthy breast cells. That's why radioactive iodine could be effective for treating these types of tumors. Estrogen- and progesterone-positive tumors, along with those that are also HER2/neu positive, appear to have the greatest amount of NIS.

Although no guidelines have been established for breast cancer prevention, the Food and Nutrition Board of the U.S. National Academy of Sciences recommends that normal healthy adults take 150 micrograms (mcg) of iodine a day. Higher amounts are recommended for certain disease states. (Approximately 1½ teaspoons of seaweed has about 225 mcg of iodine.)

Seaweed has several additional ways that it protects against breast cancer. In 2009, researchers at the University of South Carolina Cancer Center conducted a double-blind placebo-controlled trial of a seaweed supplementation, Alaria, with and without soy. The researchers found that there was an inverse and linear relationship between the dose of seaweed and serum estradiol. In other words, the more seaweed the women consumed, the lower was the amount of estradiol in their blood. When soy was added to the seaweed, the women were noted to have much higher levels in their urine of the "good" type of estrogens (2-OH) compared to the "bad" type (16-OH)—the major way that cruciferous vegetables also lower your risk.

Korean researchers found yet another type of seaweed commonly consumed in their country called gim (*Porphyra sp.*) which appears to decrease the risk of both pre- and postmenopausal breast cancer. Women who consume this seaweed were found to have much lower incidences of breast cancer compared to those who did not.

MORE NATURAL DEFENSE

Most plants contain substances that protect against and fight cancer. The anti-cancer properties of some plants, such as soybeans and flaxseeds, have been well recognized for decades. But there are many other plants, especially herbs and spices, with excellent abilities to ward off breast cancer. Isaac Cohen, a doctor of oriental medicine, licensed acupuncturist, and one of the leading authorities in the field of cancer treatment and Traditional Chinese Medicine (TCM), reported in the book *Breast Cancer: Beyond Convention* that several Chinese herbs, including ginseng, show good anticancer activity against breast cancer. He points out that it is not unusual for plants to be effective against cancer—in fact, more than 60 percent of the chemotherapeutic drugs currently being used are derived from natural substances.

Other researchers concur that many of the herbs used in TCM are effective at stopping the growth of breast cancer cells in the laboratory. For instance, in 2002 researchers at the Cancer Research Laboratory in Indianapolis, Indiana, found that licorice root (*Glycyrrhiza glabra*)—a shrub native to southern Europe and Asia and one of the Chinese herbs used in the prostate cancer herbal mixture PC-SPES—showed strong activity against highly invasive breast cancer cells. Another study published in 2002 in the journal *Anticancer Research* found that of seventy-one extracts of Chinese medicinal herbs, 21 percent (fifteen) of the extracts demonstrated greater than 50 percent growth inhibition on at least four of the five breast cancer cell lines. In 2000, researchers at Memorial Sloan-Kettering Cancer Center in New York found that Huanglian, a Chinese herbal extract used in the treatment of gastroenteritis, also inhibits the growth of human gastric, colon, and breast cancer cells.

Some common cooking spices have excellent cancer-fighting properties, too. For example, research shows that the spice rosemary protects against the initiation of breast tumors. When rats were fed rosemary before the administration of breast cancer–inducing chemicals, they developed 74 percent fewer tumors than the rats that weren't fed rosemary. Another study published in the *European Journal of Cancer* in 1999 found that rosemary, like green tea, improves the concentration of the chemotherapeutic agents (doxorubicin and vinblastin) in breast cancer tumor cells. That means that this aromatic spice may be helpful as a complementary treatment for women with tumors that are resistant to these drugs. Researchers at Columbia University in 2012 found that carnosic acid in rosemary inhibits the growth of estrogen receptor-negative breast cancer and has synergistic effects with curcumin.

According to researchers at the New York College of Osteopathic Medicine, extracts of several weak estrogenic herbs including hops, black cohosh, and chaste-tree berry also inhibit the growth of breast cancer cells in the laboratory. In addition, cranberry extract has been shown to suppress the growth of breast tumors and kill breast cells through apoptosis. Noni juice also inhibits breast cancer cell growth and can even cause precancerous cells to turn back into normal cells.

GINKGO BILOBA

Ginkgo biloba, best known for its ability to enhance cognitive function, has recently been shown to also lower the risk of and dramatically deter the growth of breast cancer in a diversity of ways. A study published in 2006 in the *Journal of Steroid Biochemistry and Molecular Biology* found that ginkgo has several anti-estrogen effects which reduce the risk of breast cancer.

- **Ginkgo decreases the amount of estradiol,** the strongest and most abundant form of natural estrogen in our bodies (and the one most associated with an increased risk of breast cancer), by speeding the rate at which our bodies break it down and eliminate it.

- **Ginkgo inhibits estradiol synthesis**, decreasing how much our bodies make.

- **Ginkgo activates a special receptor** (AhR) on the breast cell membrane, which dampens the stimulatory effect that estradiol has on the estrogen receptor.

The researchers in this study concluded that the various influences that ginkgo has on estrogen also makes it an excellent potential alternative to HRT for menopausal symptoms. They emphasize that ginkgo may help alleviate symptoms, and instead of dangerous side effects, it provides side benefits. For instance HRT, prescribed for decades for menopausal symptoms, has fallen out of favor because it also increases the risk of breast cancer and a variety of other serious disorders, whereas ginkgo actually has protective effects against breast cancer.

Another study conducted at Georgetown University School of Medicine and published in the journal *Anticancer Research* in 2006 found that ginkgo reduced the aggressiveness of breast cancer and slowed its growth by 80 percent! In an earlier study from the same institution, ginkgo was found to work specifically by affecting a protein receptor (PBR) plus 36 other genes involved in various pathways regulating cell proliferation. In addition to gene-regulating actions, ginkgo also inhibits cancer growth with powerful antioxidants and by shutting off the blood supply to tumors. Korean researchers in 2012 found that ginkgo kills tumor cells by impeding an enzyme found in tumor cells called fatty acid synthase (described in Chapter 8 under GLA). Ginkgo also blocks the aromatase enzyme from making estrogen, and stops the growth of and kills estrogen-negative breast cancer cells. In addition, it protects against some of the side effects of chemotherapy, including cognitive dysfunction and damage to the heart.

GINSENG

With a history of use that goes back 5,000 to 7,000 years, ginseng is the most famous of all the Chinese herbs because of its remarkable medicinal qualities. Best known for its ability to improve stamina and protect against the damaging effects of stress, this root—which often grows in the shape resembling a man—also holds powerful anticancer properties.

- **Ginseng kills cancer cells.** Dozens of studies conducted in the last decade consistently show that *Panax ginseng* not only stops breast cancer cells from growing, but also kills them through apoptotic cell death. One such study was conducted in Seoul, Korea, and published in the journal *Cancer Research* in 2005. Another study published in *Life Sciences* in November 2004 found that ginseng killed cancer cells more effectively than several chemotherapeutic agents including epirubicin, 5-fluorouracil, and cyclophosphamide! Researchers at the National Institutes of Health in 2009 reported that heat-processing American ginseng through steaming caused some of the anticancer components, called ginsenosides, to increase significantly. As a result, the tumor-killing activity of the heated ginseng is much greater than untreated ginseng. Ginseng also has strong anti-inflammatory actions, including shutting off the COX-2 enzyme and preventing metastasis.

- **Ginseng enhances chemotherapy.** You may want to seriously consider taking ginseng if you are currently undergoing chemotherapy treatment. There are numerous studies showing that ginseng increases the tumor cell killing abilities of chemotherapy. For example, a study conducted at the University of Cambridge in the United Kingdom found ginseng enhanced the ability of mitoxantrone to kill human breast cancer cells. Another study published in 2004 and conducted at the University of British Columbia found that ginseng could make tumor cells that were multi-drug resistant much more sensitive to chemotherapy. A third study from Harvard Medical School found American ginseng (*Panax quinquefolius*) used concurrently with breast cancer therapeutic agents resulted in "a significant suppression of cell growth for most drugs evaluated." They concluded that American ginseng worked synergistically with breast cancer chemotherapeutic drugs to stop cell growth.

- **Ginseng improves quality of life.** Ginseng has also been found to improve the quality of life of breast cancer patients. In a study published in the *American Journal of Epidemiology* in 2006, researchers at Vanderbilt University studied ginseng and breast cancer patients in China. One thousand four hundred and fifty-five breast cancer patients were recruited for the Shanghai Breast

Cancer Study from August 1996-1998 and were followed through 2002. Twenty-seven percent of the patients were ginseng users before their cancer diagnosis. Compared to those women who had never used of ginseng, their death rate was significantly lower. The women who began ginseng after their cancer diagnosis tested much higher than nonusers for Quality of Life (QOL) scores. Psychological and social well-being and overall quality of life improved as cumulative ginseng use increased. A 2011 study confirmed the ability of ginseng to help the QOL of breast cancer survivors, especially by improving fatigue and hormone-related symptoms.

How to Take Ginseng

Ginseng comes in standardized doses in capsules that you can purchase at most health food stores. The recommended dose is 1 to 2 grams daily. It is possible to overdose on ginseng, so don't take more than what is recommended. Massive overdoses can bring about Ginseng Abuse Syndrome characterized by hypertension, nervousness, insomnia, hypertonia (muscle rigidity), edema, morning diarrhea, inability to concentrate and skin eruptions.

COFFEE

The correlation between caffeine consumption and an increase of benign breast disease is well known. So it may surprise you to learn that when it comes to breast cancer, studies show that caffeinated coffee *does not* increase your risk and may in fact, have a protective effect. Nowhere in the world is more coffee consumed per capita than in Sweden. A 2002 study of over 59,000 Swedish women, ages 40 to 76, found that drinking caffeinated coffee had no correlation on breast cancer risk.

Several more recent studies however, take coffee's effect on this dreaded disease far past neutral. For instance, a 2006 Canadian study published in the *International Journal of Cancer* found that for women who are at high-risk for breast cancer because they carry the BRCA1 mutation, the more coffee they drank per day the lower their risk of breast cancer was. In this study, 1,690 women with the BRCA1 or BRCA2 mutations from forty centers in four countries were analyzed. Women (with the BRCA1 mutation, not the BRCA2 mutation) who habitually drank 1 to 3 cups of caffeinated coffee a day, 4 to 5 cups, or 6 or more cups had a 10 percent, 25 percent, and 69 percent reduction in their risk of breast cancer, respectively, compared to women who didn't drink coffee.

Other studies confirm coffee's protective effect and shed light on specifically how it lowers the risk of breast cancer. In the study above, researchers explain that coffee is an important source of phytoestrogens—weak plant estrogens that have a beneficial effect by blocking the ability of strong estrogens to bind to the estrogen receptors in the breast. Researchers at the Roswell Park Cancer Institute in Buffalo, New York, point out that coffee also contains substances called polyphenols which have anticarcinogenic effects.

In their study, published in the *Journal of Nutrition* in 2006, they found a direct linear relationship between the amount of coffee premenopausal women drank a day and their risk of breast cancer. In other words, the more coffee these women drank, the lower their risk was. For those who drank over 4 cups a day, their risk dropped by 40 percent!

Researchers are Harvard Medical School in 2009 found another good explanation for the lower risk: Caffeinated coffee increases the number of sex hormone-binding globulins (SHBG) in the blood and lowers free estradiol. Sex hormone-binding globulins are a serum protein that binds estradiol—the most abundant and strongest form of natural estrogen in the body and the one most associated with an increased risk of breast cancer. When estradiol is attached to a SHBG, it cannot attach to and turn on the estrogen receptor in breast cells.

Yet, another breast cancer defensive effect of coffee was found in a 2006 study published in the journal *Molecular Genetic Metabolism*. Women who drank 3 or more cups of coffee a day were found to have a significantly higher ratio of 2-hydroxyestrone (2-OH or a "good" protective type of estrogen) compared to 16-alpha-hydroxyestrone (16-OH or a "bad" cancer-promoting type of estrogen).

Coffee also lowers the risk of breast cancers that are not estrogen dependent. In a study published in the journal *Breast Cancer* in 2011, high daily intakes of coffee (greater than 5 cups) were found to be associated with a 57 percent decrease in estrogen receptor-negative breast cancer among postmenopausal women.

It appears that the health benefits of coffee go far beyond inhibiting cancer. A fifteen-year study published in the *American Journal of Clinical Nutrition* in May 2006, which collected data on 27,312 postmenopausal women who took part of the Iowa Women's Health study, discovered that postmenopausal women who reported drinking at least one to three cups of coffee daily were 24 percent less likely to die of heart disease compared to those who didn't drink coffee. They were also 28 percent less likely to die of other non-cancerous inflammatory diseases. Coffee, according to many other studies, may also prevent gallstones; lower the risk of cancers of the colon, kidney, bladder, uterus, esophagus, pancreas, prostate, skin (basal and squamous), brain (glioma), and liver (hepatocellular); and decrease the risk of Alzheimer's and Parkinson's diseases, and strokes. Coffee drinkers have a lower risk of liver diseases, including cirrhosis and fibrosis, and experience a slower progression of hepatitis C. For every cup of coffee that is consumed a day, there is an additional 7 percent reduction in the risk of type 2 diabetes. Two other reasons to enjoy your morning cup of joe, is that it improves brain function and athletic performance.

But, before you decide to significantly increase your Starbucks budget, keep in mind that coffee can have some drawbacks. Caffeine can trigger anxiety attacks, jitteriness, impatience, mood swings, and insomnia. It also increases the amount of calcium your body excretes in your urine and decreases the amount you absorb from your intestines putting you at higher risk for osteoporosis. Because caffeine is a mild stimulant, it can raise your blood pressure. Certain types of coffee—especially non-filtered, such as Turkish coffee or that made in a plunger pot—may contain substances that increase your cholesterol and put you at higher risk for heart disease. If you are pregnant, you will want to avoid consuming large amount of caffeine because it increases your chances of having a miscarriage. Nonorganic coffee usually contains pesticides and other potentially health-damaging substances added for processing, so always drink coffee that is organically produced.

Everyone is different and it is important for you to use your own judgment when it comes to consuming coffee or other caffeinated beverages. If you don't feel good when you drink it—don't! But if you love coffee and have worried about it damaging your health, research shows you can relax a bit. It may not really be as bad a vice as you might have thought. Coffee does have some significant health benefits, especially when it comes to your risk of breast cancer.

We have just begun our exploration of the vast and wondrous intelligence contained in plants. As more research is completed, the array of anticancer herbs will assuredly continue to grow.

Part Three

Secret Weapons for Your Warrior Goddess

An Arsenal of Nutritional Supplements

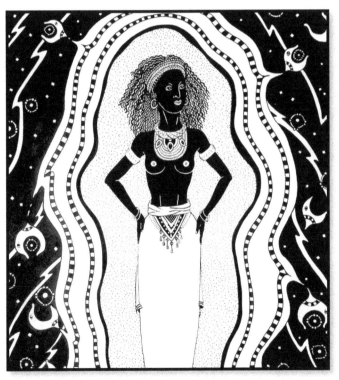

Goddess of Dynamic Defense

Chapter 12

Mighty Micronutrients
Vitamins That Defend

*J*ust like the old saying, "Some of the best things come in small packages," some of the best weapons you can give your Warrior Goddess to help her successfully fend off breast cancer are very tiny. But don't let their size fool you. Only small amounts of these tiny molecules are needed because they pack a mighty wallop against breast cancer.

In biology, it's normal for microscopic structures to contain immense potential. For instance, think of a single cell: It's so tiny that it can be seen only with a powerful microscope. Yet, contained within the nucleus of that cell is your DNA. Imagine how tiny the double helixes are, and they contain the potential to manifest a complete human being—trillions of cells, a multitude of specialized organs and structures, and a mind-boggling number of functions, all working in perfect coordinated harmony!

If you give your Warrior Goddess a few micrograms (mcg) of certain micronutrients, such as folic acid and vitamins B_{12}, D, E, and A every day, she gains enough power from these "special forces" to provide you with significant protection against breast cancer. By definition, vitamins are organic compounds that you need only in very small amounts, but they play a big role in keeping you healthy. Vitamins aren't metabolized for energy—they don't supply any calories—but some of them are important in energy production. The primary function of vitamins is to assist enzymes, which are tiny, vitally important proteins that drive all the chemical reactions in your body. Because enzymes play such a critical role, it is vital to take vitamins in the proper daily amounts to maintain your health.

The word "vitamin" originally meant a nutrient that your body can't make. This definition isn't always appropriate because your body can make some vitamins, such as vitamin D. The vitamins you can't make—or don't make enough of—you should get from your food. Most vitamins are absorbed and assimilated more effectively if you consume them in foods, especially fresh, organically grown vegetables, fruits, nuts, and whole grains. But under certain circumstances—for instance, if you don't eat enough of these nutrient-rich foods—taking supplemental vitamins is a good idea. Vitamin supplements derived from whole foods are more readily absorbed and assimilated by the body than those made synthetically. (You may have to call the manufacturer to find out if the supplements you are considering purchasing are derived from whole foods.)

FOLIC ACID

Folic acid (also known as folate) is involved in the process of making proteins. It is a crucial element in constructing and repairing DNA and in normal cell division. Without it, cells can't divide properly and can turn cancerous. Folic acid helps to prevent DNA from making the mistakes that can lead to cancer. Think of it as a built-in proofreader. Certain chance mistakes can turn the messages of DNA traitorous. For example, instead of dispatching communications for health, the DNA may accidentally spawn messages for cancer. Folic acid can prevent this from happening. This may explain why low levels of folic acid in the body are associated with a significantly increased risk of breast cancer.

In a 1992 study from the University of Vermont, researchers found that DNA mistakes or mutations increase with age and cigarette smoking. They also discovered that folate helps to prevent those mutations, including mutations that increase the risk of breast cancer. Folate is a methyl donor, meaning that it can "donate" methyl groups to DNA, which has the effect of directly influencing gene expression—in other words, turning genes on or off. According to an article published in the *International Journal of Molecular Sciences* in 2012, folate is able to prevent damage to DNA caused by bisphenol A (BPA) found in plastics by donating methyl groups to DNA.

Alcohol consumption causes folate levels to drop. (The perils of alcohol with regard to breast cancer are discussed in Chapter 18.) Women who drink alcohol and have low folate levels may be at high risk of developing breast cancer. Harvard University conducted a very large prospective study, called the Nurses' Health Study, which followed 88,818 women from 1980 to 1996. (A prospective study is one that follows the subjects into the future; it is considered one of the best study designs for obtaining significant and reliable information.) The study found that women who had the highest risk of breast cancer drank at least 15 grams (about a half ounce) of alcohol a day and had low folate levels.

Researchers at University of Bristol in the UK performed a meta-analysis of twenty-two past studies and found that taking higher amounts of folate did not decrease the risk of breast cancer. Their study was published in the November 15, 2006 issue of the *Journal of the National Cancer Institute*. In the January 3, 2007 issue of the same journal, Susanna Larsson of the Karolinska Institute in Stockholm, Sweden reported on another meta-analysis she performed, this time using nine prospective studies and fourteen case control studies regarding folate and the risk of breast cancer. Again, no association was found between folate intake and breast cancer unless a woman had moderate to high alcohol consumption. The Prostate, Lung, Colorectal and Ovarian Cancer Screening Trial recently reported that taking more than 400 mcg of supplemental folate a day may actually *increase* the risk of breast cancer by 20 to 32 percent. However, in this study they also found that women who consumed alcohol and had low folate levels had the greatest risk. So if you drink more than one or two servings of alcohol a day—which I definitely advise against doing—taking supplemental folic acid is highly recommended. But if you don't drink moderate to high amounts of alcohol, there is no need to take additional folic acid.

You might be wondering, how is it possible that too much of a simple B vitamin might increase the risk of breast cancer? The reason lies in the fact that folate is an excellent methyl donor. If you would like to review what methyl groups are and what they do, turn back to the last chapter and read the section on Cleaning Your Genes with Tea (page 113). Polish researchers published a study in 2013 that found increasing concentrations of folic acid appeared to increase the methylation of the DNA involved with the tumor-suppression genes, decreasing their expression. Said more simply, excess folic acid may shut off a beneficial gene that suppresses the growth of tumors, thereby making it easier for tumors to grow.

According to Canadian researchers, the risk of excess amounts of this B vitamin seems to only be associated with taking too much supplemental folic acid—not from consuming high amounts of folate-rich foods. So don't worry, enjoy your foods. But, only take supplemental folic acid (400 mcg a day) if you drink moderate amounts of alcohol or your doctor recommends you take it for some other condition. Birth control pills and non-steroidal anti-inflammatories (such as aspirin, and ibuprofen) can also lower folate, so if you take any of these medications regularly you might want to consider taking folic acid.

Good Sources of Folate

Folate is found in eggs, asparagus, whole wheat, dark-green leafy vegetables, and brewer's yeast. It's also found in certain meats and fish. But eating large amounts of meat and fish is a double-edged sword, since the toxins in these foods considerably increase the risk of breast cancer.

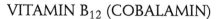

VITAMIN B$_{12}$ (COBALAMIN)

Vitamin B$_{12}$ is known as "Nature's most beautiful cofactor," because its crystalline structure is a stunning dark red, like that of a rare ruby. Vitamin B$_{12}$ works *with* folic acid, so it's also a fundamental part of the DNA construction and repair team. Without it, the quality of DNA would never pass inspection. Vitamin B$_{12}$ is vitally important for keeping your DNA messages correct and free from cancer-inducing mistakes. Research shows that women with the lowest B$_{12}$ levels in their bodies have the highest rates of breast cancer.

Vitamin B$_{12}$ may also be very valuable for women who already have breast cancer. In the laboratory, scientists found that when vitamin B$_{12}$ was applied directly to breast cancer cells, it stopped them from growing.

This vitamin is also essential for a healthy nervous system and energy production.

The richest sources of vitamin B$_{12}$ are certain animal organs—especially liver, brain, and kidney. Clams, oysters, sardines, and salmon have significant amounts of this vitamin, too. It is also found in egg yolks and fermented soy products, such as tempeh. Because eating meat and fish *increases* your risk of breast cancer, getting B$_{12}$ from other sources is probably a good idea.

It's not uncommon for those who follow a vegetarian diet to be deficient in vitamin B$_{12}$ since it is found mostly in animal products. Although a vegetarian diet is the most healthful of diets and is associated with the lowest risk of breast cancer, it's important that vegetarians (and others who avoid meat and shellfish) take B$_{12}$ in supplement form. About 3 to 30 mcg a day—about the weight of one-tenth of a water droplet—is all you need for B$_{12}$ to perform its miracles.

To be absorbed into your body, vitamin B$_{12}$ requires "intrinsic factor," a substance secreted by the cells in your stomach. As you age, you make less intrinsic factor and, therefore, absorb less B$_{12}$. So, you must consume more B$_{12}$ as you age to absorb amounts similar to what you got when you were younger. For this reason, supplemental B$_{12}$ is a great idea for everyone who is over age sixty. If you have certain conditions, such as the autoimmune disorder pernicious anemia, or if you have had partial or total surgical removal of your stomach, the amount of intrinsic factor you make will be low. Pancreatic insufficiency, disorders of the small bowel, certain drugs, and a variety of other conditions can also interfere with B$_{12}$ absorption. In all these situations, it's very important to take supplemental vitamin B$_{12}$.

VITAMIN D

Most famous for making bones and teeth strong by helping the body to effectively use calcium and phosphorus, vitamin D has another notable talent. Research shows that this vitamin protects against and fights breast cancer in a number of ways. It helps to make your breast cells more resistant to toxins; decreases the ability of breast cells to divide; stops tumor cells from growing; decreases the ability of tumor cells to invade into surrounding tissues and spread to other areas of the body; causes the death of tumor cells; prevents new blood vessels from growing into a tumor; and boosts the immune system, especially the activity of natural killer (NK) cells. Vitamin D also decreases the activity of the COX-2 inflammation enzyme and IGF-1—two big promoters of breast cancer. It modifies estrogen in the body too, by reducing the aromatase enzyme so that less estrogen is created and by turning down the volume on the estrogen receptor.

Low vitamin D levels may trigger weight gain according to researchers at Kaiser Permanente Center for Health Research. Obesity, as you are aware, is a risk factor for postmenopausal breast cancer, and therefore is another way that vitamin D may have an impact on the risk. With all the ways that vitamin D defends against breast cancer, it is easy to understand why numerous studies have found that low vitamin D levels are associated with a higher risk of breast cancer. In fact, the impact of having deficient amounts of vitamin D can be quite significant. In a study published in 2013, Australian women with the lowest levels of vitamin D compared to women whose levels were optimal, had up to a 2.5 times higher risk of breast cancer.

Women who are deficient in vitamin D when they are diagnosed with breast cancer have a worse prognosis. A study presented by the American Society of Oncology found that women low in D were twice as likely to have their cancers spread and 73 percent more likely to die compared to women who had healthy levels of this vitamin.

Vitamin D is unique because your body can make its own supply. The secret catalyzing agent is not from this world; it comes from a star—the sun. Sunlight reacts with chemicals in your skin to produce vitamin D. Specifically ultraviolet B (UVB) radiation transforms 7-dehydrocholesterol in your skin to vitamin D_3 (see the inset "The Biology of Vitamin D" on page 138.) Just fifteen to twenty minutes of sunlight a day makes enough vitamin D to reduce your risk of breast cancer by as much as 40 percent. This may be one reason why breast cancer rates are higher in women in northern climates compared to areas that get plenty of sunshine, such as the southwestern United States. Of course, too much sunlight isn't a good thing, either. Here is another example of the ancient principle of *balance*. Too much of a good thing can cause imbalances and lead to health problems, just as too little can. The ultraviolet radiation in sunlight damages the DNA in skin cells. If you get too much sun, especially if you have lightly pigmented skin, the damage can be severe. Serious ultraviolet-radiation damage to your skin can cause premature aging, leathery skin, deep wrinkles, discolored spots, and potentially deadly skin cancer.

The Biology of Vitamin D

The vitamin D_3 that is manufactured in the skin, called cholecalciferol, is not biologically active. It must go through two more conversions: one in the liver, and the other in the kidney. Vitamin D_3 is first converted to 25(OH)D, or 25-hydroxycholecalciferol—the major circulating metabolite—by enzymes in the liver. Next, 25(OH)D has another hydroxyl group (OH) added by an enzyme in the kidney, converting it to 1,25(OH)D, or 1,25-dihydroxycholecalciferol, also known as calcitriol. Interestingly, the breast tissue has the same enzyme system that the kidney does, so the most active form of vitamin D can be manufactured locally in the breast where it can immediately offer its protection!

Both the 1,25(OH) and the 25(OH) forms of vitamin D can attach to vitamin D receptors on cell membranes. But the 1,25(OH)D is 1,000 times more powerful. Because 25(OH)D hangs out in the blood for weeks and 1,25(OH)D only lasts for a few hours, blood tests designed to measure vitamin D levels are actually checking only the less biologically active form 25(OH). That's why the blood tests for vitamin D may not be completely accurate regarding how much of it really is in the body. Another reason that blood tests for vitamin D don't give the full picture is that vitamin D is fat soluble. What this means is, this vitamin will store in your fat. Blood levels of 25(OH)D do not measure the

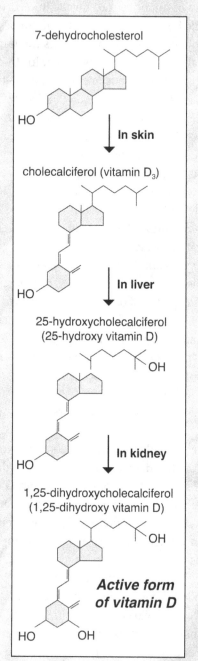

7-dehydrocholesterol

↓ **In skin**

cholecalciferol (vitamin D_3)

↓ **In liver**

25-hydroxycholecalciferol
(25-hydroxy vitamin D)

↓ **In kidney**

1,25-dihydroxycholecalciferol
(1,25-dihydroxy vitamin D)

Active form of vitamin D

amount of stored vitamin D that is in your fat. So it is possible to get too much of vitamin D and not know it, because the excess amount is being stored in your fat. Despite these issues, 25(OH)D blood tests do show a significant correlation with overall health, and the risk of breast cancer.

Serum blood levels of 25(OH)D below 20 nanograms per milliliter (ng/mL) are considered seriously low. Levels between 20 and 55 ng/mL are considered normal, although many experts believe that the ideal range should be much higher and between 50 and 80 ng/mL.

But a little sunlight is important to enable you to make enough health-promoting and health-protecting vitamin D. According to a 2013 study published in the *European Journal of Cancer*, sunlight's anticancer effects also work through different mechanisms than vitamin D production. They theorize that it may have something to do with an influence on the immune system, circadian rhythms, and folic acid. In the past, it was recommended to get your exposure to sunlight in the morning or late afternoon when the sun's rays aren't so intense. But now, the recommendation has shifted. Instead, to get enough of the sun's beneficial rays, it is recognized that getting out in midday—yes that's right, exactly the time when we were told not to be out—and without sunscreen—will give you the best medicine that sunlight has to offer. Combine your sun time with a brisk walk, and you double your benefits. Taking daily walks is an ancient *Ayurvedic* recommendation. It is called your "constitutional" walk. *Ayurveda* recommends *a brisk walk in the morning and another in the evening to maintain good health*. And now it appears that adding another one at noontime is even better yet.

If you live in a climate that doesn't see much sun, especially during the cold winter months, taking supplemental vitamin D is a must. Fatty fish (for example, salmon and mackerel) egg yolks, and certain mushrooms are about the only foods with natural vitamin D. Most of the vitamin D in our diet comes from foods that are fortified with it, for example, certain dairy products and breakfast cereals. Most multivitamins contain the minimum recommended daily amount of vitamin D_3, about 400 international units (IU). However, scientists have discovered that we actually need much more of vitamin D_3 for optimal health. In fact, for healthy people, about 2,000 IU units of vitamin D_3 are recommended each day. How much you should take depends on many different factors, including your age, weight, percentage of body fat, skin color, use of sun block, the season of the year, the latitude of where you live, and your state of health. If you are sick, you might need megadoses of vitamin D_3 for a while to get your levels back up.

Taking megadoses for a prolonged time, however, is not a good idea because you can get too much of vitamin D and have toxic side effects. As mentioned in the inset on page 138, checking serum blood levels of vitamin D does not measure the amount of vitamin D in your fat. It is possible to go from levels that are considered optimal to suddenly toxic when your fat stores become full.

An explosion of research on vitamin D in the last few years has shown that this vitamin is critically important for countless functions in our body. It activates over 200 genes that manage cell growth, differentiation, and apoptosis cell death. There are thousands of other genes it is thought to interact with as well. Low levels of vitamin D are found to contribute to dozens of diseases, including Alzheimer's disease, high blood pressure, cardiovascular disease, metabolic syndrome, autoimmune diseases, diabetes, obesity, multiple sclerosis, rheumatoid and osteoarthritis, gout, infertility, PMS, Parkinson's, chronic fatigue syndrome, fibromyalgia, premature aging, and early death. Breast cancer isn't the only cancer that low vitamin D levels play a role. There are over seventeen others, including cancers of the prostate, colon, pancreas, lung, ovary, bladder, uterus, skin, and blood (leukemia). Increasing your vitamin D levels with sunshine and with supplements has been shown to help prevent or improve all of the conditions associated with vitamin D deficiencies. That's why is so important to keep your levels optimal.

Large percentages of the population have vitamin D levels that are too low. Studies estimate that 30 to 80 percent of Americans are deficient. Those who live in northern climates, don't spend much time outdoors, and/or have darkly pigmented skin, which cuts down on UVB absorption, are at particular risk. Because vitamin D is so important to your health and most people run low, I recommend getting your blood levels checked. If you are too low, work with your doctor to get them back up. Taking supplemental vitamin D_3 is important for most people, and an easy way to protect your health, especially to lower your risk of breast cancer.

VITAMIN E

Vitamin E is another vitamin with special abilities to help protect against breast cancer. There are several different forms of vitamin E referred to as alpha, beta, gamma, and delta (α, β, γ, δ) tocopherols. Cancer prevention studies have previously primarily used the alpha type. Mixed results have been found because the alpha form doesn't have very strong anticancer properties. More recent studies have looked at the other types, especially the gamma and delta. These types have been shown to have a much stronger ability to reduce inflammation, stop tumor cells from multiplying, and shrink tumors. In animal models, gamma and delta have been very effective at preventing the formation of colon, prostate, lung, and breast cancers.

Scientists have found that vitamin E helps to decrease the risk of breast cancer and improve the chances of survival in at least six ways:

1. It is an excellent antioxidant.

2. It is a powerful anti-inflammatory.

3. It slows the speed at which tumor cells grow and divide.

4. It promotes tumor-cell death.

5. It prevents new blood vessels from growing in the tumor.

6. It inhibits estrogen receptor-positive cell growth by altering the cellular response to estrogen.

Each of these wonderful anticancer properties has a significant impact when it comes to preventing breast cancer. Research shows that women who regularly eat foods rich in vitamin E, such as avocados, almonds, sweet potatoes, leafy green vegetables, wheat germ, and salmon, have a lower risk of breast cancer.

You can also take vitamin E as a supplement, but research shows that you don't absorb vitamin E in supplement form as well as you do the vitamin E in your food. This is a perfect example of another *Ayurvedic* principle: *Fresh wholesome foods are the best medicines.* If you do take supplemental vitamin E, make sure it's made with a natural form of vitamin E, rather than a synthetic one. It should be a mix of the various tocopherols and not made of just one, especially the alpha type that doesn't have significant effects against cancer. Synthetic vitamins absorb very poorly and probably won't do you much good. The recommended daily dose of vitamin E is 400–800 IU. By the way, researchers have found that other antioxidants, such as vitamin C and CoQ_{10} (see Chapter 13), make the antitumor effects of vitamin E even stronger. If you are taking Tamoxifen, be aware that several studies show that the synthetic alpha-tocopherol may interfere with its effectiveness, so you definitely should *not* take this form. However, the gamma and delta types have been shown to have synergistic reactions with Tamoxifen, increasing its effectiveness. So again, when choosing a vitamin E supplement be sure to only take one that contains natural mixed tocopherols.

VITAMIN A

Vitamin A, like vitamin E, is a fat-soluble vitamin. Known for its powerful antioxidant powers, vitamin A comes in many different varieties and has the ability to reduce the risk of dozens of different diseases, including breast cancer. A review study of fifty-one studies published in the journal *Cancer, Causes and Control* in 2011 found that those women consuming the highest amounts of vitamin A-rich foods reduced their risk of breast cancer by 17 percent. Research shows that vitamin A—also referred to as retinoid—has many antibreast cancer actions, including decreasing tumor cell growth, causing tumor cell death, stopping the aromatase enzyme from converting androgens into estrogen, and interacting with genes affecting the function of the alpha-estrogen receptor.

As you may recall, scientists have discovered that breast cancer may recur due to the presence of breast cancer stem cells. Retinoids (vitamin A-based substances) can help to prevent relapses by causing the stem cells to mature into normal cells—a process called differentiation. This action along with all of its other anticancer properties helps to explain why women with low retinol levels have a higher risk of breast cancer and a poorer prognosis if they have been diagnosed with it.

When retinoids are combined with various other substances with anticancer actions, their tumor-suppressing effects synergistically increase. For instance, combining retinoids with omega-3 fatty acids, melatonin, and the chemotherapeutic drugs Tamoxifen and Herceptin (used for HER2/neu tumors) greatly enhances the tumor-killing capabilities of each. There has been quite a bit of research in this area and scientists believe that the role of retinoids in cancer treatment is so promising that it should definitely be developed.

Foods rich in vitamin A include mango, broccoli, butternut squash, carrots, tomatoes, sweet potatoes, and pumpkin. I recommend eating vitamin A-rich foods and not taking supplements. Supplemental vitamin A isn't necessary if you pay attention to eating delicious fresh fruits and vegetables every day. If you are diagnosed with breast cancer, then taking supplemental vitamin A may be of benefit. Be sure to work with your doctor about what form and the dose that may be best for you.

Chapter 13

Defense Shields
Preventing Damage
with Antioxidants

*T*here is a phenomenal class of natural substances that act as the body's antiaircraft and missile-defense system against oxygen free radicals, the enemy's smart bombs. Oxygen free radicals are unstable molecules of oxygen normally created as byproducts of cellular metabolism. You need them to drive all the chemical reactions in your body. But if there are too many of them, they turn into ammunition for the enemy, causing biological devastation. Excess oxygen free radicals seek out and attack their preferred targets: your cell membranes and DNA.

In the aftermath of their deadly assault, the body sends in a repair and reconstruction team. But if the damage is too extensive, the repair teams can't keep up. The DNA wounds that are left unattended can initiate and fuel chronic degenerative diseases, such as atherosclerosis, heart disease, strokes, emphysema, diabetes, arthritis, senility, accelerated aging, and cancer. Pollution, pesticides, tobacco, alcohol, and grilled red meat are just a few of the things that can penetrate your defenses by pouring excess oxygen free radicals into your body and, thus, are good things to avoid.

The only defenses against this unstable oxygen enemy are antioxidants, special weapons favored by your Warrior Goddess. She uses them to create a dynamic defense shield around every cell in your body. Unlike metal shields, which are inert and static, this shield is alive and composed of swarms of molecules, each acting like the protagonist in the old video game Pacman, gobbling up oxygen free radicals as fast as they can.

Your body makes its own antioxidants, but it can't usually create enough to win the battle. It needs a constant supply. Fresh organic fruits and vegetables hold an army of antioxidants. Research shows that a diet rich in antioxidants significantly lowers your risk of breast cancer. Each plant contains specific antioxidants, and each antioxidant has unique abilities to fend off chronic diseases, including cancer. For example, lycopene, the antioxidant responsible for the red color in fruits and vegetables such as tomatoes, is especially effective at lowering the risk of breast and prostate cancer.

Those fruits and vegetables with the most antioxidants ("antioxidant powerhouses") are listed below.

- Beets
- Blackberries
- Blueberries
- Broccoli
- Brussels sprouts

- Cherries
- Garlic
- Kale
- Kiwi
- Oranges

- Plums
- Red grapes
- Red bell pepper
- Spinach
- Strawberries

Although fresh organic fruits and vegetables are excellent sources of antioxidants, in this age of widespread pollution, toxins, and stressful lifestyles that fuel an ever-increasing attack of oxygen free radicals, you need a more powerful supplemental defense—beyond what you can get from even the best food—to keep the enemy at bay.

That's where antioxidant supplements come in. Selenium, vitamin C, vitamin E, CoQ$_{10}$, and an *Ayurvedic* herbal preparation called *Amrit Kalash* are all potent antioxidants. Research has proven that taking supplemental amounts of these antioxidants better equips you with the ammunition you need to fight the battle against breast cancer.

SELENIUM

Selenium is a mineral and micronutrient that your body needs for a number of very important functions. It plays a big role in preventing several different kinds of cancer, including cancers of the breast, prostate, lung, colon, bladder, stomach, esophagus, and liver. Research shows that most women who have breast cancer have much lower selenium levels than those who don't have the disease.

One of the reasons selenium is so effective in lowering the risk of cancer is that it causes your body to make more of its own powerful antioxidant—an enzyme called "glutathione peroxidase." Selenium makes up a fundamental part of the structure of this enzyme and, therefore, affects its function. Without selenium, the enzyme can't work.

Selenium helps to fight cancer in a dozen other ways, as well. Research has shown that it can prevent cancer cells from growing, cause cancer cells to die, foil the formation of new blood vessels needed for cancer to grow, and detoxify the body of cancer-inducing heavy metals. It can also boost toxin-neutralizing phase II enzymes in the liver; turn down the response of hormone receptors; handicap the ability of tumor cells to invade into surrounding tissues and metastasize; and enhance the immune system, especially natural killer (NK) cells and T-cell function. In addition, selenium has anti-inflammatory effects. When selenium is combined with other anticancer fighters, such as iodine found in seaweed, genistein in soy, or tea polyphenols (see Chapter 11), it becomes even more effective.

With all these anticancer effects, it's easy to understand why a growing mountain of evidence asserts that consuming selenium can be enormously helpful in preventing and treating cancer. In a legendary double-blind, randomized prospective study published in 1996 and conducted at the University of Arizona, patients were given 200 micrograms (mcg) of supplemental selenium every day. After six years, the patients taking selenium had only half as many deaths from cancer as the patients who weren't taking it. In other words, in this study the number of people who died of cancer in the group taking selenium was 52 percent lower than the number of people who died in the group that wasn't taking selenium. The subjects who were taking selenium also had 35 percent fewer new cancers diagnosed. So, taking selenium not only lowers the risk of developing cancer, it also appears to lengthen the lives of those who already have it.

Since 1996, numerous other studies have confirmed these same impressive statistics. The conclusion of the vast majority of studies looking at the relationship between selenium and cancer is that taking supplemental selenium or eating a selenium-rich diet reduces your risk of most types of cancer, including breast cancer, by as much as 50 percent and improves your chances of survival if you already have it.

There have also been a number of clinical trials studying the effects of giving supplemental selenium with mixed results: some showing benefit, others showing no benefit, while still others showing the possibility of harm. A 2009 large prospective study, referred to as SELECT (Selenium and Vitamin E Cancer Prevention Trial), created a lot of confusion when no benefit was found from supplemental selenium or vitamin E alone, or in combination, at preventing prostate cancer. Vitamin E was found to actually increase the risk by 17 percent. Needless to say, results like these cause lots of misunderstanding and media attention. Experts have spent a lot of time analyzing this study and have come up with several explanations. First, the type of supplemental vitamin E that was given was synthetic alpha-tocopherol only. As you learned in the last chapter, this form of vitamin E does not have strong anticancer properties. The natural form containing all the mixed forms of tocopherols, especially the gamma and delta types, is what shows major health benefits. Similarly, there are three major forms of selenium (sodium selenite, L-selenomethionine, and selenium-methyl L-selenocysteine) and each has different anticancer effects. You guessed it—the SELECT study only used one form. There were other potential problems with the design of the study that may have contributed to the unexpected results. Another factor is—just like folic acid reported in the previous chapter—taking too little or too much of a good thing can cause problems. Researchers refer to this pattern of influence as a U-shaped curve and when it comes to vitamins and minerals, it seems to especially hold true.

Taking Selenium

Getting your daily selenium from plant sources is ideal. Selenium is found naturally in soil and is absorbed by plants as they grow. But the amount of selenium in the soil varies considerably from region to region. If there isn't much in the soil, there won't be much in the plants growing there. Research shows that the amount of selenium in the soil and the rate of cancer in that location are inversely proportional. In other words, the areas of the world that have the *highest* selenium levels in the soil have the *lowest* rates of cancer. On the other hand, those with the lowest levels of selenium in the soil have the highest rates of cancer.

The best food source of selenium is Brazil nuts. Just one ounce of Brazil nuts a day gives you 1,200 percent of the recommended daily allowance. Other foods high in selenium include garlic, onions, leafy green vegetables, mushrooms, and whole grains, especially whole wheat. If you choose to take selenium in supplement form, make sure it contains all three types. About 200 mcg a day is recommended.

Don't take megadoses of selenium—or of any vitamin or food supplement for that matter. Remember that your body requires a delicate balance. The prudence of choosing just the right amount to achieve balance was introduced to most us of at a very early age by the fairytale "Goldilocks and the Three Bears." (Fairytales often reveal profound archetypal wisdom.) Goldilocks is remembered for one prominent personality trait: She evaluated the size or amount of anything she needed, from a chair to porridge, and always chose whichever was not too big and not too little, but "just right." Goldilocks lived her life according to the most important principle of *Ayurveda:* balance.

Ayurveda teaches that good health is *only* achieved and maintained by making choices that bring balance. In other words, always doing or taking the proper amount of the right things, at and for the ideal time, is the key to good health. In the case of selenium, if you take too much of it, you can develop the syndrome selenosis. Symptoms include hair loss, gastrointestinal upset, white blotchy nails, and mild nerve damage. To prevent these problems, don't take more than 400 mcg of supplemental selenium a day.

VITAMIN E

Vitamin E is another excellent antioxidant that helps to lower your risk of breast cancer. Chapter 12 discussed the details about this vitamin and how it battles this disease.

COENZYME Q_{10} (CoQ_{10})

CoQ_{10}, also known as ubiquinone, is a vitamin-like substance that is found in every cell in your body. It is absolutely essential to the process of cellular energy production. It's also a powerful antioxidant. Research has shown that CoQ_{10} levels are much lower in tumors than they are in normal tissues. When CoQ_{10} has been given to cancer patients, some spectacular results have been seen.

In a study from Denmark published in 1994, thirty-two patients with high-risk breast cancer were treated with antioxidants (vitamins C and E, selenium, and beta-carotene), essential fatty acids (gamma linolenic acid and omega-3 fatty acids), and 90 milligrams (mg) of CoQ_{10}. The breast tumors shrank in six of the thirty-two patients.

The researchers wondered what would happen if they increased the dose of CoQ_{10}. So, they decided to raise the daily dose of CoQ_{10} to 390 mg in just one of the six patients. They got a big, pleasant surprise. In one month, the tumor in this patient had become so small that it could no longer be felt. In another month, a mammogram showed that the tumor had completely disappeared. With these startling results, the researchers wanted to see if these higher doses of CoQ_{10} would shrink tumors in other breast cancer patients. They selected a woman with breast cancer, gave her 300 mg of CoQ_{10} a day, and waited with great anticipation. In just a few months, her tumor disappeared. In the eighteen months that the patients in this study were treated with CoQ_{10}, none of them died or showed further signs of metastases. The number of women who had been expected to die, as predicted by the stage of their tumors, was four.

Encouraged by these results, the researchers continued their study of CoQ_{10} in breast cancer patients and published a report the following year. They gave all their breast cancer patients 390 mg of CoQ_{10} each day. One patient was a forty-four-year-old woman with numerous metastases of her breast cancer to her liver. After a few months of taking CoQ_{10}, *all the metastatic tumors disappeared!* After six months of taking CoQ_{10}, another breast cancer patient, who had had a metastatic tumor to the lining of her lung before taking the CoQ_{10}, had no

The Story of CoQ₁₀

CoQ$_{10}$ (ubiquinone) was discovered by accident in a research lab at the University of Wisconsin in 1957 when a group of postdoctoral students was performing experiments on beef-heart mitochondria. (Mitochondria are the structures in your cells where energy is produced. They are considered the power plants of your cells. CoQ$_{10}$ is used by mitochondria to help drive the chemical reactions that produce energy.)

The students noticed a yellow frothy substance that kept rising to the top of their test tubes. When they looked at it under a microscope, these graduate students were viewing CoQ$_{10}$ for the first time. Incidentally, Peter Mitchell, the scientist who figured out specifically how CoQ$_{10}$ is used by the cells for energy production, received the Nobel Prize in 1978 for this discovery.

Although CoQ$_{10}$ is found in nearly every cell in your body, its highest concentrations are in the cells that make up the organs that need lots of energy, such as the heart, kidneys, liver, and lungs. Your body makes its own CoQ$_{10}$, but you also get additional amounts of it from outside sources—foods such as broccoli, spinach, and fish.

As you age, your levels of CoQ$_{10}$ begin to drop. If the amount of CoQ$_{10}$ in your cells falls too low, you can develop serious health problems. Certain disease conditions, such as congestive heart failure, are commonly associated with CoQ$_{10}$ deficiencies. When patients with congestive heart failure are given supplemental CoQ$_{10}$, their symptoms sometimes improve dramatically.

The Japanese were the first to find a way to make CoQ$_{10}$ in large enough quantities for commercial use. They began to use it extensively to treat hospital patients and soon discovered that the patients with diseases associated with low CoQ$_{10}$ levels, such as congestive heart failure, got a lot better. The Japanese now routinely treat all heart patients with CoQ$_{10}$.

Over the past few decades, there have been hundreds of studies documenting the significant health benefits of supplemental CoQ$_{10}$ for the treatment of many conditions other than heart disease. Some of these disorders are high blood pressure, periodontal (gum) disease, type 2 diabetes, male infertility, chronic fatigue syndrome (CFS), immune-system disorders such as AIDS, sickle-cell anemia, cancer, and neurological disorders including Parkinson's disease.

signs of the tumor left. Other researchers have not seen these kinds of dramatic results with CoQ_{10}. More research is needed to determine the effectiveness of CoQ_{10} in stopping the growth of breast cancer, but the results of these studies look very promising.

CoQ_{10} has been shown to help prevent the organ damage caused by chemotherapy, and it may even improve a woman's chance of surviving breast cancer. Chemotherapeutic drugs kill cancer cells, but they also kill normal cells. Certain drugs, such as Adriamycin, are toxic to the heart, and it's not uncommon for them to cause heart damage. The damage Adriamycin causes to this vital organ can be so severe that, if given to elderly patients with hearts already compromised by disease, it can kill them.

The reason Adriamycin damages the heart is directly related to CoQ_{10}. Normally, CoQ_{10} is found in high concentrations in the heart. Adriamycin causes CoQ_{10} levels to drop. Apparently, this drug can only damage the heart if the amount of CoQ_{10} in its muscle cells is low. So, when patients on Adriamycin are given a CoQ_{10} supplement, the levels in the heart muscle remain normal, and heart-muscle cells with normal CoQ_{10} levels aren't damaged by the drug. In a study published in *Molecular and Cellular Biochemistry* in May 2005, $CoQ_{10}$was found to enhance the effectiveness of Tamoxifen at stopping tumor growth. Later studies found several reasons why. CoQ_{10} helps to shut off the growth of new blood vessels, and reduces the production of a key molecule that helps tumors to invade and spread.

A 2010 study from the University of Hawaii concluded that higher CoQ_{10} levels in postmenopausal women may be associated with an increased risk of breast cancer. But a later prospective study reported that the higher the circulating CoQ_{10} levels were in women, the lower was the risk of breast cancer. Possibly CoQ_{10} may behave like other nutrients, such as folate and selenium, where either very low or very high levels may increase risk for breast cancer. Because there has only been one study showing a possible increased risk with for women with the highest levels, more studies need to be done to see if this can be confirmed. Serum blood CoQ_{10} levels in the range of 500 to 800 nanograms per milliliter (ng/mL) appear to have the lowest risk of developing breast cancer.

(For more information on CoQ_{10}, see the inset "The Story of CoQ_{10}" on page 148.)

Taking CoQ_{10}

CoQ_{10} is fat soluble. In other words, it's more easily absorbed when it's in fat. When CoQ_{10} is taken in a soy-oil suspension contained in a soft-shell capsule, it is more readily absorbed than if it's taken in a dry tablet or capsule. That means you need a higher dose of the dry form of CoQ_{10} than you do of the oil suspension to attain the same level of it in your body. If your goal is to lower your risk of breast cancer, 30–100 mg of CoQ_{10} a day is recommended. If you already have breast cancer, you'll need to take more.

Case studies from Denmark showed that breast tumors shrank in women given 300–390 mg of CoQ_{10} a day. If you are taking chemotherapeutic drugs that decrease CoQ_{10} levels, such as Adriamycin, you'll definitely want to take higher doses of CoQ_{10} to combat any potential organ damage caused by these drugs. Most CoQ_{10} is synthetically made. But a few companies produce a naturally fermented form of CoQ_{10} made from whole foods that studies show your body absorbs and uses much more efficiently. A study from the University of Scranton found that fermented CoQ_{10} had twenty times more antioxidant activity than the standard synthetic preparations of CoQ_{10} and that only 22 mg of the fermented CoQ_{10} was equivalent to 400 mg of synthetically made CoQ_{10}.

In healthy human blood, more than 90 percent of coenzyme Q_{10} exists in its reduced form called ubiquinol. Research shows that ubiquinol is a more biologically active form of CoQ_{10}—meaning that it absorbs better into our cells and its actions are stronger. Most CoQ_{10} supplements, however, contain the ubiquinone form because it remains stable longer in capsules. Ubiquinone is converted to ubiquinol in the body—so both forms work and research confirms this. Many experts are now recommending ubiquinol because it doesn't require conversion and ubiquinone does. The recommended dose of ubiquinol is the same as ubiquinone, about 100–300 mg a day. My opinion is that both forms work and it doesn't make that much difference which you chose. If you choose to take ubiquinone, a fermented product is definitely superior to a synthetic one.

Be sure to tell your doctor that you are planning to take this supplement. Let him or her help you determine how much to take. Also, because supplemental CoQ_{10} improves heart health, a person who takes heart medication may need his or her dosage adjusted while taking this supplement.

High blood pressure medications such as propranolol (Inderal), statin cholesterol-lowering drugs, and red yeast rice (a cholesterol-lowering dietary supplement) bring CoQ_{10} levels down, so you should always take supplemental CoQ_{10} when taking these substances.

AMRIT KALASH

Dr. Yukie Niwa, a Japanese researcher, studied more than 500 different antioxidants over a period of thirty years. He found that the most powerful and effec-

---

An Ancient Anti-Aging Formula

Thousands of years ago, *Ayurvedic* physicians created the anti-aging formula *Amrit Kalash*. *Ayurveda* considers *Amrit Kalash* to be a *rasayana*—"that which negates old age and disease." Research has shown that *Amrit Kalash* can indeed slow the aging process because it's such a powerful antioxidant. As you've learned, aging is accelerated by oxygen free radicals, and antioxidants neutralize them. It's incredible that science only recently discovered free radicals and antioxidants but these *Ayurvedic* physicians instinctively "knew" how to create this anti-aging formula—a formula with the most potent synergy of antioxidants of any substance ever tested.

Research shows *Amrit Kalash* may actually *reverse* aging. In a double-blind placebo-controlled study published in the *International Journal of Psychosomatics* in 1990, patients who received MAK-5 improved significantly on an age-related alertness task. Performance of this task is known to highly correlate with age. The older you are, the worse you normally do on this test. This study showed that MAK-5 could enhance the capacity for attention and alertness that predictably declines with age.

---

tive antioxidant of all those tested is an ancient *Ayurvedic* herbal preparation called *Amrit Kalash*. Research shows that the antioxidant capabilities of *Amrit Kalash* are at least 25,000 times more powerful than those of vitamins C and E. Taking it is like supplying your Warrior Goddess with a *Star Wars* deflector shield. This astounding ambrosia is composed of forty-four different herbs and fruits that seem to work synergistically, enhancing the natural strength of one another's antioxidants. The phenomenon of synergy, where each substance makes the other more effective, is a beautiful example of another marvel of Nature and *Ayurvedic* principle: *The whole is often greater than the sum of the parts.*

Due to its extraordinary antioxidants (and countless other health-protecting and wellness-enhancing nutrients), *Amrit Kalash* defends against cancer in significant ways. Research shows that it prevents tumors from starting, slows down tumor growth, and even shrinks tumors.

Several notable studies have been conducted at Ohio State University showing that *Amrit Kalash* is highly effective against breast cancer. *Amrit Kalash* is actually a two-part formula referred to as MAK-4 and MAK-5. In these studies, the two compounds were studied individually and then together. In one study, animals were fed MAK-5 before they were exposed to chemical carcinogens that often induce breast cancer. After eighteen weeks, 67 percent of the control animals (the animals not given MAK-5) had developed breast cancer. Of the animals that were given MAK-5, only 25 percent developed breast cancer.

The researchers then tested the other part of the *Amrit Kalash* formula, MAK-4, to see if it would have similar anticancer effects. The animals that were given MAK-4 before being exposed to chemicals known to cause breast cancer had 60 percent fewer tumors than the control animals. The tumors that *did* grow in these animals were only about 12 percent of the size of the tumors that grew in the control animals.

In another experiment, animals with fully formed tumors were given both MAK-4 and MAK-5. Researchers found that all the small tumors (less than 1 centimeter in diameter) in the animals shrank in size but that there was no change in the larger tumors. The conclusion of this study was that *Amrit Kalash* seems to be very beneficial in stopping the growth of small tumors.

There are other dramatic and valuable benefits of *Amrit Kalash,* as well. For one, it's an effective anti-aging supplement (see the inset "An Ancient Anti-Aging Formula" on page 151). For another, it alleviates many of the horrendous side effects of chemotherapy. In a 1994 study, breast cancer patients undergoing chemotherapy treatments were also given *Amrit Kalash.* For most of these patients, many of the side effects they were experiencing from the chemotherapy—especially nausea, vomiting, weight loss, dropped blood counts, and fatigue—went away or significantly diminished. These patients also reported that their overall sense of well-being improved when they took this supplement. Most important, *Amrit Kalash* alleviated all these side effects *without* interfering with the effectiveness of the chemotherapy.

In another study published in February 2005, *Amrit Kalash* Nectar tablets were found to significantly reduce the mortality of animals treated with Adriamycin, and reverse the toxic effects of Cisplatin on the liver and kidney.

THE ANTIOXIDANT/CHEMO CONTROVERSY

There's some controversy surrounding the use of supplemental antioxidants during chemotherapy and radiation. Why? Because certain chemotherapeutic agents (especially alkylating agents such as cyclophosphamide) and radiotherapy are known to generate and use oxygen free radicals to kill cancer cells. Theoretically, taking supplemental antioxidants could interfere with the effectiveness of these drugs at killing cancer cells. (Please take note that consuming antioxidants in foods is not at issue here; levels in whole foods are much lower than they are in supplement form.)

An extensive review of hundreds of studies on this subject was published in 1999. In it, researchers Davis Lamson and Matthew Brignall concluded that the vast majority of studies found that taking antioxidants "produces beneficial effects in many cancers with very few exceptions, and human studies show no reduction in the efficacy of chemotherapy or radiation when given with antioxidants." Lamson and Brignall felt that the argument that antioxidants might interfere with chemotherapy was too simplistic and probably untrue. Most studies showed an "increased effectiveness of many cancer chemotherapeutic agents, as well as a decrease in adverse effects, when given concurrently with antioxidants." The exact mechanisms of how these drugs work aren't yet fully understood.

After reviewing several hundred studies, Lamson and Brignall had only three cautions regarding the use of supplemental antioxidants during cancer treatments:

1. Routine use of N-acetylcysteine (NAC) with the chemotherapeutic agents cis-plantinum and doxorubicin should be avoided.

2. The flavonoid tangeretin found in citrus fruits should not be taken with Tamoxifen.

3. Beta-carotene should not be taken with 5-FU (Carac, Efudex) until the nature of their interaction has been clearly determined through research.

A highly quoted study from Finland shows that when beta-carotene was given to smokers, their risk of lung cancer went up. The theoretical explanation is that there are 500 different naturally occurring carotenoids, or plant pigments. If you take high doses of one of them, it doesn't allow you to get enough of the others. In the *Ayurvedic* view, getting your carotenoids from your food—in the proportions and amounts Nature provides—is the ideal way to consume these natural cancer-fighting substances because it brings balance and enhances health.

Certainly, more investigation needs to be done on all the antioxidants to determine exactly what their effects are on every type of cancer and every anti-cancer drug. By the preponderance of evidence, it certainly seems that taking a combination of different antioxidants cautiously and judiciously and eating foods high in antioxidants in conjunction with chemotherapy is very beneficial. In the vast majority of studies, antioxidants have been shown to actually *enhance* the effectiveness of these drugs, to protect against damaging—and sometimes fatal—side effects, such as organ damage, and to lengthen life expectancy. If I ever had to have chemotherapy, I would definitely—and selectively—take antioxidants at the same time.

Chapter 14

Smothering the Flames
The Anticancer Power of Anti-Inflammatories

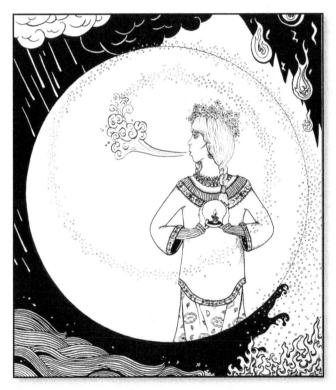

Nordic Goddess That Cools the Fires

If you have faith in the cause and the means and in God,
the hot sun will be cool for you.

—Mahatma Gandhi

*I*nflammation is a normal process created naturally by your body, and it serves an important role. It helps to get rid of unwanted bacteria and other invaders. It also assists your body in cleaning up dead cells from trauma or infection. When inflammation rises to assist your inner healing intelligence in these particular kinds of situations and then quietly wanes when it's no longer needed, no harm is done. But if the inflammation remains beyond its original purpose and becomes chronic (that is, continues as an ongoing process in your body), it turns into a lethal firestorm, breaking down cells and destroying the natural architectural boundaries of the body's tissues, making it easier for tumors to invade and grow.

Your Warrior Goddess can use inflammation as a tool to keep you healthy. It's like having a fireplace in your home where she can build a fire on a cold winter's night to keep you warm. But if you throw too much fuel on the fire, it can quickly grow out of control. Your Warrior Goddess then has to work frantically to keep the fire from burning down your house, destroying everything you own, and killing you in the process. Similarly, if inflammation is not kept under control, it can destroy your health and increase your risk of diseases that can potentially kill you, such as breast cancer.

Researchers have found that chronic inflammation not only plays a key role in the commencement and progression of many types of cancers, it also fuels a wide variety of chronic disorders, including heart disease, arthritis, and Alzheimer's disease.

One major reason why chronic inflammation acts as such a powerful destructive force is because it doesn't act alone. It creates additional destructive ammunition: oxygen free radicals. The cells in your immune system use oxygen free radicals like cosmic ray guns to shoot down bacteria and other offenders. In the presence of inflammation, these cells release showers of oxygen free radicals. And excess oxygen free radicals can cause the kind of DNA damage that can lead to cancer.

Stress and certain foods promote inflammation. Refined carbohydrates, sugar, and certain fats—especially trans fats—are some of the worst offenders. On the other hand, a diet rich in the antioxidants found in fresh, organically grown fruits and vegetables and omega-3 fatty acids reduces inflammation. Taking supplemental antioxidants (see Chapter 13) and practicing stress-reduction techniques (see Chapter 25) are also very beneficial in preventing and reducing inflammation.

THE COX-2 ENZYME

One of the best ways to reduce inflammation is to block the activity of an essential key enzyme in the inflammatory process called "cyclooxygenase-2," (COX-

2). The COX-2 enzyme is stimulated by inflammatory proteins released by cells in the immune system, growth factors, specific types of fat (such as omega-6 fatty acids), and a variety of other substances that encourage tumor growth. When activated, certain genes called "oncogenes" stimulate the growth of cancer. These oncogenes also increase the activity of the COX-2 enzyme.

A class of pharmaceutical anti-inflammatories targets the COX-2 enzyme and blocks or inhibits it. Celebrex and Vioxx are two examples. But pharmaceutical medications are hard on the body and create imbalances that can result in potentially serious side effects. For instance, COX-2 anti-inflammatory drugs have been shown to increase the risk of strokes, and potentially fatal heart attacks. This is precisely why Vioxx was taken off the market in the fall of 2004. When reaching for COX-2 anti-inflammatories, the wisest choice is to choose those made by Nature. Herbal COX-2 inhibitors not only block the enzyme with as much force as the synthetic pharmaceuticals, but they also import intelligence and balance into the body.

Nature's COX-2-inhibiting pharmacy includes dozens of herbs. The standouts are green tea, turmeric, holy basil, rosemary, ginger, oregano, skullcap (*Scutellaria*), barberry, and the Chinese herbs *hu zhang* and Chinese goldenthread. Researchers at Columbia University were the first to study the effectiveness of the herbal product Zyflamend, which is a mixture of all ten of these potent herbal anti-inflammatories, against prostate cancer. The details of their research, along with the results of studies from other institutions, are discussed in the inset "Zyflamend and Cancer" on page 158. Leading complementary and alternative physicians, such as Dr. Andrew Weil, prescribe Zyflamend for their patients with inflammatory conditions. It is also used at the Cleveland Clinic Spine Center in Ohio. If you want learn more about the properties of the herbs in Zyflamend, I recommend *Beyond Aspirin: Nature's Challenge to Arthritis, Cancer & Alzheimer's Disease,* an excellent book by Thomas M. Newmark and Paul Schulick.

Cancer and the COX-2 Enzyme

Researchers have found that inflammation isn't the only process that the COX-2 enzyme takes part in. It also plays a key role in the initiation and growth of several different cancers, including colon, prostate, and breast cancer. The COX-2 enzyme stimulates normal breast cells and breast cancer stem cells to start dividing and growing. It also prevents tumor cells from undergoing normal cell death, so more tumor cells remain alive, accelerating the growth of the tumor. The more tumor cells there are, the faster the tumor grows and the bigger it becomes. The COX-2 enzyme also encourages new blood vessels to grow into the tumor.

Zyflamend and Cancer

Researchers at Columbia University in New York were the first to study the effectiveness of Zyflamend against prostate cancer. This cancer, like breast cancer, can overexpress the COX-2 enzyme. The researchers found in laboratory tests that Zyflamend strongly inhibited the growth of prostate cancer cells by causing the cancer cells to die (a process technically called "apoptosis") and by stopping new blood-vessel growth. The COX-2 inhibiting effects of the ten combined herbs in Zyflamend were found to be greater than those of curcumin, a powerful COX-2 inhibitor and the active ingredient in turmeric. In another study, published in *Nutrition and Cancer* in 2005, Zyflamend was found to not only drastically decrease COX-1 and COX-2 activity, but it also worked through other mechanisms independent of the COX enzymes to suppress cell growth and induce apoptosis.

A phase 1 clinical trial was conducted at Columbia University and published in 2009 that investigated the influence of Zyflamend on men diagnosed with "high-grade intraepithelial neoplasia" (HGPIN). HGPIN is a premalignant condition associated with a high risk of developing invasive prostate cancer in the future. About 30 percent of men with HGPIN go on to develop invasive prostate cancer. HGPIN can be compared to ductal carcinoma in situ (DCIS) in the breast, also considered a premalignant condition that warns of a much higher risk of invasive breast cancer developing in the future.

In this study published in the *Journal of the Society of Integrative Oncology* in 2009, men diagnosed with HGPIN were given Zyflamend and evaluated for the next eighteen months. Every three months, blood tests were done measuring the level of prostate-specific antigen (PSA), a substance that increases with the presence of prostate cancer. Biopsies of the prostate were done every six months. Almost half the men (48 percent) had a 25 to 50 percent decrease in their PSA after eighteen months. Biopsies at eighteen months revealed that 60 percent of the men had normal tissue—the HGPIN had gone away! A biopsy of the prostate usually involves taking many samples of tissue called cores, and HGPIN was found in only one core of the biopsies in 26.7 percent. Prostate cancer was found in 13 percent.

Dr. Aaron Katz, director of the Center of Holistic Urology at Columbia-Presbyterian Medical Center and chief investigator of the studies on Zyflamend and prostate cancer, has written an excellent book on prostate cancer that I highly recommend: *Dr. Katz's Guide to Prostate Health: From Conventional to Holistic Therapies.*

All the herbs or isolates of active ingredients in the herbs in Zyflamend have been studied individually to determine their effects in reducing the incidence and growth of cancers. One of the herbs in Zyflamend is turmeric (see Turmeric—A Potent Anti-Inflammatory on page 161). Another is green tea (see Green Tea—The #1 Anticancer Beverage on page 110). In addition, many studies also document the impressive COX-2-inhibiting effects of holy basil, rosemary, ginger, *hu zhang*, Chinese golden-thread, barberry, oregano, and skullcap (*Scutellaria*).

Zyflamend has now been studied extensively by researchers at other institutions, including the renowned MD Anderson Cancer Center in Houston, Texas. Prostate cancer isn't the only type of cancer it deters. This herbal supplement has also been found to inhibit the growth of melanoma and pancreatic cancer. Its numerous anticancer skills include suppressing the growth of tumors, preventing invasion and spreading of the tumor, killing tumors through apoptosis, and preventing new blood vessels from growing into tumors. To gain even greater insights to Zyflamend's anticancer effects, researchers are currently mapping out the specific genes and cellular processes it activates.

New blood vessels are constantly required to deliver enough nutrients and oxygen-laden blood to feed an expanding tumor. The more nutrients and oxygen that are supplied to the tumor, the bigger and faster it grows.

Tumor cells can invade normal tissue more aggressively in response to the COX-2 enzyme. This seemingly malicious enzyme also enhances a tumor's ability to metastasize to other areas of the body, especially to lymph nodes, bone, bone marrow, and the brain. The COX-2 enzyme suppresses the immune system so that it can't fight off cancer cells as effectively, and steps up the production of mutagens (substances that cause mutations in your DNA that can lead to cancer). When you add them all together, these hazardous effects of the COX-2 enzyme powerfully promote tumor growth. It's no wonder studies show that taking anti-inflammatories to block the ill effects of the COX-2 enzyme can reduce your risk of breast cancer by as much as 70 percent.

Some tumors show an "overexpression" of the COX-2 enzyme. This means that these tumor cells have a lot more active COX-2 enzyme in them than normal tissue usually does. Cancers of the breast, prostate, and colon frequently display this overexpression, which is why the COX-2 enzyme plays such a big role in their growth compared to other types of cancers. Not all breast cancers overexpress the COX-2 enzyme, but researchers have found that a significant number do. In a 2007 study conducted by Emory University School of Medicine, 95 percent of breast cancers tested showed COX-2 expression. The amount that COX-2 expresses in each tumor, however, can vary significantly—ranging from small amounts to very high. Several studies report that about 50 percent of tumors overexpress or produce excessive amounts of the COX-2 enzyme.

Because the COX-2 enzyme has so many ways that it powerfully promotes tumor growth, those tumors that have high amounts of the COX-2 enzyme are more aggressive, come back in a short period of time after treatment, and have a far less favorable prognosis. At the time of initial diagnosis, tumors overexpressing COX-2 tend to be larger, have a higher or aggressive tumor grade and incidence of the less favorable HER2/neu receptor, and have spread to the lymph nodes.

COX-2 ENZYME INHIBITORS

COX-2 inhibitors lower the risk of cancer in two major ways: They reduce inflammation and block the expression of the COX-2 enzyme in tumors. Inflammation creates an abundance of oxygen free radicals, and it destroys natural tissue boundaries making it easier for tumors to grow. The COX-2 enzyme has an unsurpassed talent for promoting the inception and cultivation of tumors because of the impressive array of cancer-promoting techniques that it holds, but COX-2 enzyme inhibitors can block every one of its tumor-fostering processes.

Certain anti-inflammatory pharmaceutical medications, such as Celebrex, are designed to work by blocking or inhibiting the COX-2 enzyme. All the herbs found in Zyflamend inhibit the COX-2 enzyme, too. Not surprisingly, research has shown that all COX-2 inhibitors have powerful anticancer properties because they block every cancer-promoting action of the COX-2 enzyme. In experimental animals, they have been found to significantly reduce the formation of breast tumors and the number of tumors that grow in response to a carcinogen. COX-2 inhibitors also slow the growth of tumors once they have formed.

In a study published in 2001, researchers at Ohio State University found a direct inverse relationship between the amount of COX-2 inhibitor that was given and the number of breast tumors that formed in the test animals. The higher the dose of COX-2 inhibitors was, the lower the risk of breast tumors. Researchers at the Ohio State College of Medicine conducted a study on 323 breast cancer patients and 649 cancer-free controls to evaluate the use of COX-2 inhibitors such as Celebrex and Vioxx. The results appeared in the January 30, 2006 issue of *BMC Cancer.* They found that women who used one of these drugs for two years or more had a 71 percent reduction in the risk of breast cancer.

ANTI-INFLAMMATORIES AND BREAST CANCER— THE WOMEN'S HEALTH INITIATIVE STUDY

The largest ongoing national study of women's health, called the Women's Health Initiative (WHI), found that women who had taken aspirin or ibuprofen (a type of nonsteroidal anti-inflammatory drug; NSAID) an average of three times a week for ten years had a significantly lower risk of breast cancer. Those who took aspirin had a 28 percent lower risk, and those who took ibuprofen had a 50 percent lower risk.

Since aspirin and ibuprofen have the potential for some serious side effects (107,000 people are hospitalized and more than 16,500 people die in the United States alone each year from bleeding complications related to NSAIDs), many natural-medicine doctors, including Dr. Andrew Weil, and I recommend that you take a safe herbal anti-inflammatory such as Zyflamend instead. Research shows that it works just as well, and rather than causing side effects, it brings a multitude of wonderful side benefits.

TURMERIC—A POTENT ANTI-INFLAMMATORY

Let me say again that the amazing Asian spice turmeric is one of the most brilliant secret weapons against breast cancer that you can give your Warrior Goddess. The broad healing power of this extraordinary rhizome was introduced in Chapter 11, but it has other remarkable attributes, as well. When it comes to natural COX-2 inhibitors, none is as powerful as turmeric. A study published in the *Indian Journal of Medical Research* compared the anti-inflammatory effects of oral curcumin (one of the active ingredients in turmeric and the source of its bright yellow-orange color) against two powerful anti-inflammatory medications: cortisone and phenylbutazone. The study found that curcumin was *just as effective* as these two potent anti-inflammatory medications!

The anti-inflammatory intelligence contained in turmeric enhances your body's anti-inflammatory intelligence in three different ways. First, it stimulates your adrenal glands to release natural, powerful anti-inflammatory substances called corticosteroids. Second, it prevents the breakdown of cortisol, so more of this natural anti-inflammatory stays in your body. Third, it makes your body's cortisol receptors more sensitive. When the receptors are more sensitive, it only takes a small amount of cortisol to produce big anti-inflammatory effects.

Turmeric can also be used as a topical anti-inflammatory and analgesic (pain reliever). When applied over strained muscles, pulled tendons, and arthritic joints, turmeric can help to reduce swelling and pain. It depletes substance P, a chemical produced at nerve endings that causes the sensation of irritation and pain.

Another reason why turmeric is such a powerful anti-inflammatory is because it's also a strong COX-2-enzyme inhibitor—even more grounds for turmeric to be considered the number-one anticancer spice!

Part Four

Poisoning Your Warrior Goddess

Toxins That Destroy Your Healing Intelligence

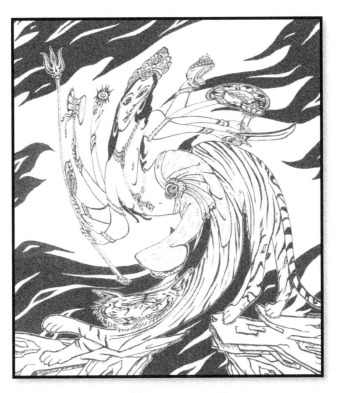

Goddess in Turmoil

Chapter 15

The Four Perils of Red Meat

Your Goddess Is an Herbivore

Nothing will benefit human health and increase chances for survival of life on Earth as much as the evolution to a vegetarian diet.

—ALBERT EINSTEIN

*T*his is the first of seven chapters that put a spotlight on breast cancer's covert allies: the foods and substances that trigger and support its growth. These factors are proven enemies to your breast health. Avoiding them lowers your risk of breast cancer. These "forces of darkness" are the foods, habits, and toxins that destroy your body's inner healing intelligence, help to midwife the cancer monster, and support cancer's rapid growth. These are the things that weaken your Warrior Goddess, strip her of her power, and obstruct her ability to keep you well. They are like Kryptonite to Superman.

Research has shown beyond a scientific doubt that eating red meat is a serious risk factor for breast cancer. You can think of it this way: Breast cancer is a carnivore; your Warrior Goddess is an herbivore. Many studies have shown that women who eat the most red meat have an 88 to 400 percent increased risk of this deadly disease. A German study published in 2002 found that women who consumed the most red meat had an 85 percent greater risk of breast cancer.

Several studies, including a 2008 study by Harvard Medical School, reveal that red meat consumption during adolescence is associated with a higher risk of premenopausal breast cancer. A 2011 study from China found that one reason for increased risk is because eating greater amounts of red meat as an adolescent increases the risk of adult breast density—a known risk factor for breast cancer.

Researchers at the Harvard School of Public Health have been conducting a very large prospective study of premenopausal nurses, called the Nurses' Health Study II. This ongoing study is gathering a multitude of health information from the participants and analyzing the effects of diet and lifestyle on health. One subject that is being studied is the relationship of eating red meat and the risk of breast cancer. More than 90,000 women, ages twenty-six to forty-six, were entered into the study beginning in the 1980s. The results of the study, published in the November 2006 issue of the *Archives of Internal Medicine,* found that women who ate more than one and a half servings of beef, lamb, or pork per day had almost double the risk of developing breast cancer compared to women who ate three or fewer servings per week.

Seven years later, another paper was published in the same journal with the latest results regarding red meat consumption and risk of mortality. In April 2013, the Harvard School of Public Health researchers combined data from the Nurses' Health Study with 37,698 men who are being followed in a prospective study called the Health Professionals Follow-Up Study. The researchers reported that those who ate red meat regularly had an increased risk of type 2 diabetes, coronary heart disease, stroke, and certain cancers. Not surprisingly, the total mortality rates, and mortality from cancer and cardiovascular disease were much higher for meat eaters. Just one serving a day of unprocessed meat was associated with a 13 percent increased risk of mortality, and one daily serving of processed meat (one hot dog, two slices of bacon) increased the risk by 20 percent. Reducing one serving of total red meat with a healthy protein significantly reduced the risk of dying. For instance, fish reduced the risk by 7 percent, nuts by 19 percent, and legumes by 10 percent.

Breast cancer isn't the only cancer that is more prevalent in those who eat high amounts of red meat. Scores of studies report that eating red meat is also associated with an increased risk of cancers of the esophagus, larynx, stomach, colon, and lung.

PERIL #1: ANIMAL PROTEIN

The meat of animals is composed primarily of protein, which is made up of smaller subunits known as "amino acids." It also contains creatine, an important substance that muscle cells use for energy. As you know, protein and amino acids are essential to health, and so is creatine. However, when animal protein is cooked, especially at high heat, structural changes occur in the protein, amino acids, and creatine—changes that create dangerous new carcinogens. A study from Uruguay found that red-meat protein is associated with a *220 to 770 per-*

cent increased risk of breast cancer! Other researchers have identified the type of iron found in red meat as a possible contributing carcinogen.

PERIL #2: SATURATED ANIMAL FATS

Saturated animal fats (a type of lipid) from red meat and dairy products are very harmful to your body. These lipids make the cells in your body more resistant to insulin. As a result, your insulin levels go up. High insulin levels can be lethal. Not only do they increase your risk of diabetes, but they also speed up the growth of tumors. In fact, they are one of the biggest risk factors for breast cancer. Research shows that women with the highest insulin levels have up to a 283 percent greater risk of breast cancer.

There are two other ways that saturated animal fat can raise your risk of breast cancer, as well. First, saturated animal fat is converted into a carcinogenic substance by the bacteria in your colon. Second, oxygen free radicals have a tendency to attack and damage these types of fats, changing them into powerful stimulators of inflammation, and inflammation fuels the growth of breast cancer. Worse yet, inflammation and oxygen free radicals engage in a deadly dance with each other, each one increasing the numbers and power of the other. Inflammation produces more oxygen free radicals, and oxygen free radicals, in turn, spark the fires of inflammation.

PERIL #3: CONCENTRATED TOXINS IN RED MEAT

Red meat is a storehouse of concentrated toxins including pesticides, antibiotics, hormones, and growth stimulators. Hormones such as melegestrol acetate, progesterone, testosterone, trenbolone, and zeranol—all known to disrupt the body's natural hormone balance and contribute to diseases such as breast cancer—are routinely injected into over two-thirds of the cows in the United States. John Verall, a member of the British Veterinary Products Committee and chemical expert stated in an article for www.newstarget.com on July 16, 2006 that according to recent studies, children are particularly sensitive to these hormones, which can cause "sudden growth or breast development, even at levels which are difficult to detect in the laboratory." He stated that these growth and sex hormones in beef not only promote the growth of breast and prostate cancer, but are also the chief cause of genital abnormalities in boys and early-onset puberty in girls. Within this lethal mix is insulin-like growth factor-1 (IGF-1), which, as you've learned, is vile and murderous at higher concentrations. IGF-1 is an extraordinarily potent stimulator of breast cancer. In fact, some scientists believe it may be *the most* potent stimulator of breast cancer known.

Eating conventionally raised beef and dairy products is the principal way that excessive amounts of IGF-1 get into your body. In the United States, live-stock are regularly fed and injected with growth hormones and stimulators to make them grow bigger and faster and to increase their production of milk. (For more information on IGF-1 and its role in breast cancer, see Chapter 8.)

Environmental toxins, such as pesticides, herbicides, chemical fertilizers, and industrial chemicals, accumulate and are stored in animal fat. Many of these toxins have estrogenic effects. In other words, they act like estrogen in the body and accelerate cell division. Many studies have shown that these pesticides can trigger breast cancer and that those women who have high levels of these pes-ticides in their bodies have a much higher risk of breast cancer.

PERIL #4: DEATH BY GRILLING

When red meats are cooked at high temperatures, additional carcinogens known as "heterocyclic amines" are formed. These sinister molecules attack DNA, destroying its vital code in a way that seriously increases the risk of cancer. Frying and grilling are the methods of cooking that use the highest temperatures to cook meat, and they are associated with the highest risk of breast cancer. The higher the cooking temperature, the more carcinogenic heterocyclic amines form. How long you cook your meat makes a difference, too. The more well-done your meat is, the more heterocyclic amines it will have, and the more carcinogenic it will be. British researchers discovered in 2007 that a type of heterocyclic amine created from red meat had potent hormonal activity, includ-ing mimicking estrogen and increasing the production of prolactin from the pituitary—another hormone that speeds up cell division of breast cells.

Research shows that of the women who eat red meat, those who eat both the most grilled and the most well-done red meat have the highest risk of breast cancer. In a 2009 review study published in the journal *Nutrition and Cancer*, researchers reported that women who consistently ate well-done meat had a 4.6 times higher incidence of breast cancer. A study from Vanderbilt University pub-lished in 2002 also found that women who consumed large amounts of red meat, especially cooked well-done, had a significantly higher risk of breast can-cer. If the women were also overweight, their risk was even greater.

Another study, done at the Medical College of Ohio and published in the journal *Carcinogenesis* in 1999, found that an enzyme in breast tissue called "N-acetyltransferase" activates the carcinogens in well-done red meat and in ciga-rette smoke. The study also identified several different subtypes of the N-acetyltransferase enzyme. The risk of breast cancer in women who had one particular subtype of this enzyme was extremely high. The women who had this dangerous subtype and who also smoked, ate a lot of red meat, or ate well-done red meat were found to have a 400 percent higher risk of breast cancer. In short, eating well-done red meat is always risky, but it is exceptionally risky for certain women.

SAFE ALTERNATIVES—MEAT MIMICKERS

If you love the taste and texture of red meat, don't think you have to give it up. The ever-growing and surprisingly delicious vegetable-based meat-substitute cuisine has come a long way. Even committed carnivores will find many of the meat mimickers to be a culinary delight. For instance, when my son was a rebellious teenager he couldn't tell the difference between a Boca Burger (made with soy protein) and an actual hamburger! Also, some vegetarians (I, for one) think some meat substitutes taste too much like the real thing!

If you do like the taste of meat, however, there are delicious substitutes for hamburgers, frankfurters, salami, lunchmeats, chicken, turkey, jerky—you name it. The next time you're at your local health food store, experiment and give one a try. I think you'll be pleasantly surprised. Many chain grocery stores carry them, too. However, keep in mind that processed foods aren't the best sources of nutrition, so don't make them your main course of every meal. They are best reserved as occasional "treats." Fresh, whole, organically produced plants—vegetables, fruits, whole grains, legumes, nuts—are always your best choice when it comes to nourishing your body.

The list below shows some good substitutes for your old meaty favorites.

- Instead of bacon, try Morningstar Veggie Bacon Strips or Lightlife Smart Bacon.

- Instead of chicken, try Gardenburger Chik'n Grill or Boca Chik'n Nuggets.

- Instead of hamburgers, try Boca Burgers, Amy's Organic Texas Burger, or Morningstar Farms Grillers Prime.

- Instead of hot dogs, try Yves Veggie Cuisine Good Dog.

- Instead of turkey, try Tofurkey.

You can find an extensive list of other vegan choices on www.peta.org.

Chapter 16

A Dangerous Foe in a Sweet Disguise
Sugar: Breast Cancer's Favorite Food

*I*t is estimated that the average American eats almost his or her entire body weight in sugar every year. The average teenage boy eats 34 teaspoons of sugar a day, and the average teenage girl consumes 24 teaspoons. When you add up the amount of sugar in various foods, it's easy to see how this is possible. Sugar is added to virtually all processed foods, especially soda pop. The average can of cola, such as Coke or Pepsi, contains 10–12 teaspoons of sugar! There's a breakfast cereal with a whopping 18 teaspoons of sugar *per serving;* that's one-third of a cup, or the equivalent of forty-eight Hershey's Kisses.

If you want your Warrior Goddess to stay in top cancer-fighting condition, this sticky substance is one of the worst things you can give her. It's like wrapping her in a spider's web of cotton candy. Caught in this gummy trap, her ability to oppose her mortal enemy, breast cancer, is dramatically hampered.

As Dr. Christiane Northrup says, for some women, chocolate is a food group. If you can limit your chocolate intake to a small amount of organic dark chocolate, that's actually good for your health. But if you prefer milk chocolate or have a sweet tooth for candy and confectionaries, what I'm about to share with you won't be good news for you: the distressing facts about sugar and cancer. But before you become totally dejected, be aware that there are good all-natural sugar alternatives—one, in particular, that tastes great and is good for you.

INSULIN—SUGAR'S ESCORT

Cancer cells love sugar. It's their preferred fuel. The more sugar you eat, the faster cancer cells grow. Your pancreas responds to sugar by releasing insulin, the hormone that escorts sugar into your cells. When you eat refined simple sugars, such as white table sugar, candy, cookies, or other sugar-laden foods, your blood sugar levels rise very quickly. Your pancreas responds by releasing a lot of insulin. That's not good. High insulin levels are one of the biggest risk factors and promoters of breast cancer. Women with high insulin levels have up to a 283 percent greater risk of breast cancer.

Insulin is capable of extraordinary evil, and the biggest reason is due to the fact that both normal breast cells and cancer cells have insulin receptors on them. When insulin attaches to its receptor, it has the same effect as when estrogen attaches to its receptor; it causes cells to start dividing. The higher your insulin levels are, the faster your breast cells will divide; the faster they divide, the higher your risk of breast cancer is and the faster any existing cancer cells will grow.

There's another wound that insulin can inflict, too. It attacks a portion of the estrogen cycle, making more estrogen available to attach to the estrogen receptors in breast tissue. Insulin regulates how much of the estrogen in your blood is available to attach to estrogen receptors. Look back at Figure 3.1 on page 42. When estrogen travels in the blood, it either travels alone seeking a mate (an estrogen receptor), *or* it travels with a partner (a protein binder, or carrier) that prevents it from attaching to an estrogen receptor. Insulin regulates the number of protein binders in the blood. So, the higher your insulin levels are, the fewer the number of protein binders there will be. Fewer protein binders mean that there's more free estrogen available to attach to estrogen receptors.

In other words, when your insulin levels are up, free-estrogen levels are up, too. And both of them speed up cell division. That's why high insulin levels increase your risk of breast cancer so much.

DANGER—SUGAR!

Eating sugar increases your risk of breast cancer in yet another way. It delivers a major blow to your immune system with the force of a prizefighter. Your immune system is your natural defense against such invaders as bacteria, viruses, and cancer cells. Research shows that right after you eat a high-sugar meal, the function of the cells in your immune system drops drastically. In the case of one type of cell in particular—the T lymphocyte (a type of white blood cell)—sugar knocks its defense abilities down by at least 50 percent. This effect lasts for a minimum of five hours! Another researcher found that the function of T lymphocytes dropped by *94 percent* after a high-sugar meal! This means that right after you've eaten a lot of sugar, your body's ability to fight off invaders or destroy cancer cells is tremendously weakened for several hours.

Over a period of time, eating too much sugar can create imbalances that lead to two more deadly diseases: obesity and type 2 diabetes. Both of these diseases dangerously increase your risk of breast cancer, and both have increased alarmingly in the United States in the past two decades. An estimated 60 percent of American adults are overweight, and 5 percent have diabetes. Of those people who have diabetes, 90 percent are also overweight. Not only do these diseases increase your risk of breast cancer, but they also increase your risk of heart disease, high blood pressure, poor circulation, stroke, and infection.

It All Adds Up

All of these cancer-promoting effects of sugar add up. In a 2004 study published in the journal *Cancer Epidemiology, Biomarkers, and Prevention*, Mexican women who ate high amounts of carbohydrates had over twice the risk of breast cancer compared to those who did not. Other studies from around the world including Asia, Europe, North America, and South America have found smaller, yet significant associations between high-glycemic index foods (foods that cause blood sugars to soar, such as refined carbohydrates and sugars) and the incidence of breast cancer. Consuming a diet that is high in refined carbohydrates and sugars has been found to also increase the risk of other cancers, particularly cancers of the prostate, colon, uterus, and pancreas. It increases your risk of other chronic diseases, including heart disease, diabetes, obesity, depression, and Alzheimer's disease.

In a meta-analysis published in the *American Journal of Clinical Nutrition* in 2008, researchers reviewed a multitude of studies in the medical literature that focused on the relationship of chronic diseases and high blood glucose levels. After pooling all the data, they concluded that "high blood glucose is a universal mechanism for chronic disease progression." In other words, eating too many refined carbs and sugars fuels the progression of *every* chronic disease!

A study conducted by Harvard Medical School and published in 2004 found that women who, as teenagers, ate foods with a high glycemic index had a higher incidence of breast cancer later in life. So, encouraging your teenage daughter to cut back on sugar will help her to lower her risk of breast cancer for the rest of her life.

STEVIA—SWEET RELIEF

Now, the good news: If you have a sweet tooth, you'll be relieved to know that you don't have to suffer. There's a natural sweetener that tastes great, and better yet, research has shown that instead of being dangerous to your health, it actually has several wonderful health-supporting qualities. It's called stevia, and it comes from the South American plant *Stevia rebaudiana*. What's interesting about this semi shrub, indigenous to Paraguay, is that every part of it tastes intensely sweet. The dried leaves, however, are the only parts that are used for medicinal and commercial purposes. Scientists have found that stevia's delightfully sweet flavor comes from a group of substances in it called "glycosidal diterpenes."

Compared to sugar, only *very* small amounts of stevia are needed. That's because stevia is 300 times sweeter than sucrose, the type of sugar found in table sugar. Stevia hasn't yet been approved by the FDA as a food additive—write your senators and Congressional representatives!—so at this time you won't find it in any processed foods in the United States. In this country stevia is considered a dietary supplement. Health food stores and national-chain grocery stores that specialize in organic foods, such as Sprouts and Whole Foods, usually carry stevia.

Stevia comes in multiple forms: a fine white powder, a green powder, or a liquid. I found that certain brands of stevia have a bitter taste or leave a strange aftertaste if you use too much. There's one brand, however, that solved this problem by adding some fiber to the stevia. It is called Stevia Plus by SweetLeaf (see the Resources section). It dissolves well and leaves no bitter aftertaste.

Stevia can also be used in cooking, but it's a little tricky. The amount you should use can vary a lot from brand to brand, so you definitely should use a stevia cookbook. Many of the companies with stevia products have their own cookbooks. There's a stevia product made especially for baking called More Fiber Stevia Baking Blend by NuNaturals. Many sites on the Internet sell it and certain health food stores carry it as well. (See the Resources section for a list of these companies and their websites.)

Stevia has been used for hundreds, if not thousands, of years by the native tribes in Paraguay and Brazil to treat high blood pressure and diabetes. Modern research has shown that it *does* help both conditions. Stevia causes blood vessels to dilate. When the diameter of a blood vessel increases, the blood pressure in it goes down. A double-blind placebo-controlled study was published in the *British Journal of Pharmacology* in 2000 documenting stevia's ability to lower blood pressure. Researchers found that after only three months, patients with high blood pressure who were given stevia three times a day had a significant decrease in both their systolic (the upper number) and diastolic (the lower number) blood-pressure.

Stevia is a great sugar substitute for people who really need to avoid sugar, such as diabetics. In addition, stevia has an added benefit for type 2 diabetics: It seems to have an effect opposite to that of sugar on their bodies; it causes blood sugar to go *down*. Many recent studies have focused on finding out exactly how stevia reduces blood sugar. This is what has been discovered so far: Stevia increases the insulin sensitivity of insulin resistant cells, enhances insulin secretion from the beta-cells in the pancreas, improves insulin utilization in cells, and slows gluconeogenesis or glucose production in the liver. Research has also discovered several more health benefits of stevia. First, it can kill certain bacteria and viruses. In a Japanese study published in 2001 by Taka Hashi, et al., in the journal *Antiviral Research,* stevia was found to have antiviral effects against the rotavirus. This virus can cause severe diarrhea and dehydration, especially in infants. Second, stevia shows a strong ability to kill a wide range of food-borne bacteria. Third, stevia has anti-inflammatory properties. Fourth, it has antitumor effects.

Another healthy natural substitute for sugar is also available. It's made from *Luo Han Guo,* the round green fruit of the Chinese plant *Siraita grosvenori. Luo Han Guo* has been used in China as a medicine since the thirteenth century, but it didn't become popular as a remedy for coughs, sore throats, and upper respiratory-tract infections until the twentieth century. In southern China *Luo Han Guo* is also used to enhance longevity. Like stevia, *Luo Han Guo* is about 300 times sweeter than sugar and is processed into a fine, white crystalline powder. WisdomHerbs makes a sugar substitute using a blend of *Luo Han Guo* and fructose called Sweet & Slender. It can be purchased at most health food stores or on the Internet.

XYLITOL: ANOTHER NATURAL SWEET ALTERNATIVE

Used as a food additive since the 1960s, xylitol is another natural sweetener that appears to be safe and, in addition, sports several health benefits. It is naturally found in fibrous fruits and vegetables, and a variety of hardwoods. The main sources of commercially produced xylitol come from wood scraps and corncobs. Research shows that xylitol is not just an excellent substitute for sugar, it also reduces plaque deposits on teeth, lowers the incidence of dental caries by 80 percent, promotes remineralization of tooth enamel, reduces infections in the mouth and nasopharynx, and decreases bone loss. Xylitol is also good for people with diabetes or who are trying to lose weight. It contains 40 percent fewer calories than sugar and is incompletely absorbed. The portion of xylitol that is absorbed enters the bloodstream very slowly and causes negligible rises in blood sugar and insulin levels. More than 2,800 studies have been published on xylitol confirming its safety. Xylitol was declared to be safe for humans and approved as a food additive by the Federation of American Societies for Experimental Biology (FASEB) in 1986.

ARTIFICIAL SWEETENERS

Artificial sweeteners were created with the good intention of helping you to lower your consumption of sugar. However, most of them are synthetic and not

Soft Drinks: Deadly Sugar Delivery Devices

Soft drink consumption has increased by 300 percent in the past twenty years according to a 2008 study conducted at Wayne State University School of Nursing in Detroit, Michigan, and 56 to 85 percent of school-children consume at least one soft drink daily. Numerous studies, including a study published in the *World Journal of Gastroenterology* in 2010, show that soft drinks are the leading source of added sugar worldwide and are associated with obesity, diabetes, high blood pressure, metabolic syndrome, coronary heart disease, nonalcoholic fatty liver, and cancer. According to Dora Romaguera-Bosch, Ph.D., M.Sc., of Imperial College London in England, consuming an additional 12 ounces of sugar-sweetened beverages—a standard size can of soda—daily is associated with a 22 percent increased risk for diabetes, and an extra can of artificially sweetened beverage raises the risk by 52 percent.

High fructose corn syrup (HFCS), a combination of 55 percent fructose and 45 percent glucose, is a major ingredient in soft drinks and is thought to be the primary culprit in promoting those diseases. But, it isn't the only potentially dangerous ingredient. Soft drinks also contain phosphorus, which gives them their effervescence pop. Harvard scientists found in a study published in April 2010, that high levels of phosphates accelerate the signs of aging, including infertility, skeletal muscle wasting, bone-mineral density loss, skin tone laxity, and a shortened lifespan. Soda comes in cans that are lined with plastic-containing bisphenol A (BPA) (see Chapter 21), which has been linked to reproductive problems, heart disease, obesity, and cancer.

Colas appear to be a special category with even more associated health problems than other carbonated beverages. Just three colas a week increases the risk of dental erosions threefold, and bone mineral loss. A study from Singapore found that just two colas a week almost doubled the risk of pancreatic cancer! In 2012 a British study found that just one serving a day increased the risk of aggressive prostate cancer in men.

Researchers from the Harvard School of Public Health reported in 2013 that sugary drinks are responsible for an increase in global death rates. An estimated 200,000 deaths worldwide in 2010 are thought due to the increased incidences of diabetes, cardiovascular diseases, and cancer caused by excessive sugary drink consumption. Of those deaths, 25,000 occurred in the United States. Mexico—which holds the dubious distinction of being the country with the highest per-capita consumption of sugary beverages in the world—ranks number one in deaths related to sugary drinks. Because people in China and Japan consume the least amounts of these unhealthy drinks, the mortality rates in these countries are the lowest.

Think diet colas are a better choice? Think again. Research shows that these drinks have a boatload of health problems associated with them, too. Carbonated water, caramel color, aspartame, phosphoric acid, potassium citrate, natural flavors, citric acid, and caffeine are the typical ingredients in a diet soda—none are ingredients for good health. "Wait a minute," you say, "they help to make you thin!" Sorry, but you are mistaken. Instead of making you thin, they are much more likely to make you fat. Just two drinks a day can actually raise your chance of becoming obese by 57 percent, and increase your waistline by 500 percent! In fact, a study from the University of Texas Health Science Center found that the more diet sodas a person drank, the higher was his or her risk of becoming overweight.

There are health consequences linked to this drink that are much worse than increasing your girth. The Nurses' Health Study suggests that diet sodas can hurt your vital organs, especially your kidneys. Just one diet soda a day is linked to a 34 percent increased risk of metabolic syndrome. A 2012 study found that strokes and heart attacks occur more often in daily diet soda drinkers. Depression can also be a consequence of consuming too much of these artificially sweetened beverages.

Diet drinks may raise your risk of cancer. Animal studies show an increased risk for a variety of tumors, including lung cancer. A 2013 study published in the *Journal of Clinical Nutrition* found that men who drink more than two diet colas a day—aspartame-sweetened—have an increased risk of several types of blood cancers.

What's most important for you to remember? Soft drinks are not health drinks. Instead of popping open a soda—sugar-laden or "diet" and chemically laden—reach for a glass of delicious purified water. Water is life. Without it, we cannot live. One of the most important daily habits you can embrace for good health is drinking plenty of purified water. *Ayurveda* says that taking sips of hot water throughout the day is one of the more powerful ways to detoxify and rebalance your body. Give it a try and I'm sure that in a short time, you will be astounded by how you look and feel.

natural to your body. Not surprisingly, a variety of health problems, ranging from the minor to the serious, have been reported by people who have used artificial sweeteners. Saccharine was the only artificial sweetener available on the market through the 1970s. The FDA proposed a ban on this product after a study showed that saccharine caused bladder cancer in male rats. But congress put a moratorium on the ban and, instead, required a warning label on all saccharine-containing products. After several human clinical trials, researchers concluded that with normal usage, the risk posed by saccharine is small. So in 1991, the FDA withdrew their proposal to ban saccharine and President Clinton signed a bill into law in December 2000 removing the required warning label from saccharine products.

More recently, aspartame has become the artificial sweetener of choice. However, it has been reported to cause severe headaches and allergic symptoms and to exacerbate mood disorders such as depression in some people. Aspartame contains aspartic acid, phenylalanine, and methyl alcohol. Methyl alcohol is the chemical that breaks down into formaldehyde and diketopiperazine (DKP), a known carcinogen and neurotoxin. In 1997, eleven-year-old Jennifer Cohen conducted a science experiment in her sixth-grade class that was reported in *The Journal of the American Medical Association* (*JAMA*). Jennifer found that the aspartame present in Diet Coke breaks down into formaldehyde and DKP *at room temperature.*

In 1998, C. Trocho and a team of Spanish researchers found that formaldehyde derived from aspartame binds to DNA and appears to accumulate in tissue proteins and DNA. The problem with formaldehyde interacting with your cells, according to Japanese researchers U. Oyama, et al., in a study published in 2002 in the journal *Cell Biology and Toxicology,* is that it causes cell death and reduces glutathione, one of your body's most powerful natural antioxidants. Lower glutathione levels mean more damage from oxygen free radicals and, consequently, a higher risk of chronic disorders, including cancer. But so far, no clinical studies on humans link any serious health problems to aspartame.

In 1998, the FDA approved the artificial sweetener sucralose (Splenda), which is made by adding chlorine to sucrose. No independent long-term human studies have been done on this product, so we don't know whether it is safe. Before a company can bring an edible product to market, it must conduct "preapproval" research. According to the Sucralose Toxicity Information Center website, preapproval studies on sucralose were found to cause shrunken thymus glands and enlarged liver and kidneys in test animals. Despite this, sucralose is now used in numerous products, including baked goods, chewing gum, salad dressings, processed fruit and fruit juices, tea, and frozen dairy desserts. A case report in the journal *Headache* in September 2006 found that sucralose can be a trigger for migraine headaches.

From my point of view and that of *Ayurveda,* you should *favor substances made by Nature.* Your body was designed to consume and thrive on the natural plants growing on this planet, not on synthetic chemicals. If you have a choice—and you do—always choose the gifts of the Earth in their most natural form.

With all that bad news, I want to leave you with a bit of good news—sweet news! Chocolate lovers rejoice! Dark chocolate has been shown to have numerous health benefits—in small amounts. It does have some sugar and is high in calories, so you don't want to overdo it. Milk chocolate isn't a healthy choice—it has too much fat and sugar. The dark variety does not. In fact, research shows dark chocolate is high in antioxidants and other health-promoting properties that can lower your risk of heart disease, high blood pressure, and certain cancers. Eating dark chocolate can also cause your stress hormones to drop, your mood to elevate, and give a boost to your immune system. So it is okay to keep this guilty pleasure!

Chapter 17

Losing Your
Goddess-Like Figure
Obesity and Breast Cancer

K
eeping your body fat low reduces your risk of breast cancer as well as your risk of developing many other diseases. You can think of it this way: Your Warrior Goddess likes to keep the figure of an athlete, or at least a Goddess-like figure. It gives her the strength and power to fight off such killer beasts as breast cancer. When she carries too much weight, it slows her down and she can't ward off enemies. For instance, women who are obese—that is, have a body mass index (BMI) over 30—have a much higher risk of postmenopausal breast cancer: up to 400 percent higher! (See the section below on Defining Obesity to learn how to calculate your BMI.)

Weight increase and obesity have been identified as the most important risk and prognostic factors for breast cancer in postmenopausal women. Interestingly, however, this is not true for African-American women where there appears to be no link. The American Cancer Society estimates that there are 60,000 new cases of breast cancer each year in the United States that are linked to obesity. At least 40 percent of all postmenopausal breast cancers are thought to have obesity as a major contributing factor. A 2013 study in the *Journal of Epidemiology* reported a linear relationship between BMI and postmenopausal breast cancer risk. In other words, the more extra weight you carry, the higher your risk is. For a BMI ranging from 24 to 29, your risk is twice as high, and if your BMI is greater than 29 then your risk may be increased up to four times higher! For every 5 kilograms per meters squared (kg/m2) increase in BMI, the risk goes up by 12 percent. Central obesity, or those with larger waist measurements and waist-to-hip ratios, is also associated with an increased risk.

Believe it or not, weighing more at birth has been shown to be associated with an increased risk of breast cancer. Baby girls weighing more than 4,000 grams or 8.5 pounds have a small, but statistically higher risk. There are many health reasons to not gain excessive weight when you are pregnant. This is another. Gaining only the appropriate amount will help ensure that your child does not weigh too much at birth.

If you gain weight as an adult, your risk of breast cancer is higher than if you've been overweight all your life. Studies show that adult weight gain is associated with an increased risk of primarily estrogen and progesterone receptor-positive (ER+/PR+) breast cancers. In a 2010 study published in the journal *Breast Cancer Research and Treatment*, the women who had the highest weight gain compared to those with the lowest, had twice the incidence of ER+/PR+ breast cancers. Obesity is generally not associated with premenopausal breast cancer, except for those that are ER-/PR- or "triple negative." According to a study published in the *Journal of the American Medical Association* which evaluated data from the Nurses' Health Study (a study that followed 87,000 postmenopausal women for up to twenty-six years), a weight gain of just 2.0 kg (4.4 lbs) or more since the age of eighteen increased the risk of developing breast cancer by 15 percent after menopause, and the same weight gain or more after menopause increased the risk of developing breast cancer by 4.4 percent.

Being overweight at the time of diagnosis of breast cancer is fraught with far worse outcomes. Early stage breast cancers have a poorer prognosis. Overweight breast cancer patients have a higher incidence of recurrence and a 30 percent higher mortality rate. In a study published in December 2006, women who had been diagnosed with breast cancer were more likely to develop a second primary cancer (breast, ovarian, endometrial, or colorectal) within seven years if they had a higher body mass index or had adult weight gain. In addition, studies show that obese women with breast cancer are more likely to have advanced breast cancer at the time of their diagnosis and to die from the disease.

There are many other serious reasons why you should avoid gaining too much weight. An estimated 300,000 adults die in the United States each year from obesity-related causes, such as heart disease, high blood pressure, diabetes, and other types of cancer, including cancers of the esophagus, pancreas, colon and rectum, endometrium (lining of the uterus), kidney, thyroid, and gallbladder. That number grows every year.

One big reason why obesity is associated with an increased risk of breast cancer is because fat cells produce estrogen. If you look at the estrogen pathway again (Figure 3.1 on page 42), you'll see that estrogen isn't created just by the ovaries. It's also made by fat cells. After menopause, fat becomes the primary site where estrogen is manufactured in your body. So, the more excess fat you have, the more estrogen your body will produce.

For Those of You Who Like the Nitty-Gritty Details

There is an enzyme, called the aromatase enzyme, which is found principally in a primitive type of cell called "undifferentiated adipose (fat) fibroblasts"—not mature fat cells. Aromatase converts a hormone called androstenedione to a type of estrogen called estrone. Estrone can be converted by another enzyme to estradiol—the strongest and most abundant form of estrogen, and the type that is most associated with breast cancer.

When a breast cancer starts to grow, undifferentiated adipose fibroblasts circle the tumor. These fibroblasts "overexpress" the aromatase enzyme or, in other words, they make way too much of it. The excess aromatase greatly increases the production of estrogen, which then speeds up the growth of the tumor. Aromatase-inhibiting drugs, such as Arimidex, interfere with the production of estrogen from the fibroblasts. These drugs are far more effective against estrogen-positive postmenopausal breast cancers than estrogen-blocking drugs, such as Tamoxifen.

OBESITY, DIABETES, AND CANCER

Obesity is a major risk factor for type 2 diabetes—in fact, 80 percent of people with this disease are overweight. Type 2 diabetes is also a major risk factor for breast cancer. Both obesity and diabetes are associated with higher glucose, insulin, and IGF-1 levels, and other tumor-growth factors such as one that promotes blood vessel growth called vascular endothelial growth factor (VEGF). In Chapter 8, I described the very powerful influences that insulin and IGF-1 have on your risk of breast cancer. They both significantly increase your risk, and if you have the disease, they make your cancer grow faster.

Metformin

If you have diabetes, you probably are feeling some anxiety about your elevated risk. But, there may be something you can do to significantly lower your risk—right away. Researchers discovered that a drug used to treat type 2 diabetes—metformin—also has impressive antibreast cancer effects. In a meta-analysis review of eleven studies published in 2010, diabetic women taking metformin had a 31 percent reduction of breast cancer. The researchers also found a notably lower incidence of pancreatic and liver cancers in these women. If you are a diabetic taking this drug and are diagnosed with breast cancer, your likelihood of surviving is much better. For example, a 2012 study found that diabetic women on metformin, with more advanced stages of HER2/neu positive breast cancers, lived much longer than those not taking the drug. Metformin's ability to subdue breast cancer doesn't just come from its principal antidiabetic action of suppressing the genes that code for glucose production. It has many other ways that it specifically protects against breast cancer. For example, this drug directly curbs the growth of tumors, kills cancer cells, inhibits tumor cell proliferation and invasion (including those that are triple-negative), and reduces the formation of breast cancer stem cells. Metformin has also been found to make breast cancer cells more sensitive to the killing effects of chemotherapy and radiation. For all these reasons, if you have type 2 diabetes, taking metformin to reduce your risk and improve your outcomes of breast cancer is highly recommended.

Myth or Fact: Does Wearing a Bra Increase Your Risk?

Over a decade ago rumors began to spread that wearing a bra could increase your risk of breast cancer. However, the fact is that there are no well-designed peer-reviewed published studies that show a real link. The unpublished study that proclaimed the association is actually a perfect example of how a poorly designed study can draw conclusions that are inaccurate and lead to the spread of false information.

A study published in the *European Journal of Cancer* in 1991 found that premenopausal women who do not wear bras have half the risk of breast cancer compared to bra users, but the researchers stated that the statistics probably had nothing to do with the bras. Instead, the real explanation lies in the many differences between women who usually wear bras and those who don't that are known to have a huge impact on the risk of developing breast cancer. For example, women who don't wear bras are usually thinner and have smaller breasts, and research shows that both of these characteristics are associated with a significantly lower risk of breast cancer. Compared to obese women, thinner women also tend to be more active and more health conscious regarding their diet and lifestyle choices, which are additional factors that greatly lower the risk of breast cancer. Women who tend to wear bras usually have larger breasts and are more likely to be obese. Both large cup size and obesity are well-known risk factors for breast cancer. In

Active Belly Fat

Scientists have found that fat cells in the obese—particularly fat found in the belly—are "metabolically active." This means that fat cells make hormones— some of which influence the growth of tumors.

For example fat cells produce:

- Hormones called adipokines that can influence the growth of cancers. One of those hormones, called leptin, stimulates the growth of tumor cells and is much higher in those who are obese. Another, called adiponectin, is lower in obese individuals and has the opposite effect. It slows down tumor growth.

- A group of hormones called cytokines. One type of cytokine called IL-6 promotes chronic inflammation, which can fuel cancer.

- Other inflammatory- and oxygen free radical-promoting substances that help tumors in a variety of ways to grow faster, invade, and spread to other areas.

---

fact, in the above study, the women who wore bras and had the highest risk of postmenopausal breast cancer had the largest cup sizes and were obese. So obesity and cup size—not the bra—are the major risk factors.

Simply having more breast tissue—independent of obesity—places a woman at higher risk. A prospective study published in the *International Journal of Cancer* in April 2006 found that lean women with breast cup sizes "D" or larger were at a significantly increased risk for premenopausal breast cancer. Obesity is not the explanation for these women. Instead, it may be that they have higher estrogen levels—the female hormone responsible for breast development and directly associated with the growth of breast cancer. A 2012 study found that certain genetic variants that are associated with breast size also influence breast cancer risk. Therefore, genetics may play a role too. Research also shows that reducing the volume of breast tissue surgically— commonly done for women suffering from severe back and neck pain due to the excess weight of their breasts—drops the risk of breast cancer.

The only way that the influence of bras on breast cancer risk can be accurately determined is from a large, well-designed prospective study—a study that follows women into the future for ten to twenty years—and corrects for all the other known risk factors. This hasn't been done yet.

When it comes to lowering your risk of breast cancer, it's best to focus on those factors that research shows have a tremendous influence, rather than worrying about the potential risk of one factor that is yet unproven.

THE OBESITY EPIDEMIC

If you are obese, you're not alone. Recent studies have found the number of obese people in the United States is increasing at an alarming rate. The latest statistics currently available are from 2010 and show that 36 percent of adults in the United States are obese (defined as a BMI over 30). Just a decade ago, only 22.9 percent of us were obese. The number of overweight people in the United States increased from 55.9 to 66 percent over this same time period, and "extreme obesity"—defined as having a BMI greater than 40—rose from 2.9 percent to 4.7 percent.

Obesity is more common in Blacks and Hispanics. More than half of non-Hispanic Black women over age forty are obese, and 80 percent are overweight. Children are suffering from much higher rates of obesity, too. The number of overweight Black and Hispanic children has more than doubled over the past twelve years. For White children, the numbers have increased by 50 percent. In the past, it typically took thirty years for the number of overweight people in the United States to double.

Defining Obesity—Body Mass Index (BMI)

Researchers use very specific measures to define a body as being overweight or obese. The measures include the BMI or body mass index and the percentage of body fat (percent BF). Your BMI is traditionally calculated by dividing your weight in kilograms by your height in meters squared. It can also be calculated by dividing your weight in pounds by your height in inches. Then, that number is divided by your height in inches again, and the result is multiplied by 703. The National Heart, Lung, and Blood Institute has a BMI calculator on its website (http://nhlbisupport.com/bmi/bmicalc.htm), so you don't have to do the math yourself. If you don't know how to convert your weight and height to metric measurements, that's okay; this website can calculate your BMI using standard American measurements.

Ideally, your BMI should be in the range of 18.5 to 24.9. If your BMI is greater than 25, you're overweight. If it's greater than 30, you're considered obese. BMI, however, is not the best measure to determine if you're overweight or obese because it doesn't take body composition into account. Muscle weighs more than fat. For example, bodybuilders may weigh a lot for their height, but their above-normal weight is usually due to their large muscle mass, not excess fat. These toned athletes may have a BMI greater than 30, but they are certainly not obese.

To lengthen your life, shorten your meals.

—Proverb

Percent Body Fat

A better way to determine whether you are overweight, obese, or just "solid" is to measure your percent body fat (percent BF). This measurement is an assessment of your body composition. It evaluates how much of your weight is lean body mass (muscle, bones, and so on) and how much of it is actually fat. There are several different ways to get this measurement. The most accurate way involves completely submerging your body into a tank of water. This fairly expensive test measures the amount of water you displace in the tank and compares it to your height and weight. Fat is lighter than muscle. So pound for pound, fat takes up much more space than muscle. The more water you displace for your height and weight, the higher your percent of body fat.

Body fat can also be calculated by the method known as "bioelectrical impedance." This test is performed by passing a small, low-amp electrical current through your body and measuring the speed at which the current flows through you. Fat doesn't conduct electricity very well, but muscle does. So, the more fat tissue you have, the slower the current travels.

The simplest and least expensive way to measure percent body fat is to use a series of skin-fold measurements. However, calculating body fat using this technique has some limitations and is a lot less accurate than the other methods. The accuracy of this approach very much depends on the skill of the person doing the evaluation. Also, skin-fold measurements are unreliable for estimating the amount of body fat on people who are either extremely thin or very obese.

To calculate percent body fat using this technique, a caliper is used to measure the thickness of skin folds in several very specific areas of the body. The skin and the underlying fat are pinched into the caliper—a device that looks and feels a lot like a vice. Yes, sometimes it hurts a little. The thickness of each skin fold is read from the numbers on the caliper. After all the measurements are taken, they are added up and divided by the person's body weight. That number is then multiplied by a conversion factor to obtain the estimated percent body fat. Certified personal trainers are taught how to take these measurements as part of their certification training. Most gyms and fitness clubs have a personal trainer who can do these measurements for you. You can also make a rough approximation by yourself (see the inset "Calculating a Rough Estimate of Body Fat" on page 188).

Studies have shown that your BMI and percent BF are associated with your risk of breast cancer. A study from Sweden published in January 2003 in the *International Journal of Cancer* found that your percent BF has a higher associa-

Calculating a Rough Estimate of Body Fat

There's a quick way that you can get a rough estimate of your percent BF without using any fancy or expensive tests, and you can do it by yourself. It's not as accurate as the other techniques, but it will give you a ballpark figure. It involves a lot of simple measurements.

First, weigh yourself (in pounds) in the nude, and then multiply your total weight by 0.732. Take that number, and add 8.987. This number is your weight factor.

(your weight in pounds x 0.732) + 8.987 = weight factor

Then, measure your wrist in inches, and divide it by 3.140.
This number is your wrist factor.

wrist measurement in inches ÷ 3.140 = wrist factor

Next, measure your waist in inches at the navel, and multiply it by 0.157. This number is your waist factor.

waist measurement in inches x 0.157 = waist factor

Now, measure your hips, and multiply that number by 0.249.
This number is your hip factor.

hips measurement in inches x 0.249 = hip factor

Measure the distance around your forearm, and multiply it by 0.434. This is your forearm factor.

forearm measurement in inches x 0.434 = forearm factor

Now, to calculate:
1. Take your weight factor, and add your wrist factor.
2. From that number, subtract your waist factor.
3. Take that number, and subtract your hip factor.
4. To that number, add your forearm factor. This number is your lean body mass.

weight factor + wrist factor – waist factor – hip factor
+ forearm factor = lean body mass

Next, take your total weight and subtract your lean body mass to get your amount of fat in pounds.

weight in pounds – lean body mass = fat in pounds

Now, multiply your fat in pounds by 100, and divide by your total body weight. This number is your percent BF.

(fat in pounds x 100) / weight in pounds = percent BF

Adapted from *Dynamic Nutrition for Maximum Performance* by Daniel Gastelu and Dr. Fred Hatfield (Avery Publishing Group, 1997) with permission.

tion with your risk of breast cancer than your BMI does. The normal overall range for percent BF in nonathletic women is 16 to 32 percent; the desirable range is 18 to 28 percent.

TOXINS—NOT CALORIES

If you are active and you don't overeat, and yet you are still overweight, a slow metabolism may not be the only reason that weight stays on you. In an article published in the *Journal of Complementary and Alternative Medicine* in 2002, author Paula Baillie-Hamilton presented a new theory about the epidemic of obesity. She said that the amount of obesity that exists in the world today can't be explained by increased calories and sedentary lives alone. She contends that toxins in the environment and in the food you eat may play a significant role in disrupting your body's weight-control mechanisms.

Toxins block the intelligence of your body in many ways. The intelligence that manages weight control seems to be particularly vulnerable to toxins. Growth promoters and hormones are given to animals to fatten them up and increase the amount of milk they produce. When you eat these animals or drink their milk, you also consume the growth promoters. If these substances put weight on animals, you can be sure that they also put weight on humans.

In addition, a variety of synthetic pharmaceutical drugs, including certain antidepressants, anticonvulsants, antihistamines, nonsteroidal anti-inflammatories, antipsychotics, and hormones have been found to cause weight gain. Moreover, studies show that pesticides may cause abnormal weight gain; in fact, animals exposed to pesticides can have *huge* weight gains. In one study, despite no increase in their caloric intake, the body weight of the animals that were given pesticides doubled! Researchers cut the calories in half for other animals that were fed pesticides, and they still gained weight! Numerous studies have shown that animals exposed to environmental estrogens in utero have a higher incidence of reproductive problems and obesity later in life. Epidemiological studies support that exposure to these toxins while in the womb has the same effects in humans.

At low concentrations, all the chemicals listed below have been shown to powerfully promote weight gain.

- Carbamates (a type of insecticide)

- Heavy metals (such as cadmium and lead)

- Pesticides (organochlorines, DDT, lindane, endrin, and hexachlorobenzene)

- Plastics (phthalates and bisphenol A)

- Polybrominated biphenyls (used as a fire retardant)

- Polychlorinated biphenyls (PCBs)

- Solvents (octachorostyrene, decalin, benzene, toluene, 1,1,1-trichloroethane, and trichloroethylene benzene)

Avoiding Chemicals

The best ways to avoid these weight-promoting chemicals are to eat organically grown produce and to use nontoxic products in your home. Common sources of toxins in your home and their nontoxic alternatives are presented in Chapter 22. Eating organic foods and using only nontoxic products in your home are excellent ways to prevent excess quantities of toxins from getting *into* your body, but what about the toxins you already have in your body? Fortunately, there are ways to get most of them out.

The most effective way to cleanse your body of toxins is through *panchakarma*—a series of detoxification procedures unique to *Ayurveda*. The procedures, which are done in a medical spa-like setting, are gentle but powerful. Research shows that just one series of treatments can cut your toxin load in half. If you eat organic foods and go through *panchakarma* twice a year for about five days each time, the levels of toxins in your body will go so low that standard tests won't be able to detect them anymore. Chapter 23 goes into much more detail about this powerfully purifying and rejuvenating technique.

DOES LOSING WEIGHT HELP TO LOWER YOUR RISK?

Research shows that it definitely does. A 2013 study by researchers at the University of California, San Diego (UCSD), found that breast cancer survivors who lost more than 5 percent of their initial weight had changes in many factors that were favorable: estrogen, insulin, and leptin levels went down, and estrogen-binding proteins such as sex hormone-binding globulins (SHBG) went up. In another study published by University of California, Los Angeles (UCLA), researchers in 2012, breast ductal fluid showed a decrease of estradiol of 24 percent and IL-6 by 20 percent. They also noted that blood serum levels of leptin, estrone, estradiol, and IL-6 dropped.

If you are overweight or obese, it is very important to lose your extra weight so that you can lower your risk of all sorts of chronic diseases. Losing weight can also give you more energy and vitality, and increase your chances of living a long life. Most people find that they are able to lose weight more effectively and keep it off if they participate in a program like Weight Watchers. Enrolling your significant other, family, and friends to help you or to help each other is another great way to ensure your success.

Chapter 18

A Drink
Not to Drink

Alcohol: Thy Name Is Devil

Oh thou invisible spirit of wine,
if thou hast no name to be known by,
let us call thee devil.

—WILLIAM SHAKESPEARE,
OTHELLO, ACT II, SCENE III

*A*s Shakespeare said, alcohol has the potential for such ill effects on your physical, mental, and emotional health that it could appropriately be called a devil. Some doctors and scientists say that drinking a little alcohol is good for you—especially for your heart. But what they don't know, or aren't telling you, is that although a little bit of alcohol may be good for your heart, it's definitely *not* good for protecting yourself against breast cancer.

When it comes to your risk of breast cancer, alcohol truly *is* a devil. It has an alarming aptitude for unleashing this deadly beast. Just a small amount effectively blocks a great deal of your body's healing intelligence. Think of it this way: Alcohol is another substance that, for your Warrior Goddess, is like Kryptonite to Superman—one small drink is enough to strip her of her full power to defend. Numerous studies have found that even one drink a day increases your risk of breast cancer by as much as 11 percent. Two drinks of alcohol a day raise your risk by 22 to 40 percent. Three drinks a day adds to your risk by 33 to 70 percent. The bottom line is this: No alcohol is safe. As far as your heart health goes, a low-fat diet, high in fresh organic fruits and vegetables, regular aerobic exercise, and the daily practice of an effective stress-reducing meditation lowers your risk much more than a glass of wine ever will. And all these suggestions have only healthy side *benefits*.

THE MANY WAYS THAT ALCOHOL
FUELS BREAST CANCER

Researchers have found that alcohol increases the amount of estrogen in your blood. It also causes the release of the hormone prolactin. Like estrogen, prolactin speeds up cell division in the breast. For women who take hormone replacement therapy (HRT), alcohol is particularly dangerous. This hazardous mixture causes estrogen and prolactin levels to skyrocket. Because alcohol appears to exert its ill will predominately through the estrogen pathway, it is easy to understand why most studies have found that the cancers it endorses are estrogen positive.

Researchers at the Fred Hutchinson Research Center in Seattle, Washington, found that when it comes to allegiances, alcohol is the biggest supporter of hormone receptor-positive invasive lobular carcinoma over all others. In fact, they did not find a statistically significant association with the more common invasive ductal carcinoma. Other researchers, however, have found a link with the more common variety, including those involved with the National Institutes of Health's AARP (American Association of Retired Persons) Diet and Health Study. Regular consumption of alcohol is also associated with an increased risk of other cancers, including those found in the oral cavity, pharynx, esophagus, prostate, and colon.

A 2010 review study published in the journal *Evidence Report Technology Assessment* reported on all the possible causal mechanisms regarding alcohol and breast cancer that could be found in the medical literature. Alcohol consumption is associated with:

1. Increased estrogen and prolactin levels

2. Increased oxidative stress

3. Conversion of ethanol to acetaldehyde, which encourages tumor development

4. Direct stimulatory effects on the growth of tumors

5. Increased hormone receptor levels

6. Increased cell proliferation

7. DNA adduct formation

8. Increased cyclic adenosine monophosphate (camp)

9. Changed potassium channels

10. Modulation of gene expression

11. Increased degradation of folate

12. Increased inflammation

13. Tumor necrosis factor modulation

Not Completely Bleak

But, you say, "My doctor—the one that tells me what I like to hear, not you—said having a glass of wine or two a day is good for me!" Is your doctor wrong? Well, yes and no. Yes, research does show all the ill effects that I described above, but there's more to the story. Alcohol isn't all bad. Research actually shows that teetotalers have a higher risk of chronic diseases compared to those who have one or two servings of alcohol a day. In fact, in cultures known for extraordinary longevity, one habit they all have in common is that they drink alcohol—but not too much! When the effects of alcohol and chronic diseases are mapped out on a graph, it resembles the letter "J." The "J curve" illustrates the incidence of chronic disease in those who abstain, followed by the drop seen in those who consume one or two glasses a day. But, if an additional glass or two becomes routine, look out! The incidence of chronic disease zooms up.

Breast cancer, as you now know, is an exception—any alcohol increases the risk. But, a glass of alcohol a day—maybe even two—may not be as bad as originally thought. First, the 11 percent increased risk with one glass is actually a very small risk that in reality doesn't amount to much. Next, researchers have discovered that low folate levels seem to be the culprit for most of the breast cancer-promoting effects seen in one or two glasses. Women who have a healthy amount of folate in their bodies because they enjoy a glass of wine along with foods high in folate, such as citrus fruits, green leafy vegetables, dried beans, and peas, or who take supplemental folic acid (400 micrograms [mcg] a day)—*do not* have an increased risk of postmenopausal breast cancer.

What does all this mean? What researchers conclude is that it is absolutely fine for most women to have a glass of wine a day, but they must make sure their folate levels are adequate. More than a glass a day begins to increase your risk. So don't make a habit out of drinking more. Be careful not to overdo on the folic acid supplements. Remember what I said back in Chapter 12. Too much folic acid can increase your risk. So if you eat foods rich in folate and don't drink alcohol, you shouldn't take a folic acid supplement. If you drink a glass of alcohol every day, it's considered a good idea to take 400 mcg of folic acid a day.

GRAPES INSTEAD OF WINE

Because it contains alcohol, wine sides with the enemy. But research has shown that the sumptuous fruit that wine is made from—grapes—is a powerful ally to breast health. Grape skins contain a wonderful substance called "resveratrol," which displays a plethora of ingenious ways that it discourages the growth of cancer and promotes health and longevity. In 2013, there were over 300 published studies on this miraculous substance and the details of all the dozens of tactics it uses to prevent the inception of breast cancer cells and inhibit their growth. For one, resveratrol is an anti-inflammatory; it blocks the COX-2 enzyme. (The COX-2 enzyme and breast cancer are covered in Chapter 14.) For another, resveratrol is an antioxidant, and antioxidants prevent free-radical damage to DNA, damage that can lead to cancer. It prevents the transformation of breast cancer stem cells and normal breast cells into cancer cells; stops tumor cells from growing and dividing; decreases the production of the tumor growth factor IGF-1; kills tumor cells by apoptosis; stops new blood vessels from growing into tumors; and inhibits the aromatase enzyme, which is involved in the production of estrogen. Resveratrol prevents metastasis of tumors to other areas of the body, stops cells from sticking together, prevents them from invading into surrounding tissues, and decreases their ability to migrate.

If you have breast cancer and are being treated with radiation or chemotherapy, resveratrol has been found to assist both of these treatments with killing more tumor cells. Resveratrol helps several different types of chemotherapeutic drugs by making cancer cells more sensitive to them. For example, it acts synergistically with doxorubicin to kill both estrogen receptor-negative and estrogen receptor-positive tumor cells. Resveratrol doesn't just amp up the tumor-killing power of chemotherapy drugs and radiation, it also helps natural tumor killers, especially vitamin D_3. With all of these anticancer actions, resveratrol is able to suppress a wide variety of tumors, including lymphoid and myeloid cancers; multiple myeloma; cancers of the breast, prostate, colon stomach, pancreas, thyroid, cervix, and ovary; head and neck squamous cell carcinomas; and melanoma.

Don't be fooled into thinking that the only way you can get the health benefits of resveratrol is by drinking wine. Resveratrol and all its potent and protective medicine are also in a handful of the fresh, sweet organic grapes, fresh grape juice, and nonalcoholic wine. (See the Resource section for some nonalcoholic wine alternatives.) You can also take resveratrol in supplemental form. An area of controversy revolves around how effective these supplements are due to resveratrol's "bioavailability." Scientists have found that although resveratrol is absorbed well, it rapidly metabolizes in the body into breakdown products called metabolites. Within thirty to sixty minutes, resveratrol is converted into three or more different substances. These metabolites of resveratrol, according to French researchers in 2013, have anticancer effects too. In fact, when mixed together, the three metabolites boost the anticancer effectiveness of each other.

There have only been a few clinical trials done on humans using resveratrol supplements, but the results of all of them are encouraging. Clinical trials on patients with colorectal cancers found that oral doses of 0.5 to 1.0 grams reduced the rate of cell proliferation, caused apoptotic cell death, and sensitized colon cancer cells to anticancer drugs. In a 2010 study published in the journal *Cancer Research*, forty healthy volunteers taking resveratrol supplements of various strengths for twenty-nine days were found to have a significant decrease in circulating IGF-1. As you know, lower IGF-1 levels are associated with a decreased risk of cancer. The daily dose of resveratrol that was found to be most effective was 2.5 grams.

The seeds in grapes also possess many anticancer qualities. One class of phytochemicals in grape seeds, proanthocyanidins, has been found to have powerful antioxidant properties and a broad spectrum of protective benefits. For instance, a study conducted at Creighton University and published in 1999 found that grape seed proanthocyanidin extract (GSE) killed breast cancer cells, while enhancing the growth and viability of normal cells. According to Chinese researchers in 2009, GSE stops breast cancer cells from growing and dividing. Moreover, in 2003, researchers in California found that grape seed extract can decrease the amount of estrogen produced by the body by blocking the aromatase enzyme. A 2010 study published in the journal *Molecular Carcinogenesis* documented that GSE prevented precancerous cells exposed to environmental chemical carcinogens from becoming cancerous. It has also been shown to prevent angiogenesis or the growth of new blood vessels into tumors. Therefore, taking grape seed extract is another way to derive the benefits grapes have to offer.

Chapter 19

Sir Walter
Raleigh's Folly
Tobacco: Smoking and
Breast Cancer

*N*o one would argue with the fact that smoking is not good for your health. It's an extremely dangerous and costly habit. An article in the journal *Lancet Oncology* in 2009 reported more than 1 billion people currently smoke tobacco and its consumption is the leading cause of cancer worldwide. According to statistics by the American Heart Association, smoking-related illnesses kill an average of 442,398 Americans and cost the nation $157 billion each year. More than one in every five deaths is related to smoking.

With over 4,000 chemicals in cigarette smoke—250 of which are known to be harmful to human health—it is easy to understand why smoking is associated with many diseases. For years we have known that smoking is linked to cancers of the bladder, esophagus, larynx, lung, mouth, and throat; to chronic lung disease, such as bronchitis and emphysema; and to chronic heart disease and cardiovascular diseases, including strokes, high blood pressure, and poor circulation.

A report released by the Surgeon General in May 2004 revealed that smoking also causes a rash of other diseases: acute myeloid leukemia, abdominal aortic aneurysms, cataracts, periodontitis, pneumonia, and cancers of the cervix, kidney, pancreas, and stomach. There's also evidence that smoking may cause colorectal cancers, liver cancer, prostate cancer, and erectile dysfunction. This report said that smokers die an average of thirteen to fourteen years earlier than nonsmokers. It also estimates that smoking-related diseases have killed 12 million Americans in the last forty years, continue to kill about 440,000 each year, and cost the nation $75 billion annually to treat these diseases.

For years, it was unclear whether smoking increased the risk of breast cancer or not. Some studies found that it was difficult to separate the risk associated with cigarette smoking from the risk associated with alcohol consumption, because most smokers also drink alcohol, and, as you now know, alcohol is a significant risk factor for breast cancer. Despite some continued controversy on the link, many researchers have concluded from several well-designed studies that there is a clear and significant association between cigarette smoking and breast cancer.

For all these reasons, your Warrior Goddess despises cigarettes. If you smoke, please do everything you can to successfully stop. Tobacco clouds your Goddess's awareness, destroys her cosmic intelligence, and strips her of her remarkable ability to outsmart enemy diseases.

YOUNGER START—GREATER RISK

Smoking during the teenage years is particularly dangerous in terms of breast cancer risk. Since most smokers start as preteens or teenagers, the majority of those who smoke have a significantly elevated risk. A study from the National Cancer Institute (NCI) found that women who smoked cigarettes during their adolescence had a 50 percent increased risk of breast cancer. Many other studies confirm these findings, including a 2013 study from the American Cancer Society published in the *Journal of the National Cancer Institute*. Scientists believe that this may be because female breast cells generally don't mature until the first pregnancy (immature breast cells are more susceptible to damage from toxins). But smoking can be dangerous at any age. A German study published in 2002 in the journal *Cancer Epidemiology, Biomarkers & Prevention* found that women who smoked had a 50 percent increased risk of breast cancer. The risk for ex-smokers kept going down the longer that they abstained from smoking. But no matter how long it had been since they smoked, their risk was still 20 percent higher than nonsmokers.

These researchers also found that secondhand smoke increased the risk of breast cancer. They documented that women who inhaled passive smoke were 60 percent more likely to develop breast cancer than those who weren't exposed to it. The highest risk was in smokers who also inhaled passive smoke. In fact, scientists working for The Air Resource Board, a California agency, concluded in a 1,200-page report released in March 2005 that women exposed to second-hand smoke have a 68 to 120 percent greater risk of breast cancer! A review of secondhand smoke studies in 2008 noted that the risk of breast cancer from secondhand smoke is actually higher than the risk of developing lung cancer!

Another study published in *The Lancet* in 2002 found that very specific categories of smokers have a particularly high risk. For instance, an unusually high risk of breast cancer was found in women who had been pregnant and who had started smoking as teenagers within five years of starting their period. Women who had never had a baby and who smoked twenty cigarettes a day or more for more than twenty years also had a significantly increased risk.

Researchers at the University of Utah in 2008 found that women with certain genetic variations, called polymorphisms, involving the alpha-estrogen receptor and a tumor-promoting substance from the immune system, called IL-6, had up to a fourfold increase risk of breast cancer from secondhand smoke and a threefold increase from active smoking. Another genetic variation that has an influence on risk involves an enzyme which breaks down carcinogens, such as in cigarette smoke, called N-acetyltransferase 2. Variations are described as rapid, intermediate, slow, or very slow types. Many studies have shown that the slow and very slow types are the ones with the highest risk and are found in 50 to 60 percent of Caucasians.

One of the reasons smoking increases the risk of breast cancer is that cigarette smoke contains carcinogens. The International Agency for Research on Cancer states that twenty substances from cigarette smoke are known mammary carcinogens. A study from Albert Einstein University published in 2002 in the journal *Cancer Epidemiology, Biomarkers & Prevention* identified several key specific groups of carcinogens in cigarette smoke: polycyclic hydrocarbons, aromatic amines, and N-nitrosamines. These groups of heterocyclic amines are similar to those found in grilled red meat. Certain carcinogens, including these, don't become carcinogens until they are activated by enzymes—predominantly phase 1 liver enzymes—in your body. Breast tissue, like the liver, contains enzymes that can activate the carcinogens found in red meat and cigarette smoke. That means that carcinogens are formed locally in the breast tissue—exactly where they can do the most damage! All these groups of carcinogens can induce mammary tumors, and they have all been found in the breast tissue and breast milk of women who smoke. Researchers have also found the changes in DNA and genetic mutations that are associated with an increased risk of breast cancer in the breast cells of women who smoke.

TO HELP YOU QUIT

If you smoke cigarettes and have tried to quit, you know how hard it can be to break this habit. Of all the addictions you can have, cigarette smoking is one of the hardest to give up. In 2005, the U.S. Centers for Disease Control and Prevention reported there were 45.1 million adult smokers in the United States, 70 percent of whom said they wanted to quit. According to the American Cancer Society, only 5 to 10 percent of smokers are successful on any given attempt. Surveys find that for most people, it takes five to six tries to end their addiction for good. About 90 percent of smokers try going cold turkey without any help, which has a success rate of about 10 percent. For the 90 percent who can't quit smoking without help, there are a variety of approaches that can increase their success. These techniques include sessions with a behavioral therapist; nicotine replacement (gums, patches, etc.); certain pharmaceutical medications, such as Zyban and Chantix; and many types of alternative treatments, for example, acupuncture and hypnosis.

Research shows that the practice of Transcendental Meditation (TM) is extremely successful at breaking the addictive cycle and helping people to quit for good. In fact, of all the programs there are to help you stop smoking, the practice of TM is the most successful. People who practice this simple stress-reducing technique spontaneously quit smoking because they find their desire for cigarettes naturally decreases. Harvard-trained researchers David O'Connell, Ph.D., and Charles Alexander, Ph.D., wrote an excellent book, *Self Recovery: Treating Addictions using Transcendental Meditation and Maharishi Ayurveda*, that reports on all the research showing the impressive success that this mental technique has in overcoming addictions. You'll find out more about TM in Chapter 27.

Chapter 20

Fatally Flawed
Pharmaceuticals
Dangerous Medications

*P*harmaceutical drugs are fraught with side effects, some mild and some deadly. The number of reported in-hospital adverse drug reactions to prescribed medications is estimated to be about 2.2 million per year. About 783,000 people die each year in the United States alone from iatrogenic causes (that is, health problems inadvertently induced by healthcare workers, a medical treatment, or a diagnostic procedure). Of those deaths, about 106,000 are from side effects of a drug or combination of drugs.

One horrifying "side effect" of certain pharmaceutical medications is breast cancer. Until recently, little attention was given to the frightening increased risk of breast cancer associated with such medications as birth control pills, hormone replacement therapy (HRT), certain heart medications, various antidepressants, and many other pharmaceuticals. Each of these medications has specific ways that it increases your risk of breast cancer.

Most drugs are metabolized in the liver, and scientists have found that they may interfere with the liver's ability to detoxify carcinogens. When your liver function is impaired, more carcinogens remain in your body, and thereby increase your risk of many different cancers, including breast cancer. That's why your Warrior Goddess prefers that you supply her with foods, herbs, and other natural approaches, rather than pharmaceuticals whenever possible.

"THE PILL"

In a laboratory study published in 1987 in the journal *Cancer,* researchers found that the combination of estrogen and progestin (found in many birth control pills) stimulates breast cells to grow and divide and accelerates the growth of breast cancer. In another study, published more than twenty years ago in the *Journal of Reproductive Medicine,* premenopausal women who used the pill after age forty were found to have a 50 percent increased risk of breast cancer. More recent studies show that women who have a mother or sister with breast cancer and take the pill long-term also have a significantly increased risk of breast cancer.

A 2006 study published in the *Mayo Clinic Proceedings* found that oral contraceptives increased the risk for premenopausal breast cancer. In a meta-analysis reviewing data from thirty-four studies, the risk of breast cancer was found to be highest for women who used oral contraceptives for four years of more before their first pregnancy. A Swedish study published in 2005 found that for each year a woman with the BRCA1/2 mutations took oral contraceptives before age twenty, there was a significant increase in the risk of early-onset breast cancer. In another study published in 2012, which reviewed thirteen prospective cohort studies, the risk of breast cancer was found to increase by 14 percent for every ten years of oral contraceptive use. In other words, if a woman took the pill for ten years, her risk was 14 percent higher. If she took the pill for twenty years, her risk was 28 percent higher.

A study published by the Fred Hutchinson Cancer Research Center in 2009 found that triple-negative breast cancer—a breast cancer subtype that is more aggressive with a worse prognosis—is much higher in younger women with a history of oral contraceptive use. The risk for those taking the pill for one year or more was 2.5 times higher. Women under forty with a long-term history of taking the pill had a 4.2 times higher risk of developing triple-negative breast cancer. Results from a study involving African-American women called the Black Women's Health Study were published in 2010 showing that the incidence of estrogen receptor-negative cancer was 65 percent greater in women who had ever used oral contraceptives. The risk was even greater for women who had used the pill within the previous five years or who had taken it more than ten years.

HORMONE REPLACEMENT THERAPY (HRT)

To combat perimenopausal and menopausal symptoms, Western medicine developed synthetic hormones. Drug companies promoted hormone replacement therapy (HRT) as the long-sought-after fountain of youth. HRT, women were told, lowered the risk of heart disease, strokes, Alzheimer's disease, and osteoporosis. But in 2002, the landmark prospective Women's Health Initiative Study, found that the opposite is true: Women taking HRT have an increased risk of heart disease, strokes, blood clots, gallbladder disease, and invasive breast cancer. It is true that HRT does help to prevent osteoporosis, but not any more so than a little weight-bearing exercise and a diet high in calcium-rich foods.

Pharmaceutical companies, as well as many doctors, still downplay the level of risk associated with these synthetic hormones. But research published in the

August 2003 issue of the prestigious journal *The Lancet* found that the risk was considerable. One-quarter of all the women between the ages of fifty and sixty-four in Britain—1 million women—were followed from 1996 until 2002. Those women who took HRT had a 66 percent increased incidence of breast cancer and a 22 percent greater risk of dying from it. Those women who took a combination of estrogen and progestin had a 100 percent higher risk of breast cancer than those women who never took hormones. The women who took estrogen alone had a 30 percent higher risk. And the longer the women took these hormones, the higher their risk became.

Of the women who developed breast cancer, those who had taken hormones had more aggressive tumors than those who had never taken them. Aggressive tumors are very dangerous because they're more likely to spread throughout the body and cause early death. The researchers of this landmark study in England estimated that HRT was responsible for 20,000 cases of breast cancer over the ten-year period from 1992 to 2002.

Several other studies have also found a significant connection between HRT and breast cancer. For instance, the Nurses' Health Study, a large epidemiological study, followed 58,520 women who took HRT from age fifty to sixty. When these women reached the age of seventy, they were found to have a 23 percent higher risk of breast cancer. However, the women who took estrogen plus progestin had a much higher risk of breast cancer—67 percent. Another study published in *JAMA* in 2002 found that long-term users of HRT who took either estrogen alone or estrogen with progestin had a 60 to 85 percent increased incidence of breast cancer.

Researchers have also discovered that HRT causes an unusual type of breast cancer called "invasive lobular carcinoma." The majority of all breast cancers start in the breast ducts. They are called "ductal carcinomas." Lobular carcinoma originates in the terminal lobules or milk glands. A study published in 2003 in *JAMA* found that women who took a combination of estrogen and progestin had a 50 percent higher risk of lobular carcinoma. They also noted that the overall incidence in the United States of this far less common type of breast cancer increased from 9.5 percent in 1987 to 15.6 percent in 1999. HRT is thought to be the primary cause of this alarming escalation. Data was analyzed from the prospective cohort study, the Nurses' Health Study, from 1978 to 2002 to assess the risk of breast cancer with different types of hormonal therapies. The results, which were published in the *Archives of Internal Medicine* on July 24, 2006, showed that women who took hormone pills composed of a combination of estrogen and testosterone (Estratest) had a 250 percent higher risk of developing breast cancer than women who never took hormones.

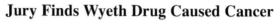

Jury Finds Wyeth Drug Caused Cancer
From *Bloomberg News,* January 30, 2007

Wyeth's Prempro menopause pill helped to cause an Arkansas woman's breast cancer, and she deserves $1.5 million in damages, jurors found Monday in the company's second trial loss over its hormone replacement drugs.

A state court jury in Philadelphia deliberated about nine hours over two days before finding that Wyeth's conduct was "malicious, wanton, willful, or oppressive," allowing plaintiff Mary Daniel to seek punitive damages. The jury will return today to consider awarding further damages.

The lawsuit is one of about 5,000 against Madison, N.J.-based Wyeth over its hormone replacement drugs, including Prempro and Premarin. Daniel was among as many as 6 million women who took the pills before a 2002 study highlighted links to cancer. Daniel, 60, took Prempro for about 16 months starting in December 1999. She was diagnosed with breast cancer in July 2001.

The jurors found that Prempro was a "factual cause" of Daniel's cancer. The panel also agreed that Wyeth failed to provide proper warnings about Prempro's cancer risk.

Wyeth lawyer Peter Grossi said the company would ask Philadelphia Common Pleas Court Judge Myrna Field to throw out the award.

Taking HRT substantially increases the risk of ovarian cancer, too. Ovarian cancer is a relatively uncommon cancer. The average woman has only a 1.7 percent chance of developing this disease over her lifetime, whereas the risk of breast cancer for the average woman is 13.3 percent. In a 2002 study published by the National Cancer Institute (NCI), women who took HRT for ten to nineteen years had an 80 percent increased risk of ovarian cancer.

Millions of women in the United States have been prescribed HRT. It was one of the top pharmaceuticals sold for many years. In 2002, an estimated 8 million women in the United States were on some form of HRT. With this extensive use, you'd think that this pharmaceutical product would have been thoroughly studied, both before it was put on the market and afterward. But a well-designed study wasn't conducted on HRT until forty years after it was put on the market! As of 2012, more than 5,000 lawsuits have been filed against Wyeth for Prempro and Premarin. (See the article above from the January 30, 2007 *Los Angeles Times* regarding the lawsuits.)

I'm not sure why the long-term health effects of HRT weren't investigated decades earlier. This tragic oversight is estimated to have caused thousands of cases of breast cancer. In other words, thousands of women were brutalized by breast cancer and had their lives cut short by it because they unknowingly took a medication that significantly increased their risk of breast cancer. With the new awareness of the dangers of HRT in 2002, doctors stopped prescribing it to their patients—the following year the incidence of breast cancer dropped by 7 percent. Researchers believe there is good data supporting a direct association with decreasing HRT use and the decline in breast cancer incidence.

Nature's Perfect Design

Prescribing hormones for menopausal symptoms is a perfect example of how the Western paradigm of health care can be so off the mark sometimes, that the consequences can be catastrophic. We seem to forget that Nature designed human beings perfectly. We can't outsmart Nature no matter how hard we try. We shouldn't try to *overpower* it, but rather *work with it*. Menopause, for example, isn't a disease or a condition that needs to be treated or controlled. The hormonal changes that women go through are perfect by design. They are part of the natural progression of life. Symptoms arise from imbalances caused by poor choices in diet and lifestyle. Restoring balance naturally is the solution; suppressing the symptoms of imbalances with supplemental hormones is not.

BIO-IDENTICAL HORMONES

Because of the health concerns with HRT, many women are now turning to bio-identical hormones. But these hormones aren't natural either and may not be safe. Although they are chemically similar to the hormones made by our body, we weren't designed by nature to take additional external hormones. A few early studies report that the side effects of compounded hormones are much less than synthetic HRT. However, no long-term prospective studies have been done. Remember, it took decades before prospective studies showed the dangers of HRT. So the truth is, we don't know how safe they are because the studies have not been done. There has been quite a bit of research that causes some concern about raising the level of various hormones, including estrogen, progesterone, and especially androgens such as testosterone.

Progesterone

There are no long-term studies showing that natural progesterone is safe and there are reasons to be concerned. Studies show that women who took HRT with progestin had a 100 percent increased incidence of breast cancer. We don't know if natural progesterone has the same effect, but it very well may. Many women develop breast cancers that are both estrogen and progesterone receptor-positive. That means that estrogen *and* progesterone will accelerate the growth of the tumor. I first became quite concerned about the possible risks of "natural" progesterone when I saw a case presentation at a medical conference of a woman who had normal breasts, started using progesterone cream, and then rapidly developed significant changes in her breasts consistent with hormonal abnormalities that put her at increased risk for breast cancer.

Researchers at the University of Porto in Portugal found that when breast cancer cells are exposed to progesterone, they produce a hormone called platelet-derived growth factor A (PDGF-A), a protein known to stimulate cell growth and division. PDGF-A stimulates angiogenesis or the development of new blood vessels, which are crucial for tumor growth and also help tumor cells to spread to other areas of the body. Polish researchers have done extensive studying on the effects of progesterone on the growth of breast cancer. In several studies they report that progesterone causes the production of various growth factors for cancer. Specifically, they noted that progesterone increased three hormones known to accelerate the growth of hormonally responsive estrogen receptor-positive (ER+) and progesterone receptor-positive (PR+) breast cancers: growth hormone (GH), insulin-like growth factor-1 (IGF-1), and prolactin. In 2011, scientists from Albany, New York, reported on the very complex response of breast tissue to progesterone involving activation of genes and factors that result in proliferation and dedifferentiation (a process that causes cells to revert to a potentially cancerous unspecialized form). In other words, progesterone encouraged cells to turn cancerous and fueled their growth.

Based on a gene panel performed on breast tumors called PAM50, there are four recognized types of breast cancer: luminal A and B, basal-like, and HER2/neu enriched—each with different a prognosis. Luminal A is the easiest to treat and has the best outcomes. Progesterone has been found to increase the risk of developing the more difficult-to-treat invasive basal-like type.

Further supporting the growth-stimulating influence of progesterone on ER+/PR+ tumors are several European studies documenting that the growth of these tumors was slightly more inhibited by progesterone-blocking drugs compared to the estrogen-blocker Tamoxifen.

Testosterone

"Bio-identical" testosterone is routinely recommended to help increase a woman's libido. Yet, studies consistently find a positive association between circulating testosterone levels and the risk of breast cancer. Italian researchers investigated the role of androgens (testosterone, androstenedione, and dehydroepiandrosterone sulfate [DHEA]) in premenopausal breast cancer by checking for these hormone levels in breast cancer patients and comparing them to healthy women. Women with the highest serum levels of testosterone compared to those with the lowest had 3.4 times the incidence of breast cancer. A Harvard Medical School study found a strong association between ER+/PR+ cancers and serum levels of both estrogen and androgens. Specifically, the risk for those with the highest quartile of circulating hormones was 3.3 times higher for estradiol, 2 times higher for testosterone, 2.5 times higher for androstenedione, and 2.3 times higher for DHEA.

These studies certainly raise concerns about the safety of elevating testosterone levels in perimenopausal and menopausal women. Because higher testosterone levels are associated with a significantly higher risk of breast cancer, supplemental testosterone should be administered with extreme caution.

The only way to know if taking supplemental hormones, such as progesterone, is appropriate for you is to have your levels checked by a physician. If your estrogen is high and progesterone is very low, for example, then progesterone may be beneficial for you. If however, your progesterone levels are normal or even high, then you shouldn't take them. The decision to take hormones of any kind should not be taken lightly and requires strict monitoring by a

Antibiotics and Breast Cancer?

A study published in the February 2004 issue of *The Journal of the American Medical Association* (JAMA) found a possible link between frequent use of antibiotics and an increased risk of breast cancer. However, because of the way the study was designed, it's impossible to determine if antibiotics really were the culprits. Infectious diseases that require treatment with antibiotics can also cause chronic inflammation, increase free-radical production, and depress the immune system—all three of which are known to promote breast cancer. It may be that the true source of the increased risk has everything to do with these well-known cancer-encouraging conditions and nothing to do with the antibiotics. Although this issue obviously requires further study, designing clinical human trials with antibiotics poses difficulties. To flush out whether antibiotics are the source of the increased risk and not the infections they are used to treat, healthy people would have to be given antibiotics. Because antibiotics pose other known health risks, a study like that would probably never be approved. I recommend taking antibiotics only when absolutely necessary and avoiding them whenever possible.

physician. My personal opinion is that it is always best to try to balance your hormones naturally. Only if natural approaches fail to achieve balance and alleviate your symptoms, and under the care of a physician, should you consider taking hormones. Taking estrogen long-term in any form (except plant estrogens that are actually more like estrogen blockers), especially if it is combined with progestin, has been shown to increase the risk of breast cancer, ovarian cancer, heart disease, strokes, and gall bladder disease.

If you suffer from menopausal symptoms and are looking for relief, or if you want to stop taking hormones, there are many safe and effective natural approaches you can take. Helping you to transition through menopause naturally is beyond the scope of this book, but there are several good books that I recommend. Dr. Nancy Lonsdorf, M.D., wrote an excellent book on the Ayurvedic approach to menopause called *The Ageless Woman: Natural Health and Beauty after Forty with Maharishi Ayurveda*. Two other outstanding books are *The Wisdom of Menopause*, by Christiane Northrup, M.D., and *Dr. Susan Love's Hormone Book*, by Susan Love, M.D.

ANTIDEPRESSANT AND HEART MEDICATIONS

Other types of pharmaceutical medications have been found to increase the risk of breast cancer, too—specifically, two groups of heart medications called "beta blockers" and "calcium-channel blockers" and several psychiatric medications. Each drug may have a number of different physiological interactions that contribute to this calamitous "side effect," but researchers think their influence on melatonin may be one of the biggest factors. Melatonin is an important hormone produced by your body that, research shows, provides powerful protection against breast cancer. People who take these medications have much lower levels of this extraordinary natural cancer-fighting hormone. (For more information on melatonin, see Chapter 24.)

A class of antidepressants called "tricyclic antidepressants"—for example, imipramine (Tofranil) and clomipramine (Anafranil)—provoke the initiation of breast cancer by triggering mutations in your genes. These mutations can lead to breast cancer as long as eleven to fifteen years after taking the drug. According to a Canadian study published in 2002 in the *British Journal of Cancer,* the risk of breast cancer for people who have a long history of taking these genotoxic medications is more than doubled. Even more alarming, another Canadian study published in 2000 in the *American Journal of Epidemiology* found that the risk of breast cancer doubled after only two years on tricyclic medication. The tricyclic antidepressant amitriptyline (Elavil) and the non-tricyclic agent fluoxetine (Prozac) were found by researchers at the University of Manitoba to stimulate the growth of breast cancer by another mechanism—binding to growth receptors. A review study published in *The British Journal of Cancer* in April 2006 found, however, that the results of their and other studies do not show an increased risk of breast cancer with antidepressants.

A Harvard Medical School study published in 2011 reviewed sixty-one studies that assessed the relationship of antidepressants and the risk of breast and ovarian cancers. They reported that 33 percent of the studies found an elevated risk and 67 percent of the studies did not. Of note was that the studies that had funding by the pharmaceutical industry were more likely to find no association. Their conclusion was that epidemiological studies suggest that there may be a modest increase in the risk of breast and ovarian cancers with the use of antidepressants, especially the popular selective serotonin reuptake inhibitors (SSRIs). At low doses, it is possible that antidepressants could increase the risk or exacerbate cancer growth in women in early stages of breast and ovarian cancer. Large prospective cohort studies need to be done to determine what the specific risks may or may not be. Clinicians prescribing antidepressants for women should carefully select which medications may be best to use, especially in women with a higher risk of breast cancer.

Natural Approaches to Relieving Depression

Fortunately, there are many alternatives to antidepressant medications that, research shows, may be just as effective. Antidepressants work by altering chemicals in your brain. These brain chemicals can also be positively influenced by many natural, nonpharmaceutical approaches. For instance, several studies have documented that regular exercise combats depression as well as many commonly prescribed pharmaceutical antidepressants. Researchers have also found that yoga, certain types of meditation, acupuncture, music therapy, and *panchakarma* all effectively relieve depression.

A variety of herbs and supplements are very beneficial for improving this common condition: omega-3 fatty acids, B vitamins, S-adenosylmethionine (SAM-e), tyrosine, DL-phenylalanine, 5-hydroxytryptophan (5-HTP), and the herbs St. John's wort and holy basil. Eating a diet high in fresh organic fruits, vegetables, and whole grains, and avoiding sugar, refined carbohydrates, caffeine, and alcohol can stabilize and lift your mood. Supplying your body with the right nutrients and avoiding the wrong ones brings balance to both your body and your mind.

If you suffer from depression, work with your doctor if you decide to try any of these natural approaches. You may find that you need less medication or a different, less harmful medication. You may even discover that some of these natural techniques work so effectively for you that you no longer require any medication at all. A warning, however: Don't go off your medication without your doctor's consent and don't take any of these supplements without getting your doctor's approval. Toxic side effects may occur if you take an herb such as St. John's wort with an antidepressant drug such as Prozac. Depression is a very dangerous condition, so be sure to work carefully with your doctor.

BE AWARE, ASK QUESTIONS

Pharmaceutical medications have their place in restoring health when necessary, but be aware that many prescription drugs, especially when taken long-term, may have serious side effects. Take the time to find out the possible side effects of your medications. Make sure that *if* you have a choice in the medications you take, you choose the one with the lowest risks.

For virtually any chronic condition, there are usually safe, natural alternative approaches that can be very effective. With the resurgence of *Ayurveda,* we have regained a wealth of knowledge about how to detect, prevent, treat, reverse, and even cure chronic disease conditions. Built on a different and highly effective paradigm of health care, *Ayurveda* teaches you how to achieve an extraordinary state of health. This ancient system holds tremendous knowledge about the normal rhythms and processes of life—what strips you of your health and what helps to enhance it and keep you well. If symptoms arise, for example, during menopause, *Ayurveda* teaches that they are due to imbalances from improper diet or from a lifestyle that works against the laws of Nature. By simply making better diet and lifestyle choices, balance is gently restored and symptoms can be alleviated.

Sometimes it's necessary to take pharmaceutical medications. But you should also make every effort to restore balance to your body at the same time by stopping those things that helped to initiate and aggravate your condition and by starting those things that will help to protect and promote your health.

*You can mop up the water on the floor, but unless you
turn off the faucet, you'll never get the floor dry.*
—AUTHOR UNKNOWN

If you take on healthy habits and stop the unhealthy ones that are contributing to your illness, the number and dose of medications you require may drop significantly, even to the point where you can stop taking them. Reversals and cures of chronic conditions are often possible. Remember, however, always work with your doctor when adjusting your medications.

Chapter 21

Portrait of an Assassin
Pesticides and Other Hidden Toxins

*P*icture an assassin. His task depends on his ability to make himself invisible and remain undetected until the last possible moment. He studies his targets to find their weaknesses. As he silently positions himself for the kill, his victims don't have even the slightest hint of what's to come. He patiently waits for just the right moment. The instant his target becomes vulnerable, he strikes.

This portrait of an assassin describes the behavior of all the toxins in your environment. These toxins are in your food and water, your home and work-place, and the products you use. You aren't aware of them, but they are there, hidden in the shadows. They find a weakness in your body and start their infil-tration. When your body becomes vulnerable due to stress, fatigue, or an emo-tional crisis, they move in for the kill.

Unfortunately, we all live in an extremely toxic world that's teeming with assassins. Fortunately, there are many ways to avoid toxins, reduce your expo-sure to them, and drive them out of your home and body.

THE CHEMICAL REVOLUTION

Chemical manufacturing began in the early 1900s, mostly with good intentions. (Remember that old expression, "The road to hell is paved with good inten-tions"?) The chemists thought that they were helping to make the world a bet-ter and safer place and that these chemicals would make our lives easier. For instance, some chemicals were developed to improve the efficiency of large-scale manufacturing plants to increase the productive output. Some chemicals were intended to increase crop production; others were created to help protect us from disease-carrying insects and pests. But what the chemists didn't know was that many of these chemicals would turn out to be extremely dangerous to our health and the environment.

A good example of a dangerous chemical created with good intentions is dichlorodiphenyltrichloroethane (DDT). This chemical, along with thousands of others, doesn't break down easily and, therefore, persists in our environment. The chemical architects didn't realize that their creations would contribute to the toxic soup overtaking our planet. They didn't know they were helping to turn Earth into a place where people, even in the most remote areas of the world, would suffer from the fallout of these toxins.

There are now toxins *everywhere*—in or over every square inch of this planet: in our water, air, soil, food, clothes, furnishings, dry cleaning, personal-care products, and cleaning products. Many of these toxins have been linked to a variety of health problems, including cancer. But the chemical assault doesn't stop there. There are also toxins in lawn and garden products, insect repellants, flea collars, paints, wallpaper, joint compound, sealers, insulation, carpet, tile, cabinets, woodwork, and, of course, home pesticides. There's not a baby born anywhere in America who doesn't have synthetic toxic chemicals in his or her body. As Bill Moyers discovered while creating his PBS documentary *Trade Secrets*, which aired on March 26, 2001, the average adult—including himself—has hundreds of different synthetic chemicals in his or her blood and fat. In December 2009, the Centers for Disease Control and Prevention issued their *Fourth National Report on Human Exposure to Environmental Chemicals* and concluded that Americans of all ages have at least 148 chemicals in their bodies—some of which have been banned for decades.

Our homes, structures originally designed to provide shelter from storms and beasts, have now *become* the storms and beasts. The air in the average American home is *four times* more polluted than the air outdoors!

The number of chemical assassins in our world is overwhelming. Why? Largely because our government does a very poor job of regulating their safety. Over 100,000 chemicals were registered in 2011 for commercial use in the world. Eighty-four thousand are registered with the Environmental Protection Agency (EPA), and only a small percentage of them have been tested for safety. The government leaves the question of a chemical's safety up to the company that manufactured it. The EPA allows any new chemical to go on the market as long as the manufacturer "thinks" it's safe. Its safety may be questioned only after the chemical is linked to serious health problems or significant damage to the environment and wildlife. Usually, a huge public outcry is required before any serious testing is done. Many animals or people must die or be seriously injured before a chemical is pulled from the market.

Of the chemicals that the EPA has tested, many have been found to be carcinogens or suspected carcinogens. Some can disrupt your endocrine system, which is made up of the glands that produce hormones, such as estrogen. Some endocrine disrupters mimic the estrogen molecule. They are called "chemical estrogens," or "xenoestrogens." Not surprisingly, they have been directly linked to causing and accelerating the growth of breast cancer.

Many other chemicals are toxic in other ways. They damage your nervous, reproductive, or immune system. Although they may not be carcinogens, they can weaken your body and make it more susceptible to cancer development and growth. Despite knowing this, many Americans use these chemicals anyway for convenience sake.

A study published in the journal *Cancer* in 2007 reviewed all the animal studies in the medical literature that tested chemicals for their potential for causing mammary cancer. In all, 216 chemicals were identified. They included industrial chemicals, chlorinated solvents, products of combustion, pesticides, dyes, radiation, drinking water disinfection byproducts, pharmaceuticals, hormones, and research chemicals. Almost all of these chemicals caused cancer in other organs, too.

Organochlorines, as well as most other pesticides and chemicals, are concentrated and stored in the body fat of the animals you eat. Not surprisingly, poultry, beef, pork, fish and other seafood, dairy, and animal-derived oils have the highest concentrations of pesticides. But don't be fooled into thinking that the amount of pesticides on fruits and vegetables is small. A sample of conventionally grown celery was found to have *seventeen* different pesticide residues, ten of which were carcinogenic. The average apple may have the residue of as many as five to ten carcinogenic pesticides! This is another reason why it's so important to eat organically grown produce.

RESEARCH FROM AROUND THE WORLD

Whether or not chemical estrogens, or xenoestrogens, can initiate and promote breast cancer has been hotly debated for years. Some studies have found a link; others haven't. Based on the most recent research, however, there is little doubt that xenoestrogens do contribute to promoting breast cancer.

Israel

During the 1970s, Israeli women, particularly young women, were found to have a much higher incidence of breast cancer than women in other countries. Given all the known risk factors at the time, their rate of breast cancer was twice as high as would be expected. In the search to find out why, it was discovered that the milk from cows raised in Israel had some of the highest pesticide levels in the world. Pesticides, such as DDT (for more information, see the section

Weed Killer Could Kill You on page 59) and benzene hexachloride (BHC), were found to be 5 to 100 times greater in concentration in cow's milk from Israel than in milk from the United States.

The Israeli women were also found to have high levels of insecticides in their breast milk. In 1978 there was a public outcry. The government responded by banning BHC and DDT. The levels of these pesticides in cow's milk began to decline rapidly. By 1980, they had dropped 98 percent. The incidence of breast cancer in young women dropped significantly, too. Within a few short years, the number of premenopausal women diagnosed with breast cancer fell 30 percent.

Denmark

Several studies from Denmark show a very strong *direct* correlation between estrogen-mimicking pesticides and breast cancer. In a study published in the journal *Cancer Causes and Control* in 2000, researchers found that Danish women with high serum concentrations of the organochlorine DDT had a 300 percent increased risk of breast cancer. The higher the concentrations of DDT that were found in the women, the higher their incidence of breast cancer was. The researchers also found that another toxin, polychlorinated biphenyls (PCBs; for more information, see the inset "What Are PCBs?" on page 84), significantly raised the risk of breast cancer, too.

A second Danish study published in 2000 in the *Journal of Clinical Epidemiology* found that another type of organochlorine called "dieldrin" also significantly increased the risk of breast cancer. The study found that as the concentration of this pesticide increased in women, so did their incidence of breast cancer. The women with the highest levels of dieldrin had twice the risk.

A third study from Denmark published in the *Journal of Clinical Epidemiology* in 2000 measured the concentration of this same organochlorine, dieldrin, in the blood of breast cancer patients and compared it to their survival rate. Researchers found a direct correlation: The higher the level of dieldrin in the blood, the worse the chances were of the patient's surviving. Their conclusion was that dieldrin raises the risk of breast cancer and lowers the chance of surviving the disease.

Germany

In 1998, a German study published in the *Journal of Steroid Biochemistry & Molecular Biology* found that organochlorine pesticides (DDT and hexachlorobenzine [HCB]) and PCBs are associated with an increased risk of breast cancer. In the study, the German women with breast cancer had higher levels of DDT and PCBs in their breast tissue. DDT was found in concentrations an average of 62 percent higher than those found in the women without breast cancer. PCBs were found to be 25 percent higher in the breast cancer patients.

DDT DETOX

A 2001 study from Westchester Medical Center in New York presented various ways in which you can lower the amounts and effects of organochlorines, such as DDT, in your body. Here are their recommendations:

1. **Eat phytoestrogen-rich food, such as soy.** The phytoestrogens found in plants such as soybeans compete with organochlorines for estrogen receptors. They can actually block the pesticides from attaching to estrogen receptors.

2. **Eat the spice turmeric.** Turmeric can inhibit the estrogenic effect of pesticides. It also has a synergistic effect with phytoestrogens. It increases the power of phytoestrogens to block pesticides from attaching to estrogen receptors.

3. **Eat cruciferous vegetables.** Estrogenic pesticides cause the production of more of the "bad" type of estrogen. The phytochemical found in cruciferous vegetables, indole-3-carbinol, reverses that effect by stimulating the production of more of the "good" kind of estrogen.

Breastfeeding Concerns

When a woman breastfeeds, pesticides are flushed out of the breast tissue, thereby significantly lowering the pesticide levels in her breasts. While it's true that the breastfeeding baby ingests these pesticides, research clearly shows that the protective benefits of breastfeeding far outweigh any negative effects on the baby's health. In fact, women who were breastfed as infants have a significantly lower risk of breast cancer than their formula-fed counterparts.

You can limit the amount of toxins your future baby will ingest by taking some precautions. For starters, *Ayurveda* recommends going through the purification procedure *panchakarma* before you get pregnant. (*Panchakarma* is discussed in detail in Chapter 23.) If you are unable to go to a *panchakarma* clinic, you can follow a modified detoxification program at home. Although you may not get the full benefit of *panchakarma* by taking this route, any toxins you manage to clear from your body will be beneficial.

Whether or not you choose to detoxify before you conceive, you can help to reduce your baby's exposure to pesticides by eating only organically produced foods and using only nontoxic products before, during, and after pregnancy.

4. **Keep your body weight down.** Since pesticides accumulate in body fat, the less body fat you have, the fewer pesticides your body can store.

5. **Low-fat and reduced-calorie diets may be beneficial.** If you eat less animal fat, you will consume smaller amounts of the toxins that concentrate in it. Also, if you eat less food in general, you'll also consume fewer toxins.

Eating only organically grown foods is the best way to prevent consuming additional doses of pesticides. Don't use home pesticides or other toxic household products, either. In Chapter 22, you'll find a table that lists nontoxic alternatives for standard toxic household products. (A list of companies that produce nontoxic products along with their websites can be found in the Resources section.)

CHEMICAL ESTROGENS

Many chemicals—not just pesticides—can act as estrogen mimickers, or xenoestrogens. Over 200 of these chemicals have been identified and include heavy metals, household products, and even pharmaceuticals. Table 21.1 below lists some of the major estrogen mimickers. Many of these chemical estrogens are also known to cause excessive weight gain. And, as you know, obesity increases the risk of breast cancer. (See Chapter 17 for more information on chemical elements involved in weight gain.) Researchers have discovered that most of these xenoestrogens also promote cancer through other pathways that are not hormone dependent. These chemicals increase the risk of other cancers too, including cancers of the testis, ovary, lung, kidney, pancreas, and brain. While all of these estrogen mimickers are of concern, a few discussions of specific chemicals follow the table.

TABLE 21.1. CHEMICALS THAT MIMIC ESTROGEN

Types of Chemicals	Specific Chemicals
Cosmetics (nail polish, perfume, deodorant)	phthalates
Dental Materials (resin-based composites and sealants)	bisphenol A
Fungicides	benomyl, mancozeb, tributyl tin
Heavy Metals	arsenic, cadmium, lead, manganese, mercury
Herbicides	alachlor, atrazine, nitrofen
Household Products (breakdown products of detergents and surfactants)	nonylphenol, octylphenol

Industrial Chemicals	benzopyrene, dioxin, PCBs
Insecticides	chlordane, dieldrin, methoxychlor, DDT, endosulfan, toxaphene dicofol, kepone
Nematocides	aldicarb, dibromochloropropane
Pharmaceutical Drugs	birth control pills, cimetidine (Tagamet), diethylstilbestrol (DES), HRT
Plastics	bisphenol A, phthalates

Beware of Bisphenol A!

In 1987, researchers at Tufts University in Boston accidentally discovered a substance in plastic that mimics estrogen and accelerates the growth of breast cancer. Alarmingly, this substance, bisphenol A (BPA), can leach out of plastic when it comes in contact with food or liquid. This endocrine-disrupting substance has been found in plastic-bottled drinking water; in canned foods (more than 85 percent of the food cans in the United States are plastic lined); in foods stored in plastic containers or wrapped in plastic food wrap; in the saliva of patients whose teeth have been treated with dental sealant and composites; and in rivers, since this chemical is also a breakdown product of detergents.

When food is heated or cooked in a microwave in plastic containers that are not "microwave safe," bisphenol A pours out of them and into your food. So, to keep your foods free of bisphenol A, don't store or cook your food in plastic containers and avoid plastic wrap.

BPA has been linked to breast cancer, more aggressive tumors, and a number of other serious health problems. According to a 2013 study published by New York University School of Medicine, children exposed to high levels of BPA from plastic bottles and aluminum cans show increased markers of oxidative stress and inflammation that are linked with a higher risk of kidney and heart disease. BPA has also been associated with infertility, uterine fibroids, endometriosis, and abnormal thickening of the uterine lining that might lead to uterine cancer. Obesity, diabetes, asthma, allergies, leiomyomas (benign smooth muscle tumors) are more common with higher levels of this toxin. Finally, BPA has been implicated in causing a syndrome called testicular dysgenesis syndrome—which is characterized by a constellation of abnormalities, including poor semen quality, testicular cancer, undescended testis, and hypospadias (a birth defect where the urethral opening has an abnormal position on the penis).

Ohio State University researchers in 2010 reported that a substantial amount of evidence indicates that exposure to BPA in the womb increases the risk for breast cancer later in life. A study conducted by Yale University School of Medicine published in 2012 found that fetal mice exposed to BPA developed changes to their genes that caused them to respond differently to estrogen. When a substance causes changes to our genes—silencing them or turning them on—it is called an epigenetic effect. When a methyl group is added to a gene in our DNA, it silences the gene. When a methyl group is removed from DNA (called "hypomethylation"), it turns the gene on causing it to "express" itself. These changes can last from birth and throughout a lifetime. There are also a variety of other complex cellular interactions that occur in response to BPA.

Whew—I bet you could use a break from all this bad news! I've got some good news for you. A study published in 2012 in the *International Journal of Molecular Sciences* reported that folic acid, as well as genistein found in soy foods, taken during pregnancy prevents some of the ill effects that BPA exposure in utero can cause. You might remember in Chapter 12 that the B vitamin folic acid is a methyl donor. Folic acid gives its methyl group to the gene section of DNA affected by the BPA, removes the toxin, and thus reverses its damage. Other studies have shown that resveratrol found in grape skins also prevents breast cancers from forming in animals exposed to BPA in utero. Yet another study found that melatonin (Chapter 24), and the nutritional supplement royal jelly (from honey bees) blocks BPA's breast-cancer promoting actions, too.

TEFLON—ANOTHER COOKING DISASTER

Cooking that Kills?

What you cook your food *in* may be dangerous to your health, in fact deadly. For example, it is well known that cooking in aluminum pans should be avoided because of the potential for aluminum to increase the risk of Alzheimer's disease. Recently, another popular type of cooking pan has been shown to have potentially serious health risks: Teflon coated. This popular nonstick surface, as well as other nonstick and stain-resistant products, has come under fire because of the potential for a multitude of health problems, including cancer.

PFOA

Perfluorooctanoic acids (PFOA) is a group of artificial acids created several decades ago by DuPont that have been used in a variety of industrial products, most notably: polytetrafluoroethylene (PTFE), or Teflon. Because they are resistant to grease, this class of chemicals is also commonly used in household surfaces, carpeting, and flexible food packaging such as microwave popcorn bags, fast food and candy wrappers, and pizza box liners. PFOA can be found in water- and stain-resistant clothing as well, especially StainMaster and Gore-Tex.

They have even been used in firefighting foams. Of all the sources of PFOA, microwave popcorn bags are thought to be the most significant. Because of high heat, more of the chemical leaches out into the food than from any other packaging. It is estimated that 20 percent of the PFOA in the average American's body is from microwave popcorn. Declared to be safe by DuPont, a plethora of animal and human studies now point to the contrary.

The Problems

In a study published in the *Journal of Occupational Medicine* in September 1993, which was conducted by 3M (another company that made PFOA, but stopped producing it in 2000 due to the health concerns), 2,788 male and 749 female workers with exposure to PFOA were found to have a significant increase in cardiovascular disease. The men were 3.3 times more likely to die of prostate cancer. Another 3M study showed that exposed workers were more likely to seek care for prostate cancer, polyps in the colon, biliary tract and pancreatic disorders, and urinary bladder infections. 3M employees working in the Cottage Grove, Minnesota plant were more likely to die of bladder cancer and were found to have 10 percent higher levels of estradiol. Estradiol is the strongest, most abundant form of estrogen in the body and it is the one most associated with an elevated risk of breast cancer and Leydig cell tumors of the testis. PFOA has been linked to changes in cholesterol, reproductive hormones, and growth hormones both in humans and in animals.

Animal studies, conducted mostly on rats, show that PFOA exposure increases prostate, testicular, breast, pancreatic and liver tumors. In a study reported in the journal *Toxicological Sciences* in November 2006, pregnant rats subjected to PFOA gave birth to lower weight animals and the mammary glands (breasts) in both the mothers and offspring developed abnormally.

Bioaccumulation

The most shocking and devastating fact about PFOA is this: It doesn't break down in the environment. That means every molecule of it that was, and continues to be manufactured, builds up and accumulates in the environment, in us, or our in wildlife—a phenomenon called bioaccumulation. PFOA is found in the blood of virtually every American and in the environment worldwide. The amount of it that is polluting us and our environment is not small. In fact, in a 2005 global survey of perfluorinated acids in oceans, this class of chemicals was found to be *the most significant* contaminate in ocean water! Worse, this class of chemicals, like most chemical pollutants, concentrates in humans and animals. A study published in April 2006 documented the "bioconcentration" of PFOA by testing the concentration of it in the water, fish and birds in New York. Researchers found the concentration of PFOA in fish was 8,850 times greater than that in the surface water. Because fish concentrate chemicals more than any other animal, it is not difficult to understand why a study of people living on the Baltic coast of Poland published in February 2006, found that those who ate the most fish had the highest load of PFOA in their bodies.

Not surprisingly, and to me a fact that is tragic and tremendously sad, PFOA is being found in significant concentrations in every fish, bird, and mammal worldwide. A study of sea otters off the coast of California from 1992 to 2002 found PFOA concentrations that were higher than in any other previously reported marine mammal. The adult females with the highest levels died more often from infectious diseases. On the southeastern coast of the USA, Logger-head and Kemp's Ridley sea turtles were tested for PFOA and according to this 2005 report, 79 percent of them had detectable levels. Alarmingly, the concentration of PFOA in the turtles was twelve times higher than what had been previously measured. Other studies published in 2005 found PFOA in significant amounts in Polar bears in East Greenland and the Hudson Bay of Canada, and all the wildlife in and around the Great Lakes including mink, bald eagles, Chinook salmon, carp, snapping turtles, and water invertebrates (which had 1,000 times the concentration of the chemical in their bodies compared to the water)!

Government Action

The EPA has finally started taking action against the manufacturing of this toxic chemical and the company that manufactures it. In 2004 the EPA began investigating DuPont for covering up knowledge of the possible ill health effects of PFOA. They fined DuPont 10.25 million dollars and an additional 6.25 million to fund environmental projects. On January 25, 2006 the EPA announced a long-term voluntary program to reduce the emissions of the chemical by 95 percent by 2010 and to completely eliminate its use in products by 2015. The following month, an advisory board to the EPA stated that PFOA should be considered a "likely carcinogen." They also recommended that the risk assessment of this chemical should include data on the potential for it to cause liver, testicular, pancreatic, and breast cancers, as well as any detrimental effects it may have on hormones, and the nervous and immune systems.

In February 2006, DuPont agreed to pay $107 million to settle a class action suit filed by West Virginia and Ohio residents over the contamination of their drinking water from DuPont's Washington Works Plant. The EPA ordered DuPont on November 21, 2006, to offer alternative drinking water to the people who live near that plant.

CONCERNS ABOUT CADMIUM

Cadmium is a heavy metal commonly found in pigments, alloys, batteries, soldering processes, the air from burning fossil fuels, shellfish, animal livers and kidneys, and cigarette smoke (2–4 micrograms per pack). In the August 2003 issue of *The Journal of Nature Medicine,* cadmium was reported to have a remarkable ability to act like estrogen. The study found that even low-dose exposure to cadmium appears to increase the risk of breast cancer.

In this 2003 study by researcher B. Martin from Georgetown University, rats that had been exposed to cadmium while in the uterus reached puberty earlier than those rats that had not been exposed to this heavy metal. What does this mean to humans? Well, beginning menstruation at a young age increases the total number of periods over a woman's lifetime. The more periods she experiences, the more estrogen is released and the higher her risk of breast cancer is. And, in fact, this is what the study showed. In rats exposed to cadmium, breast cancer rates increased.

The World Health Organization (WHO) states that the maximum safe dose of cadmium for a human is 7 micrograms per kilogram (mcg/kg) per week. However, the rats in the study were only given 5 mcg/kg. This study raises the concern that low doses of cadmium may, in fact, *not* be safe as was previously thought. Additional studies are needed to more clearly define the safety and health risks associated with this and other heavy metals.

ANTIPERSPIRANTS

For over a decade, concerns about antiperspirants and their potential to contribute to the growth of breast cancer have been raised. There have been no well-designed studies regarding this issue; therefore it is not known what role, if any, antiperspirant may have.

The limited research that has been done in this area shows mixed results. For instance, a population-based, case-control study published in October 2002 in the *Journal of the National Cancer Institute* found the risk for breast cancer did not increase with antiperspirant use, deodorants, or underarm shaving. Whereas, a retrospective study published in the *European Journal of Cancer Prevention* in December 2003 found that the frequency and earlier habit of using antiperspirants after underarm shaving were associated with an earlier age of breast cancer diagnosis. Because the designs of both of these studies do not provide conclusive evidence, the question of antiperspirant safety still remains.

In theory, antiperspirants may promote breast cancer. One of the major contributing factors to breast cancer is lifetime exposure to estrogen and there are at least two ingredients in antiperspirants with estrogenic activity: aluminum and parabens. U.K. researcher, P. D. Darbre published a report "Aluminum, antiperspirants, and breast cancer," in the *Journal of Inorganic Biochemistry* in September 2005 showing that aluminum chloride or aluminum chlorhydrate affects the function of estrogen receptors in MCF7 human breast cancer cells and therefore could play a role in the breast cancer. In 2007, British researchers performed biopsies of breast tissue from mastectomies to check the aluminum content in various locations. They found that the level of aluminum was significantly higher in the upper, outer quadrant of the breast tissue—the location where about 50 percent of breast cancers present.

Parabens (esters of p-hydroxybenzoic acid) are used as antimicrobial preservatives in underarm deodorants and antiperspirants and in a wide range of other consumer products. Parabens have been shown to have both estrogenic and progesterone related activity. In addition, they have been detected in human breast tumors indicating that they do absorb into the breast tissue. However, Golden et al published "A review of the endocrine activity of parabens and implications for potential risks to human health" in June 2005 stating that the estrogenic activity of parabens is so weak that their risk is minimal. A study published in *Breast Cancer Research* in 2009 suggested that although an individual paraben may not be strong enough to cause an issue, a combination of them could. In reality, the breast is exposed to multiple estrogenic chemicals, so parabens could potentially contribute when combined with other chemicals.

Despite the concerns raised about aluminum and parabens, there have not been any studies definitively showing an association between antiperspirants and breast cancer. When there is any doubt, as there is with antiperspirants, my approach is to always play it safe. It isn't necessary to use antiperspirants or deodorants with aluminum and parabens. There are plenty of companies that make completely nontoxic underarm deodorants. They can be found at most health food stores and grocery stores such as Sprouts and Whole Foods. Nontoxic choices are always the best choices.

A Deadly Duo: Chlorine and Dioxin

The United States manufactures huge amounts of chlorine, an elemental gas rarely found in nature. It's used to bleach fabrics and papers to a pristine shade of white, making them appear clean and pure. We pay a big price for this illusion of purity. Chlorine is added to automatic-dishwashing detergent, bleach, disinfectant, mildew remover, toilet-bowl cleaner, laundry detergent, and swimming pools. Chlorine is an irritating, corrosive, hazardous pollutant that damages the Earth's ozone layer. In fact, it is one of the main contributors to the destruction of the ozone layer.

But the dangers of chlorine don't stop there. When chlorine is released into the environment, it reacts with organic materials and creates new toxins. Some of these toxins include chloroform and organochlorines (pesticides), which can damage your reproductive, endocrine, and immune systems. One type of organochlorine, called dioxin, is formed during chlorine processing. Dioxins are released into the environment from chlorine-processing plants. They enter the air, the water, the soil . . . and then your food and, ultimately, your body.

Dioxins are deadly. They are believed to be *the most* carcinogenic chemicals known. The EPA has found dioxins to be 300,000 times more potent as a carcinogen than DDT. Recent research has shown a clear link between dioxins and cancer, suppression of the immune system, reproductive disorders in adults, and developmental disorders and deformities in children.

Don't despair—there are nontoxic alternative products for virtually everything. You'll learn that it's possible to minimize your exposure to toxins in your home, car, and workplace, and to rid your body of toxins that have already found their way into your body. So, rest assured—you *do* have the power and ability to protect yourself from these deadly foes. Read on to learn how.

Part Five

Preventing the Birth of the Enemy

Tips and Tools Against Toxins

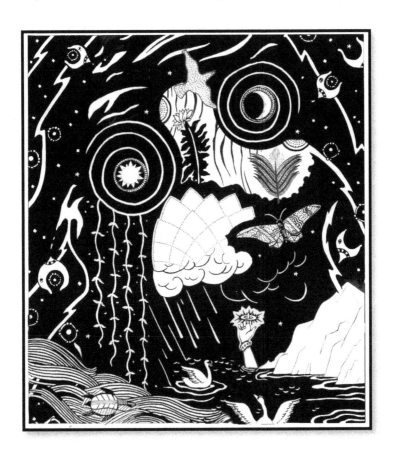

Chapter 22

Invite Friends,
Not Foes

A Treasure Chest
of Nontoxic Solutions

he best way to battle the chemical assassins discussed in the previous chapters is to avoid them as much as possible. Don't invite them home, and don't allow them into your body through food or drink. Begin by assuming that they're in everything out there. Purchase only foods and products that are labeled by the U.S. Department of Agriculture (USDA) as "certified organic" or by reputable manufacturers as "toxin-free."

In the early 1970s, a few people began to blow the whistle on some chemical assassins, exposing their identity, their hideouts, and their normal routes of entry. A large, informal intelligence network sprang up, revealing more and more of them. Then, some people really got smart. They created companies that offered toxin-free products. Now, hundreds—if not thousands—of companies make nontoxic products and offer nontoxic solutions for just about everything.

I live my life based on one primary assumption: Everything is toxic unless proven otherwise. Unfortunately, that's not too far from the truth. It's helpful to assume that everything is toxic. It keeps you aware and searching for nontoxic alternatives. Fortunately, there are nontoxic products and solutions for just about everything.

Table 22.1 on the following page lists the major categories of common toxin-containing products, the toxins of most concern contained in those products, and nontoxic alternatives, which sometimes include the manufacturer's name. (For a more expanded list of organic- and nontoxic-product manufacturers, see the Resources section.)

TABLE 22.1. TOXINS AND NONTOXIC ALTERNATIVES

Categories	Toxins	Nontoxic Alternatives
Bedding	flame retardants formaldehyde petroleum-based pillows	Organic cotton and wool box springs and mattresses, organic cotton linens
Cabinets	formaldehyde glues particleboard plywood	Medite II, wheat grass, solid untreated wood
Carpet, carpet pads	ethylene glycol glues petrochemicals styrene butadiene urethane foam volatile organic (carbon-based) compounds (VOCs)	Natural-fiber carpets (wool, cotton, jute, goat hair), wool carpet pads
Cars using internal combustion engines	carbon monoxide lead nitrogen dioxide ozone particulate matter sulfur dioxide	Hybrid electric vehicles, electric cars, fuel-cell cars, natural gas, walking, bicycles
Caulking and sealers	ethylene dichloride synthetic plastic resins toluene xylene	AMF Safecoat nontoxic caulking and natural sealers, alternative housing construction (adobe, rammed earth)
Clothing	formaldehyde hydrocarbons	Rayon, hemp, linen, organic cotton, wool, and silk
Conventionally grown foods	chemical fertilizers fungicides herbicides pesticides	Organically grown foods
Cosmetics and personal-care products	formaldehyde petroleum toluene	Burt's Bees and other natural product lines
Dry cleaning	perchloroethylene (Perc)	Professional wet clean, machine wash, steam clean, hand wash, carbon dioxide (CO_2) gas

Categories	Toxins	Nontoxic Alternatives
Flea and tick collars	neurotoxins	Herb collars, herb baths, penny royal, eucalyptus, brewer's yeast, garlic
Floor polishes	phenol	Natural oils, AMF Safecoat
Furniture	Same as above; fabrics may be treated with fire retardants, stain resistants, fungicides	Untreated natural-wood furniture, organic cotton or silk fabrics
Glues and adhesives	VOCs	Auro natural glue
Home pesticides	multitude of toxic chemicals	Nontoxic pest control, beneficial insects, Arbico
Household cleaners	chlorine phenols phosphates	Nontoxic cleaning supplies and detergents by Seventh Generation, E-cover, Country Save, Earth Friendly, Planet
Insect repellant	diethylmetatoluamide (DEET)	Neem, citronella, thyme, lemon grass, turmeric, geranium, Burt's Bees, All Terrain
Insulation	asbestos chlorofluorocarbons (CFCs) fiberglass particles formaldehyde polyurethane	Cellulose, icynene, denim
Joint compound (drywall mud)	antifungals binders dryers formaldehyde solvents (benzene)	Merco joint compound
Lawn-care products	chemical fertilizers herbicides	Organic lawn-care products (for example, Garden's Alive, Arbico)
Municipal water	benzene chlorine fluoride heavy metals pesticides	Whole-house water filters, carbon filters, distilled water, reverse osmosis, micropore filters
Paint thinners and strippers	methylene chloride solvents	Turpentine; Levos and Bioshield citrus thinners
Paints	binders solvents VOCs	Organic paints made by Livos, Bioshield, and Auro; "No-VOC" paints

Categories	Toxins	Nontoxic Alternatives
Paper	chlorine bleach	Tree-free paper, kanef, rice, other plant fibers, recycled paper
Paper towels, toilet paper	chlorine bleach	Recycled, unbleached paper (for example, Seventh Generation)
Particleboard, Oriented Strand Board (OSB), plywood	formaldehyde fungicides glues	Seal with AMF Safecoat, Safeseal
Resilient flooring, tile	polyvinyl chlorides (PVCs)	Linoleum, cork, bamboo, recycled rubber
Sealers and varnishes	Urethane	Natural varnishes made from oils and resins, Bioshield hard oil, AMF Safecoat, Oscolor
Teflon cookware	Perfluorooctanoic acids (PFOA)	Stainless steel pans
Wallpaper, especially those made from vinyl	petroleum-based adhesives PVCs	Untreated natural wall coverings, linens, plant fibers, cork, gypsum-coated fabric, pure-glass yarns by Innovative Wall Coverings, Maya Romanoff
Wood decks and deck furniture	arsenic fungicides polychlorinated biphenyls (PCBs)	Borax, salvage woods (redwood, cypress), nontoxic sealers

LIVING SAFELY WITH TOXINS

You may be concerned about all the toxic products in your home that you can't do anything about—especially the building products, such as insulation. First, be aware that building products, furniture, and carpets "outgas" immediately. This means that they release most of their toxins right away. Over time, although they continue to outgas, the rate and volume at which they do is so much smaller. If you live in an older home, these sources of toxins usually aren't much of an issue anymore. If you live in a new home, they are. You can purchase air filters to help remove the volatile organic (carbon-based) compounds (VOCs) from the air in your home, office, or car. A few examples of excellent portable air-filtration systems are listed below.

• Blueair HEPA Air Filters 501 and 402

• Healthmate HEPA Air Filter

- SilentAir 4000

- Desktop Air Filters

- UV Air Purifier (uses high-efficiency particulate air [HEPA], carbon, ultraviolet light, and ionization)

- Car ionizer (available at www.gaiam.com)

Ventilate your home well by keeping the windows open as often as possible. Don't let the temperature in your home get too warm, because heat increases the amount of toxic outgassing. If you do any type of remodeling in the future, such as painting or carpeting, be sure to use only nontoxic products.

Another way to cut down on the toxins released in a new home is to apply a product to your furniture, cabinets, or anything made with particleboard that seals the toxins in. AFM Safecoat SafeSeal is an excellent sealer; I used it when I built my home and found it to be simple to apply and very effective.

Green Builders

If you are considering purchasing a new home or if you are thinking of remodeling the home you're already in, I highly recommend that you speak with a specialist in the "green" building industry. Green builders are committed to building homes that are resource efficient and environmentally safe. There are several organizations in the United States that can put you in touch with green builders, as well as with distributors of nontoxic products for home improvements. When I built my home, I worked with several extremely helpful green builders to make my home and all its occupants as safe from toxins as possible.

Chapter 23

Cellular Housecleaning
The Power of Purification

*C*hances are you're feeling a little nervous right about now because you realize that, for most of your life, you've been unknowingly inviting toxic assassins into your home and into your body. You know that, more than likely, your body is filled with assassins just waiting to go for the kill. But just like in every Indiana Jones movie, there is a way out of this seemingly hopeless situation. You can give your body's natural detoxification system a huge boost by using the ancient purifying technique from *Ayurveda* that I've mentioned several times earlier in the book. This technique is known as *panchakarma*. Current research shows that it's very effective at getting toxins out quickly—even those that have been stored in your fat for years. It's not painful or unpleasant—quite the opposite. In fact, it's one of my all-time favorite, personal pampering experiences.

Panchakarma literally means "five actions." It is an integrated precise sequence of soothing treatments done in a spa-like setting with medical supervision over the course of several days. The treatments are gentle and deceptively simple, but their effects are remarkably powerful. The healing intelligence of the body is given such a boost through the techniques of *panchakarma* that it's capable of triggering phenomenal purification and healing.

Think of it this way: There are few things in life that Goddesses enjoy more than going to the spa. Taking time off from all your duties and responsibilities to go to a peaceful and relaxing place, free from any demands, with nothing to do but soak up the healing offerings is the essence of joy. Although spending the day at the spa may seem on the surface to be nothing more than a luxurious day of pampering, it can actually be profoundly rejuvenating and fundamental to maintaining your health and beauty. Take the revitalizing, health-promoting effects of a typical day at a spa, multiply it exponentially, and you have an inkling of the restorative effects of *panchakarma*.

DISLODGING IMPURITIES AND TOXINS

Panchakarma is especially effective at dislodging impurities and toxins and flushing them from your body. Research shows that it does this extraordinarily well. A study published by Bob Heron and John Fagen in 2002 in the journal *Alternative Therapies in Health and Medicine* found that, in test subjects, the levels of polychlorinated biphenyls (PCBs) and pesticides, including DDT, dropped by 50 percent after just one five-day series of treatments. Dr. Heron also tested subjects who had gone through *panchakarma* an average of twice a year for more than nine years. Every toxin the subjects were tested for came back negative. In other words, no toxins were present in levels high enough to be detected. The researchers concluded that regular *panchakarma* treatments are effective at removing toxins from your body and keeping your toxin load extremely low. In fact, research shows that the *only* known effective therapy that rids body fat of toxic chemicals is *panchakarma*.

As you know, your body accumulates and stores hundreds of toxins from the environment and the foods you eat. You also accumulate impurities from the waste products that are created by normal cellular metabolism. In *Ayurveda*, all toxins in the body form *ama*. Too much *ama* leads to disease. According to Ayurveda, one of the main purposes of *panchakarma* is to get the *ama* out.

Panchakarma also profoundly balances the mind/body and prevents or reverses the development of disease. Preliminary research indicates that it may slow the aging process, too. The first time I went through this series of gentle but powerful techniques, within forty-eight hours I looked ten years younger and had never felt better in my life! That experience made me a believer in the power of *Ayurveda*.

THE STEPS OF *PANCHAKARMA*

The majority of *panchakarma* is done in a medical spa-like setting over a period of time of between several days and several weeks. For the best results, you should go for a minimum of three days and ideally stay five to seven days. But before you arrive at the spa, you begin the initial steps of *panchakarma* at home. "Home prep" is designed to begin the process of softening the impurities and toxins, and mobilizing them from your fat.

1. Home Prep: Internal Oleation

This first phase of *panchakarma* is technically called "internal oleation." Oleation means saturating your body with oils. The oil used in home prep is *ghee,* or clarified butter. *Ghee* is made by boiling butter until all the milk solids precipitate out (always use organic butter). In other words, butter without milk solids and water is *ghee*. The spa you choose will give you specifics on how to make *ghee*, how much to take, and when to take it.

Ghee has very different properties from butter. First, it stays solid at room temperature and never needs to be refrigerated. Second, it lasts virtually forever without going bad. In India you can purchase 100-year-old *ghee*. Third, unlike butter, *ghee* doesn't raise your cholesterol or promote hardening of the arteries. *Ayurveda* considers *ghee* to be an extraordinarily powerful medicine that, according to ancient texts, soothes all the *doshas* (properties found in all living things— *vata* governs movement; *pitta*, metabolism and transformation; and *kapha*, structure). It improves memory and mental function, strengthens the body, promotes longevity and beauty, and protects the body from various diseases. You can purchase organic ghee in some health food stores.

During home prep, *ghee* is taken in increasing amounts every day for four days. Instead of drinking melted *ghee* straight, which can be a bit challenging, I mix it with one-quarter to one-half cup of heated organic soy, coconut, or almond milk to make it more palatable. The purpose of drinking *ghee* is to raise the level of fat or lipids in your blood to form a "concentration gradient" between the stored toxins in the fat cells in your body and the pure fat (*ghee*) in your blood. You may recall from high school biology that a concentration gradient is produced anytime there is more of a particular substance on one side of a semipermeable membrane than on the other. A law of physics dictates that the concentration of molecules on one side of a semipermeable membrane must be equal to the other. So, molecules on the side with the higher concentration will pass through the membrane to the side with the lower concentration until the amounts are equal on both sides of the membrane.

Here's how *panchakarma* uses the concentration gradient to get toxins out: During the home-prep portion of *panchakarma*, you also consume a low-calorie diet. The fat stored in your fat cells is used for energy. Your fat cells become smaller as more fat is used. The amount of space for toxins in your fat cells lessens, so the toxins become more concentrated. The pure organic *ghee* you consume contains no toxins. By introducing large amounts of toxin-free fat into the blood, you create a concentration gradient between toxin-filled fat in the body and toxin-free fat in the blood—a physiological condition that isn't normally present. The concentrated toxins will flow out of your fat into the pure *ghee* in your blood until the concentration of toxins is equal in your fat and blood. According to physics, a 50-percent reduction in the amount of toxins in your body would be expected. This is exactly what Bob Heron's research showed.

After the internal-oleation phase of *panchakarma* is completed, you should take a twenty-minute hot bath. The heat increases blood flow and the delivery of toxins to the intestines. Due to the relatively large amount of *ghee* that is ingested during home prep, not all of it will be digested. The undigested *ghee* stays in the intestines. This again sets up a concentration gradient, and toxins and impurities are drawn into the intestines. Following the bath, a mild laxative, such as castor oil, senna tea, or a special herbal mixture, is taken to eliminate the toxins in the intestines.

2. Pulse Diagnosis: Detecting Imbalances

After completing the first phase of *panchakarma,* you are ready for the relaxing and enjoyable part: the in-residence treatments at an *Ayurvedic* medical spa. When you arrive at the clinic, an *Ayurvedic* physician, called a *vaidya,* takes your pulse and asks you a series of questions. The *vaidya* picks up a lot more information from your pulse than just your heart rate. In fact, an expert in pulse diagnosis can feel, with remarkable precision and accuracy, the state of balance and imbalance in all your body systems and tissues. It may seem like magic, but the explanation for how a *vaidya* is able to do this is quite simple. Quantum physics tells us that the fundamental structure of the universe is nothing more than vibration. Every structure in your body vibrates. Blood flows through blood vessels and comes into contact with every cell in your body. The vibration that each cell emits reflects its state of health. The vibrational information from every cell in the body is transmitted to and then carried by the blood. *Ayurvedic* physicians, as well as experts in traditional Chinese medicine (TCM) and several other ancient holistic forms of medicine, are trained to "feel" and interpret this information.

A *vaidya* can also determine your body type or "constitution" from your pulse. Based on all the information from the pulse, the *vaidya* prescribes a specific series of *panchakarma* treatments customized to your current state of health. The *vaidya* has many treatments to choose from, each with its own special benefits and purposes, but all with the ultimate purpose of restoring balance.

3. Massage: Moving Toxins and Inducing Balance

The prescribed series of *panchakarma* treatments usually begins with a special procedure called *abhyanga*—an herbalized, sesame-oil massage. Two technicians apply warm oil simultaneously to each side of your body using synchronized movements designed to facilitate getting the toxins out while soothing and balancing the nervous system. The pressure is soft, and the movements are extremely relaxing.

When both sides of your body are stimulated in the same way at the exact same time, the brainwaves in the two hemispheres of your brain will synchronize. This brainwave phenomenon is also seen during the practice of Transcendental Meditation (see Chapter 27). Not surprisingly, people who practice this highly effective form of meditation report the experience of "transcending" during *abhyanga*.

Researchers have observed that there is a strong correlation between the synchronicity of brainwaves and depression. Depression is characterized by very asynchronous brainwave patterns, meaning that the brainwave patterns emitted by one hemisphere of the brain are very different from those emitted by the other side. Researchers have found that when a person experiences relief from depression, his or her brainwave patterns become more synchronized. *Panchakarma* synchronizes your brainwaves. Researchers think that this may be why it's so effective at easing depression.

Because sesame oil is the most penetrating of all the oils, it is the preferred type of oil used for *abhyanga,* as well as for many other techniques in *panchakarma.* Sesame oil is absorbed through the skin and appears in the blood within minutes. It contributes to the blood-lipid/body-fat concentration gradient, helping to flush toxins out of the body.

Herbs with special medicinal properties are usually mixed in the oil. Up to seventy-five different herbs may be added. Sesame oil, with its incredible absorptive qualities, acts as a carrier to deliver medicinal herbs into the body. Delivering medicinal herbs through the skin may seem like an unusual practice, but it's not. Western pharmaceutical companies use this route, too. Many types of medications are designed to be administered topically in patches—for example, nicotine, nitroglycerin, and estrogen. The medications are absorbed through the skin where a network of blood vessels under the skin picks them up and transports them to the rest of the body.

Research has found that sesame oil also has several other beneficial effects, including anticancer properties. It can inhibit the growth of melanoma and colon cancer cells. It also contains antioxidants. If the oil is heated, the antioxidant activity increases. That's one of the reasons why the oil is always heated during *panchakarma.*

Two other toxin-releasing, coherence-building, whole-body massage techniques may also be prescribed based on a person's specific health needs: *udvartana* and *garshan. Udvartana* is performed using a paste made of ground grains. This technique cleans the skin, increases circulation, and promotes weight loss. *Garshan* is performed using raw-silk or wool gloves to create friction, thus stimulating circulation and helping to promote weight loss.

Nasya

This technique purifies the structures in your head and powerfully balances and enhances your five senses. *Nasya* improves mental clarity and stabilizes the mind. It's especially good for people with sinus problems and headaches. The technique of *nasya* is performed by one technician. A luxurious head and shoulder massage is given while you sit in a chair. Following the massage, you gently inhale herbalized steam. Then, lying down on a bed with your head slightly tilted back, the technician places a series of drops of herbalized sesame oil in your nose. The sesame oil soothes your sinuses and helps to facilitate the release of any congestion.

Shirodhara

This procedure is designed to relax your mind, soothe and nourish your nervous system, and detoxify your body. A gentle stream of slightly warm herbalized sesame oil is applied to your forehead. *Shirodhara* is actually considered a cooling treatment. Your eyes are covered with cotton balls and a washcloth. A soft roll is placed under your neck so that your head is tilted slightly backward. The technician applies a very slow stream of sesame oil back and forth across your forehead in an infinity (or figure-eight) pattern. Most people experience deep relaxation and an expanded state of consciousness when undergoing this procedure.

Shirodhara is particularly good for alleviating anxiety, insomnia, nervousness, and worry. It also improves malaise and stabilizes the mind. And it's beneficial for your skin, too. Many people notice a distinct glow to their complexion following a soothing, relaxing, peaceful session of *shirodhara*.

4. Heat Treatments: Melting the Impurities

The next major step of *panchakarma* uses a group of heat treatments to dilate the channels in your body and increase circulation, which facilitates the flow of toxins and impurities into your intestines where they can be eliminated. Also, toxins can be removed from your body through your sweat.

There are three main heat treatments in *panchakarma: swedana, pizzichilli,* and *pinda swedana.*

Swedana

Swedana is a traditional herbalized steam treatment. It's like a steam sauna, but with a few important differences. Instead of sitting on a bench as you would in a sauna, you lie on your back in a cedar cabinet with your head *outside* the cabinet. *Ayurveda* does not advise overheating your head. To keep your head cool and comfortable, a frozen cube of coconut oil is gently applied to your head and face during the treatment. It's remarkably soothing and refreshing. To keep you well hydrated, the technician gives you frequent sips of cool water.

Pizzichilli

This is my personal favorite of all the treatments. It's considered a royal treatment, and it's easy to understand why. Imagine lying on a table while two technicians massage your body as they use a hose to continuously pour thick streams of soothingly warm sesame oil over you. The first time I experienced the sensation of the warm oil cascading in waves over my body, I actually moaned out loud. It felt like warm melting butterscotch. After the treatment, I felt deeply relaxed and I glowed from head to toe.

Pinda Swedana

The third heat treatment, *pinda swedana*, is performed by two technicians who massage your body using quick long strokes with boluses of precooked herbs and hot medicated oils in soft, smooth cloth packs. *Pinda swedana* is designed to soothe any kind of musculoskeletal problems, especially arthritis. It's also said to nourish the body, enhancing its vitality.

5. Cleansing: The Final Stage

External oleation and heat treatments are performed each day to help lift the impurities and toxins out of the tissues and transport them into the intestines. Once in the intestines, it's very important to get them out. This is facilitated by a simple procedure called a *basti,* which is a gentle internal cleansing of the colon with either herbalized water or oils. The oil-based *basti* and the water-based *basti* are administered on alternating days. You can think of a *basti* as a very gentle herbalized colonic. Getting the toxins out of the colon quickly is powerful medicine, so some people find it to be a little uncomfortable. *Ayurveda* says that the *basti* treatment is so important that it alone could cure 50 percent of illnesses.

IMMEDIATE AND LONG-TERM BENEFITS

After completing *panchakarma,* people report having greater energy, clarity of mind, and a sense of well-being. They also report relief of symptoms and improvements in disorders of both the mind and body. Research on the effects of *panchakarma* reveals that it rebalances the physiology and significantly reduces oxygen free radicals.

Oxygen free radicals increase your risk of cancer and other degenerative disorders and accelerate aging. In 1993 in the *Journal of Research and Education in Indian Medicine,* Hari Sharma, M.D., documented that patients doing *panchakarma* had an initial rise in lipid peroxidase, an enzyme that goes up in the presence of oxygen free radicals. But following therapy, lipid-peroxidase levels fell way below pretreatment levels. These findings correspond to the rise of toxins in the blood as they are mobilized during treatment and to the fall of toxins after they are eliminated from the body.

Researchers have also found psychological improvements in patients following *panchakarma*. Standard psychological tests show that these people are less anxious, less depressed, less distressed, and less fatigued. In 1988, researcher Rainer Waldschütz used the Freiburg Personality Inventory, a standardized test that measures twelve different personality scales, to evaluate patients who had just finished *panchakarma* treatments. These post-*panchakarma* patients showed improvements in six of the twelve scales: decreased body complaints, reduced irritability, less bodily strain, fewer psychological inhibitions, more openness, and greater emotional stability.

Panchakarma also significantly improves several cardiac risk factors. Blood samples taken from patients shortly after they completed *panchakarma* showed many beneficial changes. For example, vasoactive intestinal peptide (VIP)—a substance that dilates coronary arteries—increased by 80 percent. The "good" kind of cholesterol (high-density lipoproteins; HDL) increased by 75 percent, and total serum cholesterol decreased.

Nothing is more powerful than this special series of techniques for eliminating the impurities that obstruct your full strength; nothing surpasses the balancing and healing effects; nothing centers you more; and nothing recharges you more. Think of it this way, after a week of *panchakarma,* the unobstructed flow of your Warrior Goddess's cosmic intelligence becomes so powerful and so intense that you positively glow with self-luminescence and beauty.

HOME DETOX PROGRAMS

If you cannot go to a *panchakarma* clinic, you can detoxify at home. Although home detoxification programs are not as powerful as *panchakarma*, they can effectively remove toxins.

A Simple Start

Let's start with the simplest. Because your body naturally detoxifies itself, you can work with that natural ability without having to go anywhere or do anything exotic, time consuming, or expensive. Simply stop pouring in the toxins, drink plenty of pure clean water, and get some exercise—as easy as fast-paced walking will do the trick. It's amazing to me to hear about how many people don't drink water. Instead, their fluid intake each day primarily comes from coffee, sodas, and beer. No kidding! If you fall into this category—for example, if you eat lots of fast foods and sugar, and drink very little water—this might be a great way for you to help your body to begin to gently detox. Eliminate red meat, sugar, coffee, and preserved and processed foods. You'll notice that every detox program always includes eliminating major sources of toxins. Fill your plate instead with fresh organically grown vegetables, fruits, and whole grains. Lightly cooked is easier to digest and research shows it actually enhances the availability of certain nutrients, especially antioxidants.

The Power of Juice

Fresh vegetable-based juices are wonderful to consume daily and are an excellent and easy way to stimulate the detoxification process. Every time I make a commitment to juice every day, within a week or so, my skin takes on a self-luminous glow. Comments like, "What are you doing? You look amazing! Your skin looks radiant!" come from nearly everyone I encounter. There's nothing more affirming and encouraging than having the evidence of your efforts toward a better state of health radiantly displayed on your face! I haven't found any published research specifically measuring what happens when a person consumes a glass of fresh organic vegetable-based juice each day. But, it's only logical that more nutrients and antioxidants get absorbed in the body, compared to that from eating solid food, which requires a lot of digestion.

For many people, including perhaps you, making fresh juice is realistically not something you will ever do. There are blenders, such as the Vitamix and the Nutribullet, that require less time and clean up. You simply put some vegetables in the blender, push the button, and watch them magically turn into juice. Another plus with this approach is that it contains all the fiber in the whole vegetables, which is normally lost in juicing.

Supplemental Concentrates

If you know making fresh juice will never be a part of your routine. . .that's okay. There's yet another option: a variety of companies offer "green drinks" that are made of powdered concentrated greens which are packed full of antioxidants and nutrients. All you need to do is mix a scoop with water and shake it up.

One of my favorites is a product made by the Institute for Vibrant Living called All Day Energy Greens. It contains thirty-eight nutrient dense superfoods, including spirulina, barley grass, aloe vera, rose hips, parsley, chlorella, and beet juice. This concentrate not only delivers an impressive amount of nutrients, but it also encourages your body to become more alkaline, release toxins, and feel more energized. Oftentimes green drinks don't taste all that great. They can taste bitter or too "earthy." But, this one is surprisingly delicious.

Go Ruby Go! is a companion product filled with forty-two concentrated fruits, including raspberries, strawberries, cherries, cranberries, and mangos. Mix it with water in a blender and toss in some fresh or frozen organic berries to make a thicker fruit smoothie. It's one of my favorite treats in the afternoon. You can find easy blender recipes for these two super-nutritious products at www.ivlproducts.com.

Ayurveda definitely recommends consuming fresh fruits and vegetables for your best nutrition. However, if you can't get yourself to consume enough of these plants every day, research does support the benefits of fruit and vegetable supplemental concentrates. Numerous studies conducted in the lab, in animals, and in humans have shown that these concentrates increase serum antioxidants and carotenoids, reduce inflammation, and demonstrate significant anticancer effects.

Flushing Toxins Out with Herbs

Another good approach to encourage toxins out of your body is to do a modified *panchakarma*-like program by beginning with the home-prep program for *panchakarma* described earlier in this chapter. Then for two weeks following the prep, take herbs that detoxify the liver, kidneys, and colon. For example, cascara, milk thistle, dandelion, and turmeric help purify the liver and boost liver enzymes. Licorice root, psyllium seed, alfalfa, yucca root, violet leaf, cascara sagrada, and marshmallow root act as colon-cleansing agents. Horsetail, uva

---

A Word about Water

Our bodies may look solid, however, they are composed mostly of water. Estimates for how much water each of us holds range from 70 to 90 percent. The exact amount doesn't matter—what's important is to understand that our bodies are mostly composed of water. That's why it is so important for us to drink water. Consuming at least eight 8-ounce glasses a day is recommended, and much more if you are active and perspiring.

Unhappily, we are now challenged by the fact that much of our water is contaminated. I know, I know, it seems like another catch-22 situation. You need to drink water, but most sources of water are contaminated with health-destroying toxins.

Municipal tap water, for instance, commonly contains dangerous contaminants like chlorine, heavy metals, pesticides, pharmaceutical drugs, and much more. Bottled water isn't a great alternative for many reasons.

ursa, and nettles help to flush toxins from your kidneys. If you would prefer, you can work with a knowledgeable herbalist to determine which herbs to take and at what dosages.

I highly recommend an even simpler choice—you can take toxin-flushing herbal products conveniently already formulated for you. One of my favorite brands is Maharishi Ayurvedic Products International (www.mapi.com). They make three excellent detoxification herbal formulas: One for your bowel, another for your liver, and a third for your kidneys. To cleanse your bowel, take 2–5 tablets of Digest Tone or 2–4 tablets of Herbal Cleanse before going to bed each night. Take 2 tablets of Elim-Tox morning and evening to support detoxification of your liver, blood, sweat glands, and your entire elimination system. (Take Elim-Tox-O if you have any symptoms of reactive toxins such as skin breakouts or other inflammatory symptoms.) Finally, to purify your urinary tract and assist the removal of toxins, take 2 tablets of Genitrac in the morning and evening.

During your cleanse it is important to follow a pure diet consisting of lightly cooked, fresh organic fruits, vegetables, and whole grains. Be sure to avoid alcohol, sugar, chocolate, cold foods, meat, drugs, cigarettes, and canned, preserved and/or processed foods. You can boost the results by giving yourself an organic sesame-seed oil massage every morning. If you have access to an infrared or dry sauna, massage yourself with oil and sit in it for twenty minutes or so sev-

---

First, most of it comes in plastic bottles that have estrogen-mimicking molecules, including BPA and phthalates that can leach into it. Next, there's no regulation on bottled water and an estimated 40 percent is merely tap water! For those of you who would like more specific details about what's in bottled water, there is an excellent comprehensive analysis of 173 different varieties of bottled water conducted by the Environmental Working Group that can be found on their website (www.ewg.org).

So what form of water is safe to drink, and won't harm the environment? Drinking filtered tap water is thought to be the best solution by most experts. Ideally, you should have a whole-house water filtration system installed. The next best option is to use a system, such as a reverse osmosis system that fits under your sinks and/or place filters directly on your faucets and showerhead. You can also filter your water with separate filtration systems such as the Brita filters. Fill stainless steel bottles with filtered water to take with you to the gym, or wherever you go.

eral times a week. The heat treatment will enhance the absorption of the sesame oil and speed up the movement of toxins out of your body.

Sweating Out Toxins

Speaking of heat—saunas treatments alone are not only wonderful detoxifiers, but they also provide many other health benefits. Most of us are aware that the sweat our bodies produce isn't just water, it also contains salt. All of us have experienced the salty taste of sweat and felt it crust on our skin. But, what many people may not be aware of is that sweat also contains many other trace minerals, heavy metals, and toxins. Therefore, our sweat provides another channel for the elimination of toxins.

The heat causes several beneficial physiological effects. First, it increases heart rate and blood flow, which helps mobilize toxins into the organs of elimination including the colon, kidneys, and skin. Second, it causes our skin to release sweat in an effort to cool the body, and as a side benefit also releases toxins. Surprisingly, there haven't been many studies analyzing what's in our sweat. The only published studies are from the late 1970s and 1980s, which looked at the trace element concentration in human sweat. Researchers found that there was considerable variation from individual to individual. Concentrations of elements were found to vary in different body locations and between genders. The researchers consistently found that heavy metals, including copper, lead, cadmium, nickel, and zinc were released in sweat. A study published in the *Annals of Clinical Laboratory Science* in 1978 found that the concentrations of nickel and cadmium were higher in sweat than in urine.

Researchers at the University of Southern California published a study in *Archives of Environmental Health* in 1989 of firemen who were exposed to PCBs and the byproducts generated from a transformer fire and explosion. The firemen were treated with a two-to-three week detoxification program consisting of a medically supervised diet, sauna treatments, and exercise. The major symptom all of the firemen displayed was significant memory impairment. After the detoxification program, every fireman showed marked improvement of memory based on the results of three different types of memory tests.

The most common types of saunas are steam, dry, and far-infrared. Steam and dry saunas produce similar results and are a matter of personal preference. *Ayurveda* cautions that sauna durations should not be over twenty minutes to avoid excessive heat in the head. Far-infrared saunas have many more health benefits compared to the steam or dry variety. Research shows that they are beneficial for several health conditions, including cancer. For instance, far-infrared saunas improve cancer treatments by synergistically increasing the tumor-killing effects of chemotherapy and radiation. This type of sauna lowers blood pressure in patients with high blood pressure; treats congestive heart failure; reduces chronic pain; and may improve chronic fatigue syndrome, fibromyalgia, and multiple chemical sensitivities. It also aids weight loss. You should not go into a sauna if you have unstable angina, have had a recent heart attack, or suffer from severe aortic stenosis. Never drink alcohol before you go into a sauna. It increases the risk of your blood pressure dropping, and can cause cardiac arrhythmias or sudden death.

The Life Vessel

An innovative technology called the Life Vessel can help you to detoxify, rebalance, and relax. For you, it is very easy. All you need to do is lie down in a cozy relaxing chamber, close your eyes, and listen to soothing music. The magic of the Life Vessel comes from the subtle energy of light, sound, frequency, and vibration. The results have been nothing short of miraculous for a variety of ailments. The Life Vessel improves certain physiological measures, such as your autonomic nervous system, so effectively that it was certified by the Food and Drug Administration (FDA) in 2006.

Treatments are administered in four 1-hour sessions over the course of three days. Heavy metals, petroleum products, and a variety of other toxins are also mobilized and released by the treatments. The detoxification has been found to be significantly improved by combining the treatment with drinking lots of pure water—a recommended one gallon a day—along with infrared sauna sessions and colon hydrotherapy. Currently, there are just a few Life Vessel Centers in the United States with plans to distribute them across the nation. The centers are located in Scottsdale, Arizona; Santa Fe, New Mexico; Long Beach, California; with two in Colorado (one in Denver and the other in Boulder).

DETOXIFY REGULARLY

Although we are living in a toxic world, you needn't let that fact drive you to despair. Keep in mind that most of these chemicals can be removed with effective detoxification techniques. Because it is impossible to avoid exposures to potentially harmful chemicals no matter how hard you may try, it is important to make regular detoxification a part of your health routine—and it really works!

For optimum health, you should follow a detoxification program for at least a few days to a week, at least two or three times a year. Think of it this way—machines like your car need regular cleaning and maintenance to continue performing well, and so do you. There's nothing that boosts your radiant health and beauty quite like a week or two of a good detoxification program. It's a quick and very effective way to not only remove toxins and lower your risk of diseases such as breast cancer, but to also achieve a better state of balance, enhance your inner healing intelligence, and charge your enthusiasm for life!

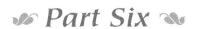

Part Six

Balancing Rest and Activity

Protection Against Breast Cancer

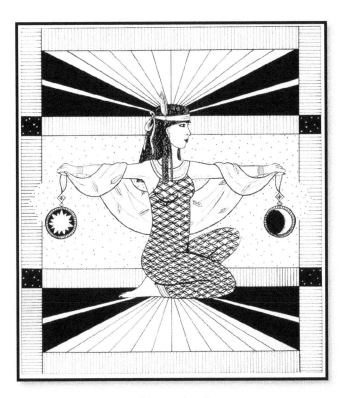

Goddess of Balance

Chapter 24

Healing Nectars of the Night

Melatonin and Other Bodyguards

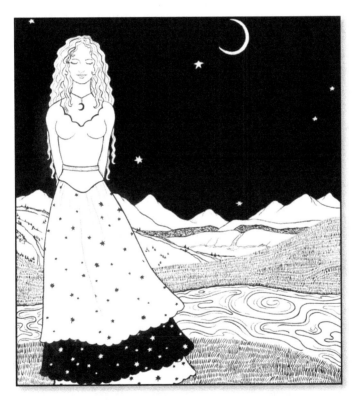

Goddess of Sleep and Dreams

Lack of knowledge is darker than the night.

—AFRICAN PROVERB

*I*t's a timeless *Ayurvedic* principle that *proper sleep and rest are fundamental to good health. Activity must be balanced with rest.* Think about a time when you have gone to bed early and enjoyed a peaceful rejuvenating night of sleep. You woke feeling fresh and full of energy, optimistic, and upbeat. When you looked in the mirror, the youthful and radiant face looking back at you took you by surprise. What you saw was the end result—the gift of proper sleep—of a multitude of complex biological processes designed by Nature to keep you healthy. When you follow the laws of Nature, these are the results you can expect to achieve. Proper sleep and rest are of supreme importance to your Warrior Goddess's health, strength, vitality, and beauty.

THE NECTAR OF SLEEP

When you sleep, your Warrior Goddess orders the nocturnal repair and purification of your mind/body to begin. She commands your mind/body to produce medicinal potions and nectars with truly magical healing properties. In scientific terms, they are known as chemicals and hormones.

The nectar of sleep is the hormone melatonin. Several years ago, researchers discovered some of melatonin's remarkable effects. This hormone subsequently received a lot of media attention, mainly for two reasons: 1) Melatonin supplements can help relieve or quicken recovery from jet lag, and 2) they are safe, natural alternatives to sleeping pills. While these effects can be quite helpful, there's so much more to know about melatonin than the media shared.

When darkness falls, the pineal gland in your brain increases its production of melatonin. In other words, as soon as the sun sets, your Warrior Goddess calls for melatonin to start flowing. As the level of this hormone rises, you start to feel sleepy. The moment you fall asleep, it starts to flow even faster. The faster it flows, the greater its power becomes. If it flows to its highest potential, its power becomes so great that it becomes a raging river of cancer protection.

Melatonin mirrors the attributes of a goddess; it gently yet powerfully seduces you into sleep, but while you're asleep, it acts as a great warrior on your behalf. It provides extraordinary protection from many of the factors that increase your risk of breast cancer.

This hormone is a very potent antioxidant, and, as you know, antioxidants are powerful defenders against the attack of oxygen free radicals. They disarm oxygen free radicals, rendering them incapable of damaging your cells and DNA—damage that could lead to cancer. Melatonin slows down the production of estrogen, prevents its overproduction, blocks its stimulatory effects on breast cells and favorably influences the BRCA1 gene as well as other estrogen-responsive genes. But melatonin's defenses don't stop there. It opposes many different growth factor threats that can increase cell division in the breast, including the hormone prolactin and "epidermal growth factor." In addition, it stops new blood vessels from growing into tumors, directly slows down the rate at which they grow and divide, and prevents tumors from invading and spreading.

Melatonin also enhances the tumor-fighting power of vitamin D and increases this vitamin's ability to stop tumor growth. In fact, it makes vitamin D's tumor-fighting abilities 20 to 100 times stronger! All of melatonin's various breast cancer-fighting capabilities can be summed up in three big points:

1. Melatonin prevents the initiation of breast cancer.

2. Melatonin slows down tumor growth.

3. Melatonin prevents metastasis.

The only thing you really need to remember about melatonin is this: It's a powerful weapon against breast cancer.

A Comrade to Chemotherapy

Taking supplemental melatonin can enhance the effectiveness of chemotherapy, such as Adriamycin, by increasing its ability to kill tumors. A 1999 study from Italy, reported in the *European Journal of Cancer,* found that breast cancer patients treated with chemotherapy lived longer if they were also given supplemental melatonin. In scientific terms, these patients increased their survival by one year. In other words, more women were alive one year following the diagnosis and treatment of their breast cancer than would normally have been expected to be. When melatonin supplements were given in addition to chemotherapy, the size of the tumors decreased significantly more than when chemotherapy was given alone.

Melatonin can also provide protection from many of the harmful side effects of chemotherapy. A 2005 study in the *Journal of Cardiovascular Pharmacology* found melatonin protected against heart damage caused by Adriamycin. Chemotherapy is commonly toxic to several components in the blood. Platelets, which have an important role in blood clotting, are particularly vulnerable. Chemotherapy usually reduces the number of platelets in the blood, thereby increasing the risk of bleeding problems. Melatonin protects the platelets and keeps their numbers up. Researchers found that when melatonin was given to patients on chemotherapy, the number of platelets in their blood remained normal. These patients also had fewer toxic side effects from the drugs, including less damage to their nervous systems and hearts, and fewer mouth ulcers. In another study, published in *Anticancer Research* in 2005, melatonin was found to reduce the toxicity of doxorubicin to bone marrow stem cells.

THE RHYTHMS OF NATURE

Whether you honor them or not, your mind/body is ruled by the natural cycles and rhythms of Nature. In other words, your Warrior Goddess has a schedule that she likes to keep to stay strong and balanced. She is very particular about the number of hours she sleeps, what time she goes to bed, and many other details. When you live in harmony with her cycles and rhythms, you enhance her strength. When she is strong and empowered, she expresses that power by increasing your body's natural healing capabilities—its inner healing intelligence. This principle is beautifully demonstrated by the profound effects that respecting or disrespecting these rhythms has on how melatonin expresses itself.

If you followed the natural rhythms of the sun, you would go to bed shortly after it sets. Research indicates that there is tremendous health value in following the cycles of the sun. Research shows that if you go to bed early, before 10:00 P.M., your melatonin levels rise to their highest possible and most medicinal levels during sleep. If you go to bed late, around midnight for instance, you are working against the natural rhythms of Nature and obstructing the flow of healing intelligence. Melatonin levels don't rise as high in this case, and you lose its full medicinal power. If you severely disrespect Nature's rhythms, you seriously impede the healing intelligence of your mind/body, and your Warrior Goddess loses her balance, becoming dull and weak. She can no longer protect you with brilliance, discriminating intelligence, and strength.

If you keep an extreme schedule that assaults the natural laws and rhythms of Nature (for example, if you work all night and sleep all day), the deleterious health consequences are spectacular. Your inner healing intelligence is dramatically weakened. For instance, researchers found that nurses who worked the night shift had a 50 percent higher risk of breast cancer. The longer they worked the night shift—that is, the longer they worked against the laws of Nature—the higher their risk of breast cancer became. In 2012, a Danish study confirmed this finding. Interestingly, the researchers found that the women working the night shift, who described their natural nature as "a morning person," had the highest risk of all. The risk of breast cancer in those individuals was almost four times higher! Other researchers found that breast cancer tumors grew seven times faster in animals exposed to constant light.

When you sleep, your melatonin level rises, but melatonin responds to more than just your change in consciousness. Melatonin is a nocturnal nectar. It loves the darkness. The darker the environment is, the better it flows. Even though you don't consciously *see* when you sleep, your eyes perceive the light. Melatonin is as repelled by light as Count Dracula is. It shies away from even the faintest glimmers of light. Any light at night—even a soft nightlight or the glow of a full moon—will prevent your melatonin from rising to its full potential. Bright city lights burning continuously through the night may be one reason for the more common incidence of breast cancer in industrialized regions.

The darker it is, the more your melatonin responds and the more freely it flows. Melatonin loves the darkness so much that it seems to prefer blindness. In women who are blind, this natural medicinal hormone expresses its protective might in full glory. Blind women have half the incidence of breast cancer that women with normal eyesight have.

If you can't make your bedroom totally dark, I highly recommend that you wear an eye mask when you sleep.

Sleep Creates Immune Ammo

Melatonin is only part of the cancer protection that you gain during sleep. Your sleep patterns govern changes in the strength of your immune system that also affect your risk of cancer. Your Warrior Goddess, empowered by sleep at the proper time, can command more immune protection. She orders your immune system to produce a powerful cancer-fighting substance called "tumor-necrosis factor," a natural biological weapon that destroys tumors.

Your immune system takes the nighttime order very seriously. When your Warrior Goddess says, "jump," your immune system jumps. It creates ten times more tumor-necrosis factor when you're asleep than when you're awake. During sleep, another cancer-fighting weapon is also called forth from your immune system—natural killer (NK) cells. You can think of these cells as gladiators who kill tumor cells and any other undesirable cells that invade your body. But if you don't get enough sleep or don't sleep during the best times, your immune system won't respond to the command to make more NK cells. Researchers have found that without enough sleep, the number of your NK cells goes down significantly.

> *There is a time for many words,*
> *and there is also a time for sleep.*
>
> —HOMER, *THE ODYSSEY*, 800–700 B.C.E.

Natural Law

Five thousand years before Ben Franklin said, "Early to bed and early to rise makes a man healthy, wealthy, and wise," *Ayurveda* understood and taught people the natural laws governing sleep. Ben Franklin was right. His astute observations are in alignment with those natural laws—laws that never change. They are true, always have been true, and always will be true. According to ancient

Ayurvedic texts, it is a law of Nature that when human beings *go to bed before 10:00 P.M. and get up by 6:00 A.M.*, they experience the most balancing and healing effects of sleep.

Modern research supports this 5,000-year-old recommendation. Scientists have found that you experience deeper stages of sleep when you go to bed by 10:00 P.M. This is partly due to the greater rise in melatonin and other hormone responses. When you get up before 6:00 A.M., you will probably notice that you feel more awake, less groggy, and more energetic than if you sleep later. Try it and see.

Sleep Is a Pillar of Health

Of all the thousands of natural laws governing your health, there are three that are considered the most important. They are described as the "three pillars" of Ayurveda. Proper sleep is one of those pillars. The other two are proper diet and lifestyle. This recommendation, *Go to bed before 10:00 P.M., and get up by 6:00 A.M.*, like most *Ayurvedic* recommendations, sounds simple but has profound health benefits. Modern research confirms that the Ayurvedic physicians were correct: The exact hours we sleep are as important as the total number of hours we sleep. Melatonin naturally begins to rise around 9:00 P.M. and peaks after midnight. If you go to bed too late, you will blunt melatonin's rise and prevent it from ascending to the height it loves to reach. The consequences of frequently thwarting melatonin's mission to reach its zenith each night can be spectacular—especially when it comes to your risk of breast cancer. The studies of night-shift workers, mentioned earlier, found that if you sleep during these recommended hours, your risk of breast cancer is 50 to 400 percent lower than if you don't.

When you don't get enough sleep, it drastically weakens your Warrior Goddess. In fact, it diminishes her power more than almost anything else. Without enough sleep, she quickly falls apart, loses her coordination, and becomes less alert and discriminative. Her reaction times slow down. It becomes impossible for her to manage all the tasks and demands placed on her—and it shows. Without proper sleep, she is too weak to protect you from making mistakes that could cost you your life.

For example, when workers are fatigued because of lack of proper sleep, the risk of on-the-job errors and accidents is much higher. Worker fatigue is credited for such major accidents as the Chernobyl nuclear meltdown and the Exxon Valdez oil spill. Research shows that 60 percent of road accidents are caused by fatigue due to lack of sleep. In one study, drivers who stayed awake for more than seventeen hours had significantly impaired coordination, reaction time, and judgment. Even more frightening, these sleep-deprived drivers were found to be *more severely impaired than drivers who are legally drunk*! The moral of the story? Without proper sleep, your inner intelligence becomes dangerously weakened, and your risk of serious illnesses and accidents goes up.

If you continually get less than the ideal amount of sleep, the hard fact is, you'll take years off your life. Sleep is so important that even one hour less of it each night can cut your life short. Research shows that people who sleep less than six hours a night don't live as long as those who sleep seven or eight hours.

The magnificent multitasking intelligence that manages your mind/body— your Warrior Goddess—needs rest to properly perform all the tasks she needs to carry out to keep you balanced and healthy. If you sleep fewer than four hours a night, she can't do her job, and diseases begin to manifest. Your risk of diabetes, high blood pressure, and weight gain increases.

Researchers have found that when you sleep only a few hours, glucose (blood sugar) is metabolized 30 percent less efficiently, and the stress hormone cortisol rises higher than if you'd gotten an adequate amount of sleep. When cortisol goes up, it causes your blood pressure to rise. It makes your cells more resistant to insulin, which increases your risk of diabetes. There is another key reason that cutting your sleep increases your risk of diabetes. Researchers discovered that your pancreas has melatonin receptors on the cells that make insulin. So, insulin production is directly tied to your circadian clock by melatonin. In a study published in 2013 based on data collected from the Nurses' Health Study, researchers at Brigham and Women's Hospital in Boston measured urinary melatonin levels of 640 women who did not have diabetes in 2000 and followed them until 2012. The women with the lowest levels of melatonin had a 2.2 times higher incidence of developing type 2 diabetes in those twelve years.

Many studies have found that the incidence of being overweight and obese is much higher in those who work the night shift. For instance, a study by Columbia University found that people between the ages of thirty-two and fifty-nine who slept only four hours were 73 percent more likely to become obese than those who slept seven to nine hours. The reasons are many, including alterations in glucose and fat metabolism; disruptions of the appetite-regulating hormones ghrelin (which causes hunger to increase) and leptin (which causes hunger to decrease); and chronic elevation of the stress hormone cortisol—all of which, encourage fat storage.

Another factor contributing to excess weight in night owls and night-shift workers, according to a study at Vanderbilt University in 2013, is that *when* you eat is just as important as what and how much you eat. At night, our circadian-clock mechanisms set us up to be inactive—to sleep, and not to eat. Our cells are more insulin resistant during the night. If you eat at night when you should be sleeping instead, the food that you eat will not be used for energy, but will be converted to fat. In their study, a group of mice were constantly exposed to light to disrupt their circadian rhythms. The mice stayed in the resting phase or metabolically inactive phase. Even though they ate fewer calories, they developed a higher proportion of body fat and gained more weight compared to the mice that had normal circadian rhythms.

Elevations in blood pressure, triglycerides, total cholesterol, and LDL (the bad type of cholesterol) are common in those who regularly work at night. So it should come as no surprise that metabolic syndrome and cardiovascular diseases are too. Researchers in Taiwan found that women, after five years of working the night shift, had a 4.6 to 12.7 times higher risk of metabolic syndrome. The notoriously bad diet and lifestyle habits of those with this schedule, researchers point out, also contributes significantly to the higher rates of chronic disease. For instance, night workers more commonly smoke tobacco, drink heavily, don't exercise, and have numerous psychosocial problems.

Not getting enough sleep is also associated with non-Hodgkin's lymphoma and cancers arising in the colon or rectum, endometrium, and prostate. It can lead to chronic fatigue, depression, accelerated aging, and even divorce.

Too Much Sleep Isn't Good Either

As you have seen, natural law says that your mind/body does its best when you retire by 10:00 P.M. and rise by 6:00 A.M. This also means that sleeping too much—sleeping beyond these recommended hours—can throw you out of balance. Although your Warrior Goddess enjoys her sleep, she has a lot of things to accomplish during the day to help protect you. When it comes to sleep, there are optimum times and amounts. Sleeping too much makes her dull and unable to function well, so much so that fatal diseases may form.

Research has found that people who sleep more than nine hours a night have an increased risk of heart disease. A Japanese study, reported in *The New York Times* on February 10, 2004, surveyed the health and sleep habits of more than 100,000 people for ten years. This study found that people who slept eight hours a night had a higher mortality rate than those who slept seven hours a night. The longer the study participants slept, the higher their risk of dying became. The researchers haven't yet determined how sleep and mortality are linked. One possible explanation for their findings is that people with serious health problems tend to sleep more than healthy individuals.

Do Not Disturb

Sleeping at the wrong times isn't the only thing that can disturb the proper flow of melatonin. A study published in October 2001 in the *American Journal of Epi-*

demiology found several other factors that can lower melatonin levels: daylight, a high BMI (body mass index; see page 186), alcohol consumption, and the use of certain medications, including beta-blockers, calcium-channel blockers, and psychotropics. Researchers reported in 2013 that the only food found in the Nurses' Health Study that lowered melatonin was red meat.

If you drink alcohol, your Warrior Goddess won't demand as much melatonin as she normally would. In a study from the University of Connecticut, published in *Epidemiology* in November 2000, researchers found that the more alcohol a woman consumed in a twenty-four-hour period, the lower her melatonin level was. One alcoholic drink didn't have any effect, but two drinks caused a 9 percent reduction in the level of melatonin, and three drinks dropped the level by 15 percent. This may be another reason why alcohol increases the risk of breast cancer.

THE DANGERS OF ELECTROMAGNETIC FIELDS (EMFS)

An electromagnetic field (EMF) is an invisible electric field that is produced when an electrical current runs through a wire. All electrical devices—both wired and wireless—emit EMFs. This includes household appliances such as microwaves, blenders, refrigerators, computers, cell phones, and hair dryers. Outdoors, dangers of EMFs are found in power lines, transformers, cell phone towers, and broadcast towers. You can't see them, hear them, smell them, taste them, or feel them, but the effects of man-made EMFs—now recognized as a new form of pollution called electropollution—can be very damaging to your health. Links have been found between EMFs and serious diseases such as breast cancer, leukemia, and brain cancer. EMFs exposure can also cause many nonspecific symptoms including fatigue, headaches, fuzzy thinking, and pain.

So why are they so dangerous for us? Think of an EKG (electrocardiogram) of the heart. What does it measure? The electrical activity of the heart. And an EEG (electroencepthalogram)? The electrical activity of the brain. Human beings are bioelectrical. So, electrical fields from electrical devices interact with our own electrical fields. EMFs interfere with our bodies in many other ways, too. In August 2006, fourteen scientists and experts from around the world collaborated on a major document called the BioInitiative report (www.bioinitiative.org), which reported on all the known health detriments associated with EMFs. The purpose was twofold: to show that the current safety standards fall far below what is safe and the urgency for revising them. The experts summarize the research by stating that there is a clear link between EMFs and an increased incidence of numerous cancers and serious health conditions, including childhood leukemia, brain tumors, acoustic neuromas, melanoma of the eye, breast cancer, Alzheimer's, Parkinson's disease, ALS (Lou Gehrig's disease), and immune system disorders.

EMFs and Breast Cancer

In a comprehensive review of the all the published studies on EMF exposure and breast cancer, a definite link between the two was found, and so we can say with certainty that EMF exposure contributes to breast cancer. In many studies, even male electricians showed an increased risk of the disease. A review of eleven occupational studies found a statistically significant increased risk of breast cancer in several categories. Overall, the risk of breast cancer doubled in pre-menopausal women who had jobs with significant EMF exposure. These jobs included telephone-line installers, repairers, and line workers. The risk was 65 percent higher for system analysts and programmers and 40 percent higher for telegraph and radio operators.

One way that EMFs interfere with your body's ability to stay healthy is by disrupting certain hormones, especially melatonin. Melatonin is known as your sleep hormone, but it is also profoundly important for general good health and breast health. Women with chronically low melatonin levels, usually caused by going to bed too late or working the night shift, have a significantly elevated risk of breast cancer. Even seemingly small amounts of EMFs like those created by the wires and appliances in your home, can disturb your melatonin levels. Researchers have found that residential 60-hertz (Hz) magnetic fields caused by normal electrical house wiring and equipment (such as clock radios, electric blankets, and televisions) depress melatonin. A German study published in *Cancer Research* in 2002 found that 50-Hz EMFs caused breast tumors to start growing and accelerated their growth—but, in this study, melatonin levels remained normal. These researchers concluded that EMFs may disrupt the body some other way. Regardless of the specific disturbance that EMFs cause in the balance of your body, we know one thing for certain: Exposure to EMFs contribute to the initiation of breast cancer and accelerate its growth.

Another way that EMFs exert damage to your body is by disturbing the signal pathways, or the ability of your cells to communicate with each other. Normally cells emit subtle electromagnetic frequencies as a form of communication that then gets transformed into the physiological processes of your body. EMFs or electropollution induces stress into your body and disrupts intercellular communication. This leads to bedlam, disorder, and breakdown of your cells and your physiology. Researchers have found that your blood-brain barrier becomes "leaky" to toxins and genetic damage occurs that can increase your risk of cancer.

Cell Phone Risk

Dr. George Carlo, an epidemiologist and principal researcher looking into the safety of cell phones, discovered after six years of intensive investigation, that cell phones are dangerous. According to Dr. Carlo, 40,000 to 50,000 cases of brain and eye cancer will have been diagnosed in 2006, and cell phones are a direct contributor. Dr. Carlo states that using a cell phone for only 500–1,000 minutes per month may increase the risk of brain and eye cancer by two or three times. The average teenager uses a cell phone for 2,600 minutes per month.

Understanding EMFs through Quantum Physics

Quantum physics has shown through the "superstring theory" that everything in the Universe including your mind/body at its most finite level is composed of vibrations. The intelligent vibrations of your mind/body create a measurable electromagnetic field around you called a "biofield." The health of your biofield influences the health of your mind/body and vice versa. Some external influences are harmonious with your biofield and support its health; others disrupt it. When you're exposed to man-made EMFs, they interact with your biofield. If the external EMF is out of harmony with your own, it creates imbalances in your biofield and obstructs the flow of its intelligence. When this intelligence is interrupted, it creates imbalances in your mind/body and causes it to malfunction. Eventually diseases such as cancer can result.

Protecting Yourself from EMFs

There are many steps you can take to protect yourself from EMFs. For example, if you're building a new house or rewiring your existing one, have your electrician install a master switch in your bedroom. Turning this switch off at bedtime will cut off all the power and, therefore, any EMFs in your bedroom. Your electrician can also use "BX electrical cable" when wiring your home. This twisted wire doesn't produce significant EMFs.

Simply standing a few feet away from most electrical appliances reduces your EMF exposure to nearly zero. Whenever you use an appliance, such as a microwave, toaster, or blender, step a few feet away from it while operating it. There are some appliances that it's not possible to use and stand a safe distance away from, such as computers, cell phones, and hairdryers. Of all the common electrical household appliances, hairdryers produce the strongest EMFs. Fortunately, there are companies that manufacture low-EMF hairdryers such as the Chi hairdryer, which is available for purchase on many websites. So, if this is something you use daily, consider purchasing one.

The other approach that offers excellent protection against the damaging effects of EMFs is to use devices that *alter how your body and biofield responds to them*. For example, a company called GIA Wellness, which is dedicated to providing effective solutions to the serious problem of electropollution, produces a variety of devices that have been shown to be highly protective against electropollution. These devices range from ones that you wear, to chips that you place on your cell phone and appliances, to "harmonizers" that you plug into the walls in your home, to nutritional supplements. When I began using these devices, I experienced a profound difference in the level of fatigue and stress I experienced, especially while working at my computer. There have been amazing case reports of improved symptoms after using these devices revealing that EMFs may play a significant role in many health problems. For instance, symptoms including headaches and pain associated with fibromyalgia have resolved. Most impressively, a health provider in Tennessee who specializes in autistic children has observed tremendous improvement in her patients using these devices. One child after using the devices for several weeks began speaking for the first time!

If you would like more information about these devices, please log onto my website www.drchristinehorner.com.

Ayurvedic Tips for a Good Night's Sleep

1. Eat three nutritious meals a day. The evening meal should be light and early.

2. Exercise regularly, preferably early in the day. If you exercise in the late evening, it may keep you up.

3. Go to bed by 10:00 P.M.

4. Eliminate or severely restrict stimulants such as caffeine and alcohol.

5. Wear comfortable clothing to bed.

6. Avoid hot, spicy foods at dinner.

7. Do not bring work-related material into the bedroom and turn off the TV.

8. Keep your bedroom dark.

9. A gentle massage of your hands, feet, and neck before bed can aid relaxation.

10. Stress can definitely interfere with your sleep. So practicing an effective stress reducing technique such as Transcendental Meditation (TM), Qigong, or yoga can be very beneficial. For example, a study of sixty-nine men and women over sixty who had sleep problems were divided into three groups:

The first group participated in an hour of yoga practice six days a week, the second group took an *Ayurvedic* herbal tonic, and the third made no change to their routine. The groups were then followed for six months. Overall, those in the yoga group experienced the best improvement in sleep. Relaxation is the key. Doing something as simple as taking long, deep, easy breaths, and letting your mind and body settle down when you first go to bed can do wonders.

HONORING THE NIGHT

The rhythms of Nature have created the night as a time of rest. It's a time when your mind/body undergoes magical repair, rejuvenation, and purification. The power and magnificence of your Warrior Goddess's healing protective powers depend upon your honoring all her desires. When you do, her ability to keep you well and balanced is extraordinary. When you don't honor her, she is weakened and loses the ability to keep you well. Honor and respect her ability to protect you by following Nature's rhythms and natural laws, and she will reward you with a great treasure—good health.

Chapter 25

The Medicine of Movement

How Exercise Lowers Your Risk of Breast Cancer

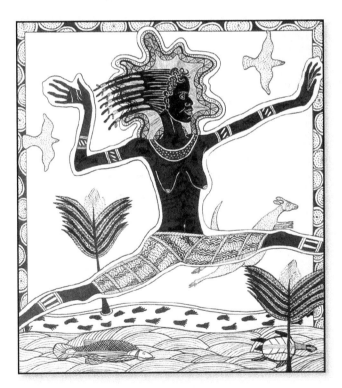

Goddess of Joyous Activity

To dance is to give oneself up to the rhythms of life.

—DR. MAYA PATEL

To Live is to Dance—to Dance is to Live.

—SNOOPY

noopy is right. The natural rhythms of life are a harmonious balance of activity and rest. When you dance with those rhythms, you can experience life to its fullest. The degree to which you respect those rhythms plays a huge role in your risk of developing or surviving breast cancer. Resting and sleeping at the proper times have powerful medicinal effects. The right type of activity at the proper times of the day is also very powerful medicine. It produces an array of health-protecting potions: magical chemicals and hormones, each expressing its own healing intelligence. When you work in harmony with Nature's rhythms, your inner intelligence is powerfully strengthened to ward off the development and progression of breast cancer in many ways.

THE IMPORTANCE OF MOVEMENT

Regular invigorating aerobic movement decreases your risk of a multitude of disorders, including your risk of breast cancer. Research shows that any type of aerobic movement for just thirty minutes, three to five times a week, decreases your risk of breast cancer by 25 to 50 percent. The more you exercise, the greater is your risk reduction. A study published in the journal *Epidemiology* in 2007 found that for every additional hour of physical activity per week done consistently— there is an additional 6 percent reduction in breast cancer risk. Other studies show that the risk of postmenopausal breast cancer can drop by as much as 80 percent for those who regularly engage in vigorous physical activity.

Vigorous activity in the teen years is particularly important because the effects are very significant and long lasting. If you were very active as a teenager, your risk of breast cancer may be as much as 30 percent lower than that of more sedentary teens. Polish researchers in 2007 found that women who were active between the ages of fourteen and twenty, and then lived a fairly sedentary lifestyle for the rest of their lives, had a lower risk than those who started recreational activities after the age of twenty!

If you have regularly exercised and develop breast cancer, your risk of recurrences, especially of estrogen receptor-negative (ER-) and progesterone receptor-negative (PR-) tumors, is much less. Moving your body after you have been diagnosed with breast cancer can significantly improve your outcome, regardless of the type or stage of your disease. According to a study published in the *Journal of the American Medical Association* (JAMA) in May 2005, if you have breast cancer and exercise during your treatment, your chances of surviving are twice as high. Just walking briskly for an average of three to five hours a week makes a significant difference. A 2011 study found that women who exercised regularly during the first three years after their diagnosis had a 40 percent lower risk of dying from their disease.

Regular invigorating movement will also benefit your quality of life during cancer treatments, including improving fatigue and depression. Active women receiving chemotherapy report fewer side effects. For example, the heart damage caused by anthracyclines (a class of chemotherapy drugs) is significantly reduced with aerobic exercise, according to a study published in 2011 in the journal *Circulation*.

Your Warrior Goddess thrives on regular movement that elevates your heart rate. It enlivens and expands her intelligence, and endows her with balance, strength, and stamina. Those gifts she then bestows on you. She becomes masterful at balancing your female hormones and regulating your menstrual cycles in a way that enhances your protection from breast cancer.

Researchers have found that aerobic exercise decreases both estrogen and progesterone levels, which contributes to lowering your risk. It also causes your menstrual cycles to lengthen—that is, the number of days between your periods becomes greater. The longer your menstrual cycles are, the fewer of them you'll have over a lifetime. In other words, you'll produce much less estrogen. Invigorating movement also produces hormonal changes that boost your immune system, making it stronger and more effective at fighting disease and getting rid of cancer cells. Changes in DNA, called methylation, are more frequent in cancer patients, and exercise has been shown to lower the levels of DNA methylation. When a methyl group is removed from the DNA, it improves the function of gene, including certain cancer-fighting genes such as a tumor-suppression gene identified as L3MBTL1. Moving your body also increases your natural production of melatonin.

Regular invigorating movement helps to keep your weight down, too. That's important when it comes to your risk of breast cancer. People who are obese have twice the risk of breast cancer as those who are of normal weight do (see Chapter 17). Weight gain during early adulthood is thought to be a major contributor to approximately one in every three cases of breast cancer diagnosed after menopause. The main reason for this is that fat creates estrogen. After menopause, your fat becomes an estrogen factory. So, if you include lively physical activity in your daily routine, you can keep both your fat stores and your risk of breast cancer to a minimum.

No matter how much you exercise, it is important to not sit too much! A 2013 study published in the *International Journal of Behavioral Nutrition and Physical Activity* found that compared to those who sit less than four hours a day, those who sit more than four hours a day are significantly more likely to have a chronic disease, including cancer, diabetes, heart disease, and high blood pressure. The more that people reported that they sat, the higher was their risk of chronic disease. The University of Sydney School of Public Health followed 200,000 adults, ages forty-five and older, for three years. Those who sat eleven or more hours a day were 40 percent more likely to die than people who sat fewer than four hours.

MENDING MATTERS OF THE HEART

Your heart beats about 100,000 times a day and about 35 million times every year. It circulates six quarts of life-giving blood to all the cells in your body three times every minute. But it is far more than just a pump. *Ayurveda* considers the heart to be the seat of your mind and consciousness. Of all the sacred spaces within your mind/body, your Warrior Goddess is most fond of your heart. It's where she communicates with you through your feelings.

When you show devotion to your Warrior Goddess by moving every day in ways that stimulate this sacred space, she expresses her gratitude by creating a powerful medicinal tonic that protects and strengthens your heart. It helps to keep your cardiovascular system strong, cuts many of the risk factors associated with heart disease and stroke, and lowers blood sugar, cholesterol, and triglycerides. It makes the good kind of cholesterol (high-density lipoproteins; HDL) go up and the bad kind (low-density lipoproteins; LDL) go down.

> *While I dance, I cannot judge, I cannot hate.*
> *I cannot separate myself from life.*
> *I can only be joyful and whole.*
> *That is why I dance.*

> —HANS BOS

Emotions are felt in the heart. *Ayurveda* says that the heart is the organ of emotion. *Ayurvedic* physicians always consider emotional causes first when they are evaluating patients with heart disease. Positive emotions can strengthen your heart, and negative emotions can weaken it. Research shows that if you have repressed anger and feelings of hostility, your risk of heart disease is higher.

A study published in the *Mayo Clinic Proceedings* in 1999 found that patients who participated in a cardiac-rehabilitation program within a month of having a heart attack showed significant improvements in feelings of hostility, anxiety, and depression. These patients also had a higher appreciation of the quality of their life. That's because the right types of movement provide your Warrior Goddess with a natural pharmacy of healing chemicals called neuropeptides. Neuropeptides relieve stress and reduce the risk of all stress-related illnesses, including peptic ulcers. Research also shows that neuropeptides soothe your emotions and ease depression as effectively as many popular antidepressant medications. That's important when it comes to your risk of breast cancer, because research shows that depressed women are much more likely to develop this disease.

AEROBIC EXERCISE

Brisk revitalizing activities are so stimulating to your Warrior Goddess that they enable her to bless you with a wide spectrum of protection. They lower your risk of type 2 diabetes and of developing cancers of the colon, ovary, uterus, and pancreas. If you smoke cigarettes—something extremely frustrating to her cosmic intelligence—exercise encourages her to forgive you somewhat by lowering your risk of lung cancer. Exercise will also reduce your risk of certain conditions, including asthma, mild emphysema, back problems, arthritis, glaucoma, and neurodegenerative diseases, such as Alzheimer's disease and senile dementia.

Those who exercise regularly tend to live much longer, too. The reason doesn't just come from preventing deaths from chronic diseases. Scientists believe it also has something to do with the fact that movement affects the segment on the end of your chromosomes, called telomeres, that directly relates to lifespan. As you age, your telomeres become shorter. An enzyme called telomerase slows down the shortening of telomeres and preserves their length, which has been shown to support a longer life. Exercise increases the production of telomerase and keeps your telomeres longer.

There are shortcuts to happiness, and dancing is one of them.

—VICKIE BAUM

Your Warrior Goddess is just waiting for you to start your sacred dance with her. She wants you to find some form of invigorating movement that speaks to you and expresses your soul. It may be dancing, bicycling, rowing, running, or a team sport. When you begin to increase your heart rate through an activity of your choosing, she will encourage you to continue. She is so grateful to you for this powerful form of protection that she will order pleasure-inducing endorphins—your body's natural morphine—to be released from your brain in return. Endorphins lift your spirits and give you a natural high. It's a great natural reward for the effort and dedication to your health.

Your schedule may be tight, but when you move your body with intentional vigor, even briefly, she loves the strength that she receives from it so much that she's willing to work around your schedule. She bestows the same protection on you no matter how you divide up the time you spend on aerobic activities. A study from the Department of Epidemiology at the Harvard School of Public Health published in 2000 found that it didn't matter whether you exercised for a long continuous period or broke it up into multiple shorter sessions. For instance, ten minutes of exercise three times a day is just as effective as one thirty-minute session.

Your Warrior Goddess appreciates every little bit of your effort. You can honor her by getting up and doing something during commercials if you're watching television. Park your car at the far end of the parking lot, and walk briskly to your destination. Get up from your desk for a few minutes every couple of hours, and climb a few flights of stairs. Remember, it all adds up. If your boss asks what you're doing, explain that you're taking a few minutes to make yourself more productive, decrease your number of sick days, and lower the company's healthcare costs! I doubt you'll hear any complaints. Even doing housework can cut your risk of breast cancer according to a study published in December 2006 in the journal *Cancer, Epidemiology, Biomarkers, and Prevention*.

STRENGTH TRAINING

Aerobic exercise isn't the only type of exercise that lowers your risk of breast cancer. Strength training with weights works, too. First, it increases muscle mass, and muscle uses more energy than fat. Therefore, your metabolism speeds up and that helps you lose even more weight. Second, strength training has been found to lower insulin-like growth factor-1 (IGF-1) levels by 15 percent. As you may recall, IGF-1 is a strong stimulator of breast cancer, so anything you do to lower the amount of it in your body will make a big difference in your risk of breast cancer.

Strength training is also the best thing you can do for your bones. It keeps them strong and lowers your risk of osteoporosis. A study conducted by Oregon State University published in 2001 followed postmenopausal women who did specific weight-bearing exercises for five years. The women had no decline in their bone density at the end of the study. Those women who didn't exercise lost density. Researchers feel that the best form of exercise for your overall health is a combination of aerobics, stretching, and strength training.

ANCIENT *AYURVEDIC* WISDOM

Ayurveda has recognized the importance of regular exercise for more than 5,000 years. It recommends that you participate in "medicinal movements" every day. But it also recognizes that too much of the wrong kind of exercise for your body type can have the opposite effect. It puts a strain on your body and can cause injuries and imbalances that increase your risk of disease. For instance, putting too much force into invigorating activities causes the release of oxygen free radicals, and that raises your risk of cancer. Extremely heavy exercise may make your muscles stronger, but the body, as a whole, may become weaker.

Ayurvedic Exercise Recommendations

1. **Exercise to 50 percent of your capacity.** If you follow this advice, you'll never overstrain your body, and it will gradually become stronger. You'll feel exhilarated and energized instead of drained. You'll be able to exercise every day instead of needing to take days off to recover. For example, if the most weight you can bench-press is 50 pounds for ten reps, do five reps instead.

2. **Exercise in the morning.** Different types of energy govern different times of the day.

   Between 6:00 A.M. and 10:00 A.M. is *kapha* time when your energy tends to be settled and slow. If you exercise during this time, you stimulate yourself out of any sluggishness, and you will feel energized all day. Incidentally, waking up in *kapha* time can make you feel lethargic when you get up. That's why *Ayurveda* recommends waking up before 6:00 A.M.

   Between 10:00 A.M. and 2:00 P.M. is *pitta* time. *Pitta* is associated with heat and digestion, and, therefore, *pitta* time is considered the worst time to exercise. When the sun is at its peak, you can easily become overheated by exercise. This is also the time of day when your digestion is at its peak. During this time you should eat your largest meal of the day, not exercise.

   Between 2:00 P.M. and 6:00 P.M. is *vata* time; *vata* governs movement. This is an acceptable time to exercise (although morning is considered best). The cycles then repeat. *Kapha* time is from 6:00 P.M. until 10:00 P.M. Only light exercise, such as walking, is recommended during this time. You should use this time to slow down and get ready to go to sleep. Vigorous activity during these hours is too stimulating and may cause you to have difficulty falling asleep.

3. **Choose movements that are right for your type.** *Ayurveda* recognizes that each of us is different. Different activities are recommended depending on your body type. Just as there are *vata*, *pitta*, and *kapha* times of day, there are *vata*, *pitta*, and *kapha* kinds of people.

   Vata people are thin and prone to anxiety and nervousness; they are usually cold and do everything fast. If this is you, slow-paced light exercises such as swimming, walking, and yoga are recommended.

   If you have a medium build, are usually hot, and have a quick temper and sharp intelligence, you are a *pitta* type. Moderate exercises such as brisk walking, cross-country skiing, swimming, cycling, weightlifting, and tennis are good for you.

If you have a tendency to be overweight, are easygoing and reliable—but possibly a little lazy—you are a *kapha* type. You need to get up and get moving as much as possible. Vigorous exercise, such as jogging, more intense weightlifting, and aerobics, is excellent for you.

4. **Perform special movements to facilitate the union of your mind/body and breath.** If you have ever wondered where yoga originated, wonder no more. Yoga got its start as unique postures prescribed by *Ayurveda*. In addition to regular exercise, *Ayurveda* recommends that you do yoga, too. The word "yoga" means union. The purpose of the exercises is to bring union to the mind and body, creating balance and promoting health. Yoga also helps to increase flexibility. Normally, you lose flexibility as you age. Yoga has been found to reduce anxiety, fatigue, tension, and stress and to improve mental function.

A Japanese study published in June 2000 in the journal *Perceptual and Motor Skills* examined the brainwave activity, as well as the level of the stress hormone cortisol, in yoga instructors during their practice of yoga. Researchers found that alpha brainwaves increased. Alpha waves correspond to a state of restful alertness. They are also the type of brainwaves found during the practice of Transcendental Meditation (TM). In addition, researchers found that blood-cortisol levels decreased during the practice of yoga. Cortisol levels go up in response to stress and go down when stress is relieved. As you can see, yoga has several powerful health-enhancing effects—especially reducing stress. According to studies at the National Institutes of Health (NIH), stress causes or aggravates approximately *90 percent* of all illnesses, including cancer, so reducing stress is *very* important.

5. **Wait at least two hours after a full meal to exercise.** It takes about two hours for your stomach to empty after a full meal. During this time, blood flow is increased to the digestive tract to facilitate digestion. If you exercise too soon after eating a full meal, you will divert the blood flow from your digestive tract to your muscles and impede the digestive process.

6. **Wait at least thirty minutes after you exercise before you eat.** When you exercise, blood flow increases to your muscles and is shunted away from your digestive tract. Therefore, if you eat while exercising, or too soon afterward, there won't be enough blood available for your digestive tract to function properly. After about thirty minutes of rest, your muscles no longer need additional blood so your digestive tract can get all the blood it needs without any interference.

7. **Don't strain when you exercise. Cut back if you start to breathe heavily through your mouth.** Research shows that over-exercising can actually be detrimental to your health. It depresses your immune system and increases free-radical production. So it's important not to stress yourself too much during exercise. Just like medications, herbs, foods, or anything else that's good for your health, there's a proper amount to take; too much or too little of these things can create imbalances that lead to disease.

8. **If you meditate, practice yoga before meditation and your conventional exercises afterward.** Yoga helps to center and relax the body and mind and prepare it for meditation. On the other hand, stimulating exercise activates the body and mind—the opposite of the effect required to foster meditation.

Everything in the universe has rhythm—everything dances.

—MAYA ANGELOU

FINDING YOUR OWN MOVEMENT

If you have never experienced a form of movement that expresses your soul, keep looking; you'll find it. You were designed to enjoy moving with vigor and dynamism. Nature created special neuropeptides to reward you with bliss when you dance and move to the individual expression of your soul. These magical molecules of movement create a feeling of exhilaration and make you naturally high on life.

There are so many different ways that you can express yourself in movement. No matter what your personal preferences are or what your physical condition is, you can find something that resonates with your soul. Consider biking, jogging, or brisk walking; you can do these activities solo or with a friend. If you like to have company when you exercise, find a partner for a two-person sport such as tennis, racquetball, or one-on-one basketball. Or you may simply want to find a buddy to work out with at the gym. If you discover that you enjoy working out at the gym but you need a more structured format to keep you motivated, make a series of appointments with a personal trainer. Last, if you like to be part of a group that meets regularly, then you may really enjoy taking an exercise class. You can find a class for just about anything: aerobics, cycling, kickboxing, martial arts, dancing, rowing—you name it.

Even if you are obese and haven't exercised in years, it's never too late to start. However, be sure to speak with your doctor before you begin any exercise program. Walking is a great activity for just about anyone who wants to begin exercising. Each day, choose a destination that's a little farther away or simply pick up the pace at which you walk. Beginner's yoga is another good starting point. Try out different activities to find the one that's fun for you and suits you best.

> To dance is to be out of yourself, larger, more powerful,
> more beautiful. This is power. It is glory on Earth,
> and it is yours for the taking.
>
> —AGNES DE MILLE

Chapter 26

Emotional Healing
Using Your Emotions
for Your Benefit

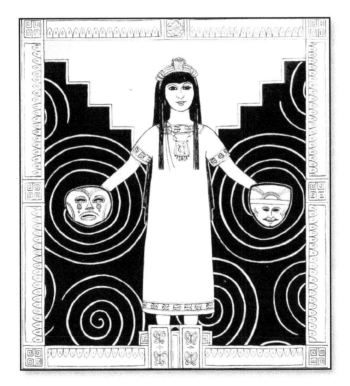

Goddess of Emotional Choice

A merry heart does good like medicine.

—PROVERBS 17:27

*E*ach feeling that you have creates a biochemical reaction in your body. When you feel up and positive, your mind/body produces the chemicals and hormones that enhance your inner healing intelligence, stimulate your immune system, and strengthen your health. When you feel depressed or angry, your mind/body produces other hormones and chemicals that obstruct your healing intelligence, depress your immune system, and weaken your health. In other words, positive emotions stimulate a surge of powerful natural chemicals that magnify your Warrior Goddess's healing might. Negative emotions and stress have the opposite effect; they depress your Warrior Goddess, dampen her brilliance, and diminish her ability to defend and protect. It's no wonder researchers have found that the chemicals released in response to your emotions can affect your risk of breast cancer.

EMOTION MOLECULES

Every emotion you feel is packaged in molecules that spread throughout your body. These molecules of emotion, in turn, cause the release of other chemicals and hormones or may stimulate impulses in your nervous system. When you feel positive and upbeat, healing chemicals are released that help to keep you strong and healthy. When you feel down and depressed, stress hormones and other chemicals that impair your immune system and your health become abundant. Negative emotions, unresolved anger, repressed and suppressed emotions, and stress can take a big toll on your health. But there are many techniques that you can use to process your emotions effectively and reduce how much your mind/body reacts to stressful situations.

In her book *Molecules of Emotion*, Candice Pert, Ph.D., documented that every thought you think, every emotion you express, triggers the release of neurotransmitter molecules that spread throughout your body. If you've ever questioned the mind/body connection, think back to a time when you just missed hitting another car or almost fell down the stairs. Your heart started racing, your breathing increased, a prickly sensation may have rushed through your body, you felt a little lightheaded, had a sinking feeling in your stomach, and maybe even started trembling. When you become angry or upset, your face turns red, your blood pressure goes up, and your skin may break out in hives. In these situations, your body is reacting to a flood of chemicals released by your brain and nervous system. The connection between mind and body is clearly an intimate one; you can't separate them.

One of the most fascinating studies I've ever read dramatically proves the point of the union between mind and body. It's a study of heart transplant donors and recipients published in the journal *Integrative Medicine* in March

2000. Researchers observed as many as five donor characteristics in a recipient after transplant.

In one case, a fifty-six-year-old heart transplant recipient began having flashbacks of seeing a Jesus-like image followed by a flash of light. He then experienced an intense burning sensation over his face. The organ donor had been a thirty-four-year-old policeman who died after being shot in the face by a drug dealer who allegedly looked like Jesus.

In another case, the donor was an eighteen-year-old introverted male who wrote poetry and music. The recipient was an eighteen-year-old female who, according to her father, had been "wild." After her transplant, she started playing the guitar and writing songs and became quiet and reserved like the donor.

Other examples include a militant gay woman who chose a heterosexual lifestyle after receiving the heart of a heterosexual woman; a five-year-old child who recognized the never-before-seen father of the donor in a crowd, ran up to him, climbed into his lap, and called him "Daddy"; and a male recipient who loved meat before the transplant, but became nauseated by it after receiving the heart of a female vegetarian.

The Science of How Emotions Affect Our Immune System

When you feel an emotion, scientists say that it's processed through the brain's limbic system and the hypothalamus. The hypothalamus releases neuropeptides, which then stimulate the pituitary gland to release hormones. All the endocrine glands, especially the adrenals, react to these hormones by producing other hormones that can weaken or strengthen the function of the immune system. Certain immune-system cells called "lymphocytes" have receptors that receive messages from the molecules released by thoughts and feelings. The hypothalamus also has receptors for peptides released by the immune system's lymphocytes.

A two-way communication takes place between your emotional center and your immune system. Anger, fear, and rage produce neurochemicals that strain your body and can damage your organs. On the other hand, laughter reduces levels of cortisol and epinephrine, stress hormones that are released by the adrenal glands. Laughter also stimulates the activity of the immune system. In a study published in *Alternative Therapies in Health & Medicine* in March 2002, researchers found that laughter increased natural killer (NK) cell function, as well as that of many other types of immune-system cells. These immune-boosting effects lasted for twelve hours after "humor intervention." Depression and suppression of strong emotions can generate such a blow to your immune system that it nearly stops functioning. Depressed women are nearly four times more likely to get breast cancer than those who have never been depressed, according to researchers at the University of Pennsylvania.

Time spent laughing is time spent with the gods.

—A JAPANESE PROVERB

To Be Human Is to Be Emotional

We are spiritual beings having a human experience. The human experience involves a wide range of feelings and emotions—from sadness, resentfulness, and hatred, to compassion, forgiveness, and love. As human beings, it is part of our journey to continually feel and process emotions. Imagine if you felt nothing—no compassion, no desire, no joy, no sense of accomplishment, no pride, no pleasure, no pain. Nothing could move you to tears—not the most exquisite beauty of Nature, not the birth of your child, not the atrocities of war. Nothing! It's hard to even imagine. Feelings and emotions were designed for a reason: They give purpose to life.

The Energy Center of Emotion

The ancient *Ayurvedic* texts describe energy centers called *chakras,* which are located in different areas of the body. The heart *chakra* is referred to as the fourth *chakra.* In Sanskrit, it's called the *Anahata chakra.* It's said to be the energy center that enables you to feel higher emotions, such as love, compassion, forgiveness, tolerance, happiness, and joy. Your heart is what allows you to "feel," according to *Ayurveda.* It is the center of your emotions and the home of your consciousness. Activating and balancing the heart expands your consciousness. The heart *chakra* is considered to be the fundamental center for your growth as a human being.

Dr. Caroline Myss, medical intuitive and author of *Anatomy of the Spirit: The Seven States of Power and Healing* and *Why People Don't Heal and How They Can,* says that the fourth *chakra* focuses on your feelings about your internal world. Your emotional responses to your own thoughts, ideas, attitudes, and inspirations, as well as the attention you give to your emotional needs, are all contained within this *chakra.* Anatomically, the fourth *chakra* is located right over your heart and breasts. Energetically speaking, everything you feel with your heart also affects your breasts.

According to Dr. Myss, breast cancer is a fourth *chakra* issue. The fourth *chakra* has to do with how you express the emotions that you feel and your capacity to form mutually beneficial, balanced relationships with others and with yourself. In Dr. Myss's experience, women who develop breast cancer have issues with hope and trust. They often suffer from hurt, sorrow, and unfinished business. In a 1995 study, women who had suffered a major loss such as divorce, loss of a job, or some other stressful trauma within the past five years were twelve times more likely to have breast cancer than those who hadn't had one. According to Christiane Northrup, M.D., in her book *Women's Bodies, Women's Wisdom,* studies that look at the different personality patterns of women with different types of cancers found some statistically significant common patterns in women with breast cancer. For example, they tended to have emotionally distant fathers; they had a greater tendency to stay in loveless marriages; and during their childhood, they most likely had the responsibility of caring for their younger siblings. These women also had a greater probability of not taking care of their own physical needs and getting proper medical care.

Behavioral studies show that women who develop breast cancer have a tendency to be caregivers. They take care of everyone else's needs before they take care of their own. Take a look at your life, and make sure you're taking care of your own needs. Don't sacrifice what you need to do to take care of yourself in order to take care of other people. Nurture yourself by doing things that make you feel good. As a very wise friend of mine says, "The best way to take care of other people is to take care of *yourself* first." In fact, it is very important to learn how to truly love yourself. There are many programs available that can help you with the process. One of my favorites is one by Christine Arylo called "Madly in Love with Me." You can download the guidebook on www.madlyinlovewithme.com.

I watched a video last year with Steve Sinatra, M.D., a holistic cardiologist, who said, "Did you ever notice that when you are in love you don't get sick?" That's because the emotions of being in love are the best immune boosters ever. I thought—why not try to generate those feelings about myself? If I do, I won't have to rely on an outside source that may or may not be there. Every day I woke up and did a meditation where I felt into my heart, focused on generating the feelings of being in love, and then repeated several times "I am in love with myself!" I did this several times throughout the day and before I went to bed at night. Within a few days I amazed at how overcome I was with joy, peace, and happiness. When I shared this with some of my girlfriends, they tried it and said they couldn't believe how peaceful and happy they felt, too. Give it a try! It's magical.

All human beings tend toward negative self-talk—I don't understand why we are designed this way, but it appears that most of us are. I call it a design flaw. But that's how it is, so chances are you have an inner "mean-committee" that needs to be gagged. You know that critical one that likes tell you that you aren't enough of something to be lovable: not skinny enough, not smart enough, not pretty enough, or whatever—you fill in the blank. Every time it has something nasty to say, thank the committee members for sharing and then tell them to go take a hike. Immediately, counteract those negative words by saying something great to yourself; for example, how kind, loving, or generous you are. Take on a practice such as the self-love exercise I mentioned above. Not only will replacing the negative thoughts with positive ones improve your immune system, but it will also bring you more peace, joy, and happiness. The more you practice self-love, the quieter the inner mean-committee becomes. Instead of constantly belittling you, eventually, it will only whisper weak criticisms every once in a while to test you.

Managing our emotions increases intuition and clarity.
It helps us self-regulate our brain chemicals and internal hormones.
It gives us natural highs, the real fountain of youth we've been
searching for. It enables us to drink from elixirs locked within
our cells, just waiting for us to discover them.

—Doc Childre

LEARNING TO COPE WITH STRESS

Arriving home from a rough day at the office, you open the door. The kids are shouting, the house is a mess, the dog ran away, and everyone wants to know what's for supper. Yes, you know what stress feels like, but do you really know the magnitude of destruction that this level of chronic stress can have on you? According to studies at the National Institutes of Health (NIH), *approximately 90 percent of all illnesses—mental and physical—are caused by or aggravated by stress!*

Dr. Hans Seyle, a pioneering stress researcher, defines stress as a psychophysiological (mind/body) event that takes place when your system is overwhelmed by any experience: physical, mental, or emotional. Stress isn't something *out there;* it's completely subjective and internal. It is a mind/body reaction.

Researchers have found that stress causes a cascade of neurochemical reactions that can lead to disease. In stressful situations, the adrenal glands release cortisol, epinephrine, and norepinephrine, otherwise known as the *stress hormones.* The pituitary releases more stress-related hormones, and as a result, the sympathetic branch of the autonomic nervous system "revs" up. The response is known as *fight or flight.* It's very useful—even essential—in an emergency, because it gives you the ability to respond quickly for your safety, for example, jumping out of the way of a New York City taxicab.

However, that fight-or-flight response is neither necessary nor appropriate if, for instance, you're at work and you receive an e-mail from your significant other saying that he wants to date other people. You can neither engage in a fight nor take off in flight under the circumstances.

The subsequent psycho-physiological response leaves behind a soup of chemicals that stick around and wreak havoc on your system. They can cause high blood pressure, insomnia, anxiety, depression, frustration, anger, and tension; they can increase risk factors for heart disease, diabetes, and stomach ulcers; they can depress your immune system; and they can even enlarge your waistline. Stress reactions also cause an increase in oxygen free radicals and inflammation—both of which are linked to most degenerative diseases including accelerated aging, wrinkles, and cancer.

As I was reflecting on stress and its effects on the body, I came to the conclusion that stress, in one form or another, is responsible for the origin of *all* disease. *Ayurveda* describes five disease stages, and the first stage begins with an imbalance. According to *Ayurveda, perfect health is all about the perfect balance of mind and body.* So, when something takes your system out of balance, it creates stress in your body, and that stress initiates disease.

You're probably familiar with the list of big stressors: death of a loved one, divorce, moving, and loss of a job. But what you may not have considered is that just about anything can create stress in your body. Too much or too little of things that are considered good for you—or even essential—can do it: good food, rest, exercise, a vacation, or any sensory stimulus. Of course, traditionally bad-for-you things can cause it, too, like eating the wrong food, eating too late at night, staying up too late, watching too much TV, or watching a violent movie. Other big stressors can be war, a drop in the stock market, toxins in your environment, a strained relationship, traffic, loud noises, and the challenges of travel. Anything can induce a stress reaction if you don't receive it in the proper way at the right time in the correct amount.

According to *Ayurveda,* the best way to prevent stress is to live life in a way that keeps your body in perfect balance. This is precisely what the techniques and recommendations of *Ayurveda* are designed to do. The most precise way to do this is to see an *Ayurvedic* physician (a *vaidya*) who will determine your physiological type (*vata, pitta, kapha,* or a mixed blend of two of these types) and prescribe the proper foods, exercises, and routines you need to keep your specific physiology in balance. Keep in mind that what brings one person into balance may induce stress in another. However, despite individual differences, there are many things that are effective at reducing stress or, at least, at decreasing your physiological response to it.

10 Stress-Reducing Techniques

1. **Get enough sleep at the proper times.** This topic is covered in Chapter 24.

2. **Eat primarily fresh organic fruits, vegetables, and grains.** Hundreds, if not thousands of studies, show that a plant-based diet—especially when the plants are organically grown, whole, fresh, and unprocessed—is loaded with protective nutrients, like antioxidants, that guard against stress and disease. Conventionally grown foods (grown with pesticides and other chemicals), red meat, processed foods, leftovers, and frozen or canned foods all have lower nutritional values, increase oxygen free radicals, and are generally toxic to your body. Chapter 5 deals with this subject.

3. **Practice an effective, stress-reducing meditation.** More than 500 research studies have shown that Transcendental Meditation (TM) is more effective at reducing the signs and symptoms of stress than any other meditation or stress-reducing technique, including biofeedback and progressive muscle relaxation. TM significantly lessens anxiety, depression, insomnia, digestive disturbances, neurotic tendencies, physical complaints, and psychosomatic problems. This mental technique also decreases the risk of being admitted to the hospital for any reason—physical or mental—by more than 50 percent. Chapter 27 contains a full discussion on the benefits of TM.

4. **Avoid assaults to your senses.** Any strong, prolonged, or otherwise caustic stimulus to your senses can induce stress: loud noises, certain forms of music (for me, the worst is the heavy-metal, head-banging variety), strong unpleasant odors, hot spices, watching TV or sitting at a computer too long, or exposure to extreme temperatures.

5. **Listen to relaxing music.** Studies show that classical music or any other soothing music of your choice can cause a significant relaxation response.

6. **Get a massage, or give yourself one.** Massage has been found to release many hormones associated with relaxation, and it boosts the immune system. The effects are enhanced when a good penetrating oil, like sesame oil, is used.

7. **Have fun.** Don't let your life become all about work and getting things done on your to-do list. Make sure you balance things out by regularly includ-

ing some of your favorite activities. Frequently participate in activities that are fun and joyful for you, such as getting out in Nature, riding your bike, going to a play, singing, playing with your kids, enjoying a day at the spa, spending time with friends, dancing, or soaking in the bathtub with a good book. Make a habit of doing something that brings you joy every day.

8. **Take an antioxidant supplement.** The many benefits of taking a good antioxidant are discussed in Chapter 13. A stress reaction creates excess oxygen free radicals, which have been linked to most chronic degenerative disorders including Alzheimer's disease, cancer, and accelerated aging. Some good antioxidants are vitamin C, vitamin E, selenium, and CoQ_{10}. The *Ayurvedic* herbal mixture *Amrit Kalash,* according to research, may be the best antioxidant of all. Dr. Yukie Niwa, a Japanese researcher, studied more than 500 different antioxidants over a period of thirty years. He found that the most powerful and effective antioxidant of all those tested was Maharishi *Amrit Kalash.*

9. **Take an herbal supplement.** Certain herbs have been shown to effectively reduce the stress response through a variety of mechanisms. They are called "adaptogens" because they help us adapt to stress. For example, research shows that an *Ayurvedic* herb called holy basil, which has a 5,000-year-plus history of use, protects against and reduces stress. It decreases the release of the stress hormone cortisol. It also enhances stamina and endurance, increases the body's effective use of oxygen, and boosts the immune system when you're under stress. In addition, it slows aging and provides a rich supply of antioxidants, as well as a multitude of other benefits.

10. **Exercise regularly.** In many studies, regular aerobic exercise has been found to be *as effective* in relieving depression as pharmaceutical medications. Yoga is also a wonderful stress reliever.

Some of these stress-reducing techniques are what *Ayurveda* would call "behavioral *rasayanas.*" As you may recall, *rasayana* is "that which negates old age and disease." *Ayurveda* recommends certain behaviors to negate old age and disease. Molecular studies have shown that uplifting activities and emotions produce molecules (neuropeptides) that strengthen your immune system and overall health. The behavioral *rasayanas* to practice, according to *Ayurveda,* are respect, love, compassion, uplifting speech, cleanliness, charity and regular donations, religious observances, being positive, moderation, and simplicity. The behaviors to avoid are anger, violence, harsh or hurtful speech, speaking ill of others, egotism, dishonesty, and jealousy.

Why not learn to enjoy the little things—
there are so many of them.
—AUTHOR UNKNOWN

Ayurveda also says that to reduce stress you should *pay attention to the rhythms of the day, week, month, and year.* If you attune yourself to the rhythms of Nature and adjust your activities accordingly, you will strengthen your immune system and enhance your health. If you keep unnatural routines, you will weaken your immune system.

Modern science has documented daily fluctuations in hormones and biorhythms. There are better times during the day for some activities than for others. The most obvious one is sleep (see Chapter 24). If you sleep during the "wrong" hours, your risk of breast cancer can increase by as much as 50 percent or more.

IDEAL *AYURVEDIC* DAILY ROUTINE

- Rise before 6:00 A.M.
- Use the bathroom.
- Give yourself a sesame-oil massage.
- Wait twenty minutes, and take a warm shower.
- Practice yoga for at least fifteen minutes.
- Practice breathing exercises (*pranayama*; see opposite page) for about ten to fifteen minutes.
- Meditate for twenty minutes or longer.
- Exercise for about a half hour (see Chapter 25 for more details).
- Eat a light breakfast of cooked fruits.
- Go to work.
- Eat your main meal at noon.
- Rest for ten minutes after your meal.
- Go back to work.
- Do your evening meditation program: yoga, breathing, and meditation.
- Eat a light dinner.
- Walk after dinner.

- Read something pleasant, enjoy pleasant conversation, or listen to soothing music.

- Go to bed by 10:00 P.M.

> *Slow down and everything you are chasing*
> *will come around and catch you.*

—JOHN DE PAOLA

PRANAYAMA—USING YOUR BREATH

Breathing is synonymous with life. If you stop breathing, you stop living. But breathing has many finer aspects than the black and white of life and death. The way you breathe can affect your health for better or worse. *Ayurveda* uses a set of breathing techniques called "*pranayama*" to enhance health and lower stress.

Prana is a Sanskrit word that means "breath," but its full meaning goes way beyond that. In *Ayurveda*, *prana* is known as "life energy," paralleling the ancient notion of "*chi*" energy in China, "vital force" for the ancient Greeks, and "*ki*" in ancient Japanese medicine. *Prana* is the life force that governs all bodily functions and influences your mind, memory, thought, and emotions. By breathing with the techniques of *pranayama*, *Ayurveda* says you can strengthen your life force and induce balance, which enhances your health and lowers your risk of disease.

Pranayama literally means "regulating the breath." The techniques of *pranayama* are numerous but usually involve breathing through alternating nostrils. The technique of breathing through alternating nostrils is said to create balance in the physiology, improve the function of the nervous system, and benefit many specific organs.

Research has documented that the regular practice of *pranayama* increases the depth and the length of time that you're able to hold your breath and enlarges the vital capacity of your lungs. It improves stress-hormone balance and decreases pulse rate, blood pressure, and blood fats such as cholesterol. *Pranayama* can also be extremely beneficial in treating asthma.

One *Pranayama* Technique

Pranayama is usually practiced just before meditation to settle the body and mind and facilitate transcending (see Chapter 27). You can also use *pranayama* to help calm yourself whenever you are upset. Here's a simple way to practice:

1. Sit upright, and close your eyes.

2. Use your right thumb to gently close your right nostril.

3. Breathe out through your left nostril slowly and naturally until you breathe your breath completely out. Don't force it.

4. Breathe slowly back in the same (left) nostril.

5. Close your left nostril with the long finger or ring finger on your right hand.

6. Release your thumb on your right nostril, and breathe out slowly and easily.

7. Breathe back in through the same (right) nostril.

Repeat this process for about five to ten minutes. You should notice an almost immediate calming effect.

There is more to life than increasing its speed.

—MOHANDAS K. GANDHI

CHANGING YOUR REACTION

Life is stressful. Many events take place every day that are beyond your control. You can't prevent them from happening, but you can change how you react to them. Remember, stress isn't something *out there*. It's purely subjective and an *internal* reaction. You can decrease the severity of your stress response by getting enough sleep at the proper times, respecting the rhythms of Nature, eating a healthy diet, avoiding assaults on your senses, participating regularly in activities that bring you joy, taking care of yourself by getting regular massages, listening to relaxing music, exercising daily, and remembering to breathe (especially using the techniques of *pranayama*).

There are also a number of very effective techniques that can help you to instantly shift or release your negative emotions—whether they have been long-standing or have just arisen. One of the simplest and best is the Emotional Freedom Technique (EFT). Nothing fancy is required—it only takes a few minutes to learn, is free, and can be done anywhere. There are some great instructional videos on YouTube. (Here is a link to one I recommend: www.youtube.com/watch?v=6i33V2EcVlY.) Finally, one of the most powerful techniques you can use to protect your health from the damaging effects of stress is the daily practice of an effective meditation—the topic of the next chapter.

Near the beginning of this chapter, I told you about a few fascinating stories of heart transplant patients which dramatically prove that memories are not just stored in the brain, but also in the body. Trapped stressful emotions and traumatic memories can be responsible for a spectrum of chronic health problems; for example, chronic pain, fibromyalgia, and recurring emotional upsets. There are several types of treatments that help to release these trapped emotions. The most effective one that I have personally experienced is called Body Memory Recall (BMR). Developed by Jonathan Tripodi, stored memories and their emotions are released from the body using a unique method of energy work and physical touch similar to myofacial release. I recommend reading Jonathan's book *Freedom from Body Memory* to learn more about this technique. He has trained practitioners in BMR all over the country. To find someone who is certified in your area, go to: www.freedomfrombodymemory.com.

> *Tension is who you think you should be.*
> *Relaxation is who you are.*
>
> —CHINESE PROVERB

Chapter 27

Turning Inward

Cranking Up the Volume of Balance

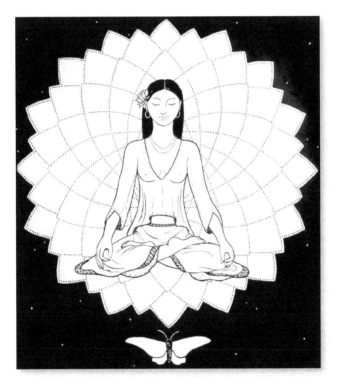

Goddess of Meditation

If the inner mind is not deluded,
the outer actions will not be wrong.

—PROVERB OF TIBET

*T*urning inward to reach that quiet part of yourself is one of the simplest and most effective things you can do to rebalance and recharge your health. At the center of each of us is our soul and spirit—the part of ourselves that is connected to all other people and all other things. It is our *true* Self. But in this plane of existence, we are often so caught up with surface activities and concerns that we forget where our true Self lies—deep within. When we take the time to quiet our mind and reconnect with our Self, we are also tapping into universal energy, because at the finest level, *that's* who we are. Uniting with the Source is like touching Nature's tuning fork—we start to vibrate with tremendous calming, rebalancing, and healing energy.

The most effective way to turn inward is through the practice of meditation. While you sleep, your Warrior Goddess—although replenished by your rest— is still actively managing all the critical purification and rejuvenation events that take place within your body. But when you meditate, your Warrior Goddess soaks much more deeply in a soothing bath of pure relaxation. She stays with you, but she also goes home to her Source. Each time you reunite with your Self, your Warrior Goddess experiences rebirth and emerges with immense strength. When you make it a daily practice to go within and reunite with your Source, your Warrior Goddess's power to keep you balanced, whole, and well becomes so vast that she remains virtually invincible.

Transcendental Meditation® (TM)

Research shows that the most effective stress-relieving, anxiety-reducing, and health-promoting form of meditation is Transcendental Meditation (TM). *Ayurveda* considers TM to be the single most important modality for inducing balance, integrating the mind and body, preventing disease, and restoring health.

THE FOURTH STATE OF CONSCIOUSNESS

To meditate means to think, contemplate, or concentrate on something. *To transcend* means to go beyond. During the practice of TM, a unique state of consciousness is reached by transcending thought. It is characterized by a state of restful alertness and deep silence. Typically, the only states of consciousness you routinely experience are waking, sleeping, and dreaming.

When you practice TM, your mind goes to a fourth distinct state of consciousness, appropriately named "transcendental consciousness," or pure consciousness. Brainwave recordings, called electroencephalographs (EEGs), reveal that this special state of consciousness produces patterns completely different from those seen when you are awake, dreaming, or sleeping. For instance, the left and right hemispheres of the brain are normally asynchronous, which means that they have very different rhythms in their brainwave patterns. During transcendental consciousness, the two hemispheres begin to synchronize and alpha waves predominate. Alpha waves are generally associated with a state of restful alertness. Practitioners of this type of meditation report that when they "transcend," they experience feelings of rest, relaxation, calmness, peace, expansiveness, and unity with the world. In essence, this mental technique is a powerful behavioral *rasayana*—"that which negates old age and disease."

Quantum Physics and Consciousness

Quantum physics has shown us that the world we perceive, the material world, is just an illusion. An atom—the smallest particle of an element—is made up of more space than matter. So, what appears solid, such as a table, is actually mostly empty space. According to quantum physicists, underlying all the diversity of the material world is the real world: a homogeneous, nonchanging, unified field composed of nothing but small vibrating strings. If you're interested in reading more about this, I recommend a wonderful book that beautifully explains the "superstring theory" called *The Elegant Universe* by quantum physicist Brian Greene.

What lies beyond these strings? What controls the vibration of all these strings and how they manifest the diversity of the material world? According to scientists (and logic), there *must* be an underlying field of intelligence or consciousness that manages these strings. Scientists have called this field of intelligence the "unified field of intelligence," or the "unified field of consciousness." This field holds the power to orchestrate Nature; therefore, it contains all the laws of Nature.

When you experience transcendental consciousness, your mind merges with this unified field of consciousness. This merging powerfully establishes balance in your mind/body. In other words, when you tap into the Source that holds the knowledge of all the things you need to do to keep your body in perfect balance and perfect health (the laws of Nature), you are immersed in this knowledge and at the same time soothed and healed by its balancing effects. Not surprisingly, when people first connect with this Source of knowledge, they discover that they spontaneously start making choices in alignment with good health. For example, their yearning to smoke cigarettes, drink alcohol, and partake in other disease-promoting activities decreases, and their desire to eat nourishing foods and engage in healthy activities increases. That's why research shows that regularly experiencing this unified field of consciousness produces powerful health benefits in mind, body, spirit, and emotions.

TM's Mind/Body Health Benefits

More than 500 studies have been conducted on TM at 200-plus independent institutions and universities in more than thirty different countries. These studies show that the health benefits of experiencing transcendental consciousness daily are nothing short of miraculous. It dramatically reduces stress and anxiety and promotes good health. (For more information on the background of TM, see the inset "The History of TM" below.)

As you may recall, according to the National Institutes of Health (NIH), stress is the cause of, or a major contributing factor in, more than 90 percent of all illnesses. Because TM radically lowers stress, it also substantially lowers the risk of most diseases. For example, research shows that people who practice this form of meditation daily have 56 percent fewer hospital admissions for all diag-

---

The History of Transcendental Meditation

Transcendental meditation is not a new technique. In India, it was passed on from teacher (yogi) to student for thousands of years. It remained unavailable to the general public until the late 1950s when concern over the deteriorating health and collective consciousness of the world's people drove one yogi into action. Maharishi Mahesh Yogi adopted the task of teaching this technique to the public. He and his lineage of masters knew that the simple mental practice of TM was so powerful that if enough people were taught how to do it, it could substantially improve health, calm the collective consciousness, and promote world peace.

In the mid-twentieth century, the practice of meditation was radically foreign to most people in the West. In order to gain widespread acceptance and to encourage as many people as possible to learn it, a focus was also placed on research to prove and document TM's many astounding benefits. Studies were initiated all over the world. Today—thanks to the proliferation of studies that show that TM is a remarkably effective approach for boosting and fostering health and peace—millions of people throughout the world have learned this technique and practice it daily.

noses, including cancer and accidents, and 87 percent fewer admissions for cardiovascular diseases, including heart disease.

The research-proven health benefits of the regular daily practice of TM are
numerous, diverse, and impressive. They include lower blood pressure, reversal of coronary artery disease, better mental capacity with improved academic
performance, enhanced creativity, and improved verbal and analytical thinking.
TM is also associated with less worry, depression, and anxiety, as well as with
fewer emotional disturbances, better relationships, enhanced job performance,
and increased satisfaction.

TM and Addictions

For many people, overcoming health-destroying addictions is one of the most
difficult challenges they will face in their lifetime. Standard treatment programs
are very successful for some, but for others, especially over the long-term, they
are not. Researchers have found that people have greater success in overcoming
addictions if they replace a health-destroying habit with another habit—ideally
one that is health-supporting, such as the practice of an effective stress-reducing meditation. A meta-analysis of 198 independent treatment outcomes for
drug, alcohol, and cigarette addictions found that the daily practice of TM was
more effective in helping people overcome these addictions than any of the standard treatment programs.

TM and Aging

One of the most astonishing findings about the regular practice of TM is that it
can *reverse* the aging process. Research shows that individuals who have medi-
tated for more than five years are physiologically about twelve years younger
than those who haven't. These conclusions were based on measurements of
near-point vision, hearing, and systolic blood pressure—all of which predictably
worsen with age.

As you age, the levels of hormones in your body also change. For example,
you produce much less of the hormone dehydroepiandrosterone sulfate
(DHEA)—the most abundant hormone found in young adults. DHEA has many
positive roles in the body, one of which is to help in the production of lean muscle mass. By the time you reach your mid-thirties, you start losing lean muscle
mass and declining DHEA levels are thought to be largely responsible for this
phenomenon. Research shows that you can slow down the rate at which DHEA
levels drop and stay physiologically younger by exercising and practicing TM.
In general, the level of DHEA in TM practitioners is the same as that normally
found in people five to ten years younger.

As a woman, maintaining youthful DHEA levels is especially important since this hormone also has a protective role against breast cancer and osteoporosis. Studies show that women with high DHEA levels have lower risks of these diseases.

Please note that I don't recommend taking supplemental DHEA because its long-term safety has not been adequately evaluated and there is some cause for concern. Raising and maintaining your DHEA levels naturally seems to have a far different effect on your body than taking supplemental DHEA. DHEA is a steroid-type molecule that is converted to testosterone and estrogen in the body. Taking supplemental DHEA may abnormally raise the levels of these hormones and has been reported to cause unwanted hair growth, acne, and mood swings.

Of even greater concern is that it may also increase the risk and accelerate the growth of breast and prostate cancer. In a study published in the *European Journal of Clinical Nutrition*, prolonged supplementation of DHEA, particularly by those who are obese, significantly increases the risk of postmenopausal breast cancer. Higher serum concentrations of DHEA are thought to increase the risk through several mechanisms. For one, a high concentration of DHEA increases the level of IGF-1, a known a breast-cancer promoter. A second mechanism involves the androgenic metabolites of DHEA, which may have a direct stimulatory effect on breast cells. DHEA may also activate estrogen receptors. If you have breast cancer, you definitely should not take supplemental DHEA.

Learning TM

You can't learn TM from a book. As my good friend and long-time teacher of this technique says, "Think of it like flying a plane." You would never try to fly a plane if your only experience came from reading a flight-instruction manual. There are many variables and subtle nuances that can make the difference in a safe flight. Similarly, awareness of the refined subtleties of TM can make all the difference in successful practice. If you don't practice TM properly, you will not reap the full health benefits.

Like flight instructors, certified teachers of TM have gone through a long, rigorous training course to become proficient at teaching this technique. To locate a certified teacher in your area, call 1-800-LEARN-TM (1-800-532-7686) or go to www.TM.org. The Transcendental Meditation program is taught in seven steps over four days.

There are a couple of common concerns people have that interfere with learning and practicing this technique. The first is time. When will they find time in their already overloaded day to meditate? Rest assured, TM is practiced for only twenty minutes, twice a day. Anyone can squeeze two twenty-minute sessions into his or her day with relative ease. Here's how: Wake up twenty minutes earlier than you usually do, or meditate on your way to work if you take mass transit, or skip one half-hour television show in the evening and meditate, instead.

Another common concern that people have is that learning to meditate is difficult because you must force your mind to stop thinking. People who believe this fear that they won't be able to meditate successfully because their mind is always racing. The TM technique is a simple, effortless, natural process that your mind easily follows. You don't have to *try* to do anything. There's no forcing, no concentrating, and no effort required.

Taking the time to learn and practice TM is one of the best gifts you can give your Warrior Goddess. There's nothing more powerful that you can do to improve your overall health and decrease your risk of disease. Practicing TM will also help you to specifically reduce your risk of breast cancer by decreasing stress, promoting hormones that reduce your risk, and helping you to make spontaneous choices that are better for your health. If you smoke or drink excessive alcohol—two risk factors for breast cancer—TM can also help you break your addictions to these substances by reducing your desire for them.

OTHER FORMS OF MEDITATION

Learning TM is expensive, and unfortunately teachers are becoming more difficult to find. So, if you cannot arrange to learn TM, consider learning another form of meditation. Although other forms of meditation may not be as effective as TM, they certainly have their benefits. Be sure to research various techniques to find one that works for you. Certain types of concentration meditation may actually increase anxiety, so be careful in your choice of technique. Other good stress-reducing and health-promoting practices, such as yoga or the breathing technique *pranayama*, can provide you with excellent health benefits.

There is a wonderful relaxation device I recently discovered that I absolutely love. Made by New Realities, guided meditations recorded on a digital iPod-looking device are listened to with earbuds or headphones. What makes this device so special is that subliminal binaural beats accompany each meditation. The unperceivable alternating beats in your ears cause your brainwaves to synchronize—just as they do when practicing TM. The device also comes with nifty goggles with light-emitting diode (LED) lights designed to stimulate your retina through closed eyelids. The LED lights help to facilitate the meditative state. The first time I tried it, I became a big fan: Anyone can use it and no training or classes are needed. It's a very simple, affordable, and effective way to receive the benefits of meditation. You can read more about the New Realities device on my website: www.drchristinehorner.com.

Chapter 28

The Spiritual Journey of Cancer

When you come to the edge of all the light you know and are about to step off into the darkness, faith is knowing one of two things will happen: There will be something solid to stand on or you will be taught to fly.

—Barbara Walters

*T*hroughout this book, you have read about all the research-proven factors that influence your risk of breast cancer: What to avoid and what to favor. These factors range from body-centered foods and supplements, detoxification, exercise, and rest to emotional issues, especially stress and relationships. There are, however, aspects of your life that play an equally important role that scientists can't quantify and measure, such as your personal relationship with a higher power. Whatever name you have for that power—God, Allah, Spirit, Source, or the Divine—doesn't matter. I'm not talking about a religion, but a personal relationship. Your relationship. Your inner life. Your journey. Whatever concept of the higher power you have—it is the right one for you. I will refer to the higher power as Spirit or God, but you can translate that into the word that works best for you.

Life gives you exactly what you need to awaken.
—T. Scott McLeod

SPIRITUAL WAKE-UP CALL

Having worked with breast cancer patients for almost twenty-five years, and having been an intimate witness to my mother's journey with this disease, I have learned that cancer isn't just a physical disease. It's also a spiritual wake-up call. Your Spirit has grabbed your attention through your body, and is pleading with you to take a look at your life. A *real* look at *every* aspect of your life: mind, body, emotions, relationships, purpose, and relationship with Spirit.

When a woman with breast cancer calls me for a consultation, I often spend the final minutes talking with her about the spiritual journey of cancer. (A convenient appointment scheduler is located on my website www.drchristinehorner.com if you are interested in a consultation.) What do I mean by the spiritual journey? I believe that we are spiritual beings going through a human experience. We are given this miracle of life and free will in order to make choices. Ultimately, the point of this life is to love, learn, evolve, laugh, feel, and fulfill our unique purpose or mission, and to become a better, more conscious person.

There are many dimensions to being human, and it is important that each of us, including you, pays attention to and nurtures all of them. If you don't, imbalances develop and eventually "something happens"—the proverbial sledgehammer from the Universe—that forces you to wake up and make some positive changes. The cancer wake-up call is an extreme attention-grabbing event that can be an expansive opportunity. It's an opportunity for you to take time out for yourself—a nonnegotiable time-out, because your life depends on it. It can be a time to authentically evaluate every aspect of your life: How are you living your life? Is it everything that you want and desire? If not, what changes do you want to make? How are you taking care of your body? What can you do to upgrade that care? Better nutrition, supplements, regular detoxification, exercise, proper rest?

Next, a cancer diagnosis can be an opportunity to look at your emotional life. Are you passionate about the work that you do? Do you feel that you are living your life's purpose? Are your relationships satisfying and fulfilling? What causes you stress? Do you have any practices to help alleviate stress? Cancer can be an opportunity to do a complete inventory of your life. Asking a close friend or a therapist to help you with this can be life-changing in and of itself. For cancer survivors who have done this type of work, it is not uncommon to hear them say that their cancer diagnosis was the best thing that ever happened to them.

After you have completed your inventory, ask yourself what is the one thing that you could do that would make the most important difference in each area. Map out your action plan. Enroll the help of your family and friends to support you with the changes you would like to make.

> I had no idea that being your authentic self
> could make me as rich as I've become.
> If I had, I'd have done it a lot earlier.
>
> —Oprah Winfrey

Being Your Authentic Self

There's a wonderful book I recommend called *Dying to Be Me: My Journey from Cancer, to Near Death, to True Healing* by Anita Moorjani. Anita was diagnosed with terminal cancer and had been given just hours to live. But, she didn't die. Instead, she says that she experienced "crossing over and coming back" with a clearer understanding of her life and purpose on the Earth. Her cancer rapidly disappeared and her health totally recovered. She describes her experience in her book and also in several YouTube videos. Anita is a living example that each of us has the potential to heal, even from life-threatening illnesses. The key for her was her extraordinary spiritual experience. From it, she learned that her cancer was a result of living her life only by trying to make others happy, instead of being the authentic expression of her unique self. For you, it may be a different issue. But, as a physician, I believe that all illnesses symbolically give us clues about emotional and spiritual issues that must be addressed for healing to occur. When we fully confront those issues, and ask for help and guidance from Spirit, the possibility of healing is profound.

Follow your heart and intuition,
they already know what you truly want to become.
Everything else is secondary.

—STEVE JOBS

Living from Your Heart

As I mentioned in Chapter 26, "Emotional Healing," breast cancer is a fourth *chakra* issue. This *chakra* is about your heart and your emotions. When you are told to live from your heart and not your head, it means to live your life guided by the feelings in your heart. If you have been diagnosed with breast cancer, this is one message that your condition is crying out for you to hear. Check in with your heart about every major aspect in your life to see if your choices "feel" right. Notice what makes your heart feel happy, loved, passionate, peaceful, and joy-filled. Let your heart be your guide.

Most importantly, your heart is all about love—giving *and* receiving love. As women, we naturally tend to give more than we receive. Studies show that this is especially true for women who develop breast cancer. Learning how to receive may be one of the more difficult and important tasks for you to master. It's tough for most of us, because we are taught by parents and religions that it is better to give than receive. Giving is thought of as noble and the highest form of altruism. We give awards and recognition to those who are the biggest givers. Receiving is thought of as selfish. But it is not; it is necessary and life-sustaining. Giving without an equal balance of receiving is life-draining. Ironically, the ability to receive is a feminine quality—so, to deny it, is to deny a part of our true feminine nature.

> The reality of all life is interdependence. We need to compose our lives in such a way that we both give and receive, learning to do both with grace, seeing both as parts of a single pattern rather than as antithetical alternatives.
>
> —MARY CATHERINE BATESON

Learning to Receive

I want to tell you the story about how I learned to receive. In 2011, I saw one of Anita Moorjani's YouTube videos and noticed a related video next to it about Wayne Dyer, bestselling self-help author and motivational speaker, and his diagnosis of leukemia. I didn't know that Wayne had leukemia. Alarmed, I clicked on the video to get the details. In his interview he spoke about the healer, John of God, in Brazil. I had known of John of God for over eight years at that time and seeing him had been on my bucket list ever since. Wayne told the story of how his cancer had been miraculously cured by John of God. Even more remarkable, Wayne was in Hawaii and John of God was in Brazil when the healing took place! In that moment, I decided I could wait no longer to see this remarkable healer. I flew to Brazil a few months later and what I experienced there was completely life-altering.

John of God—the man—is a simple individual with a powerful gift. He is a medium who has the ability to allow spirits, called entities, to use his body to help heal others. He says that he does not heal, God does. If you don't know about him, I recommend that you look him up on the Internet. Oprah and Dr. Oz have featured him on their programs. The main reason I wanted to see him was to witness an alternative reality filled with miracles. My desire was completely fulfilled.

Emma, my guide for the trip, said that only about 10 percent of people receive instantaneous healings. A larger percentage of people make many trips and experience gradual healing, because their illness is an important part of their spiritual journey. Some conditions don't improve because their illness is their spiritual path. The most important key to receive healing, Emma said, is to surrender to God and receive.

If you wish for light, be ready to receive light.

—Rumi

Rather than coming to see John of God only as an observer, I wanted to personally experience how God works through him to heal. There were a few minor conditions I requested to be healed, including a small hernia on my abdomen. After asking for the healing, I realized I didn't know how to completely surrender to God and receive. So, I cried and prayed for hours asking to be shown. I was. When I met with John of God, he told me I needed "surgery." The surgery he recommends is no ordinary surgery—it is invisible. In other words: no surgeon, no scalpels, and no physical person that touches you. Instead, you sit on what looks like a church pew with many others who are also there for invisible surgery. Prayers and invocations are given at the beginning of the session. Mediums sit in front of the room to hold a meditative state of consciousness that facilitates invisible spirits or entities to enter the room. You are instructed to close your eyes, place your hands on the affected area of your body or place them on your heart, and then receive. Trust, surrender to God, allow and receive.

I felt hands touching me, although no physical hands actually were. "They" worked on closing my hernia above my belly button and it hurt so much I felt nauseated. Waves of joy passed over me. And there was so much more . . . but the point of this story is this: Beyond a shadow of a doubt, I know that each of us has angels and beneficent guides that love us, and watch over us. Talk to your angels and guides, God/Spirit. Ask for guidance and to be shown the path to your healing. Then surrender, trust, and open yourself to receive. Even if you have an advanced stage of breast cancer and would like to live many more years, do not give up. Plenty of people, such as Anita Moorjani, who was in a coma and given just hours to live, go on to live long, productive lives.

Embracing Your Femininity

Another realization I had after returning from Brazil was that all the qualities that are important for receiving love and healing from Spirit/God, are feminine in nature. Our culture, however, in general reveres masculine qualities and views feminine qualities as weak. As a direct result, women usually find it easy to express outer attributes of femininity, but simultaneously suppress inner feminine qualities such as trusting in a higher power. Asking and receiving, and working in cooperation holds much more power than the masculine approach of forcing things to happen on your own. I wonder: Could the denial and suppression of our feminine qualities be a contributor to our breast cancer epidemic? Although impossible to prove, energetically it makes sense to me.

Finding Your Path

I find that reminding myself that I am on a spiritual journey helps with all sorts of challenges and traumas that life throws at me. Through the years, I have developed several spiritual practices that work for me. They include prayer, meditation, shamanic journeying, sweat lodges, and consulting with healers to name a few. Your spiritual journey is your journey—no one else's. Only you can decide what is right for you. Explore and find what makes you feel closer to God. Pray often. Ask for help. Your prayers will be heard. Sometimes we don't get everything exactly how we ask for it, but trust that what is delivered to you is in your best interest. You are loved. You are being guided. Listen to the guidance with your heart, and you will intuitively know exactly what you need to do in the next step of your healing journey.

Part Seven

Putting It All Together
The Plan of Attack

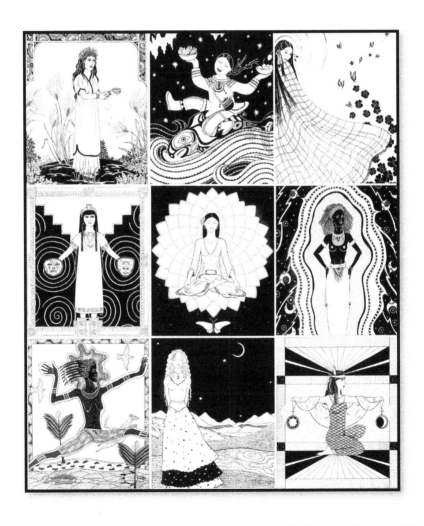

Chapter 29

Dr. Christine Horner's 30-Step Program

How to Protect Against and Fight Breast Cancer

*I*f nothing else, know this: You are far from powerless when it comes to your health and your risk of breast cancer. You have the ability to enormously lower your chances of getting this disease. And if you already have breast cancer, you can significantly improve your chances of surviving it, preventing a recurrence, and living a long and healthy life.

Okay, you're ready to begin the program! Don't let any of the information you read in the previous chapters overwhelm you. There's no need to make many radical changes all at once. Be gentle with yourself. While it's important that you eventually adopt all of the techniques and recommendations presented in this book to maximally protect your health, you don't have to implement them all at once. You don't have to start them all today or tomorrow or this week. Change your life gradually so that making these lifetime changes isn't stressful. Start with one change—one new "custom" at a time—then, when you're ready, add another. Soon, you'll be doing everything you can to enhance your inner healing intelligence and to keep your body strong and vibrantly healthy.

The only thing that has to be finished by next Tuesday is next Monday.

—JENNIFER YANE

This program was designed to give you a simple—yet inspiring—step-by-step approach to help you successfully make all the health-promoting changes discussed in this book. It's structured to be easy and stress-free. There's no *right* way to do the program, nor is there an advantage if you do the program in the order it's presented. So, if you want to mix up the order of the steps, that's perfectly fine. The first few steps aren't any more or less important or powerful than the last few steps. You may want to choose the steps that come most easily and naturally to you first, and later, choose the more personally challenging ones— or vice versa.

It's important that you choose a comfortable pace. People are usually better at sticking with a program if it is time-sensitive. So, select a time schedule, and then follow it as closely as you can. For instance, you can opt to implement a new change every day for thirty days, or each week for thirty weeks, or every month for thirty months. Although the schedule is flexible, the end result is not. You'll eventually need to make most of these changes. Making only some of them will not give you enough protection.

Don't let the fear of the time it will take to accomplish something stand in the way of your doing it. The time will pass anyway; we might just as well put that passing time to the best possible use.

—EARL NIGHTINGALE

Be not afraid of going slowly; be afraid only of standing still.

—CHINESE PROVERB

Just for fun, let's imagine that you've transported yourself 100 years into the future. The culture and its customs and habits are radically different from the place you left behind. The world is far more advanced and enlightened now, and all of the ideas in this program are part of this culture's tradition. All women—all people—here experience perfect health. Now, you must fit yourself into this world. This is your guidebook. Follow it and share it so that we can make this future world a reality.

Learning these new customs will take you on a wondrous, magical adventure that will make you feel better than you've ever felt; it will slow down your aging and nurture and protect your health. These customs will take you to a land of Warrior Goddesses, where the Goddess in every woman shines! Let's begin the adventure. . . .

Yesterday is a dream, tomorrow but a vision. But today well-lived makes every yesterday a dream of happiness, and every tomorrow a vision of hope. Look well, therefore, to this day.

—SANSKRIT PROVERB

Friendship & Support

A great way to begin this program is to invite a group of supportive friends to join you on your new health adventure. Be creative, and make it fun. For instance, you could start your own Warrior Goddess group. Structure it any way you like. I recommend monthly meetings—or even weekly meetings, if time permits. At each meeting, the members of the group implement one new custom. You can share your experiences, encourage one another, and explore new and exciting ways to integrate each step of the program into your lives. Some ideas for meetings include preparing creative vegetarian dishes highlighting a new medicinal food or spice; taking yoga or exercise classes together; hiking in Nature or taking trips to a spa; forming a community-sponsored agriculture (CSA) group; creating a buyers' group to get discount prices on supplements and herbs; and so on. The possibilities are endless.

If you or other group members have teenage daughters, invite them to do the program with you, too. Remember, teenagers have immature breast tissue that is more susceptible to toxins in the environment. Research shows that what you do during the teenage years is so important that it has lasting lifetime effects. If your teenager regularly exercises, doesn't smoke, and has healthy eating habits, her risk of breast cancer will be 30 to 50 percent lower for the rest of her life, regardless of her diet or habits later in life! But you'll want to encourage your daughter to maintain these habits. If she does, her risk of breast cancer and most other chronic diseases will be even lower.

TODAY IS THE DAY

Today is the day that you've decided to begin a new relationship with yourself. It is a sacred moment. As Antoine de Saint-Exupery said, "A single event can awaken within us a stranger totally unknown to us. To live is to be slowly born." This day is an event that will begin to awaken within you something you may not have been aware of—the extraordinary power of your inner healing intelligence—your Warrior Goddess. It is the moment of conception for the birth of a new you, an even more extraordinary woman than you already are, a woman with deep understanding and reverence for her body, a woman who experiences and honors her body's profound intelligence, a woman who possesses remarkable wisdom and knowledge about how to harness the power of Nature to achieve balance and an excellent state of health. You are becoming a woman who is not a victim to fluctuating states of health but is, instead, a powerful master of balance.

According to an old English proverb, the first step is usually the hardest. But once you commit yourself to living a life that supports your health in every way, you'll find that a universe of support will flow your way.

Begin to weave, and God will give you the thread.
—GERMAN PROVERB

DR. CHRISTINE HORNER'S 30-STEP PROGRAM

As mentioned previously, the steps in this program do not have to be done in order. In fact, as you've probably already noticed, I don't even refer to them as "steps." Instead, I present them as new customs to implement into your daily life. Unlike carrying out a step and then moving on to the next step, you will be acquiring and maintaining a healthy habit each time you move forward in the program—you'll leave nothing behind. By the time you've completed the program, you will have acquired thirty new customs that will arm your Warrior Goddess with all the ammunition she needs to keep you safe.

CUSTOM #1

Eat fresh, organically grown fruits and vegetables every day.
Include cruciferous vegetables at least three or four times a week.

This is the day that you will discover and experience the amazing medicines of organically grown fresh fruits and vegetables. Remember that they contain extraordinary intelligence and a phenomenal, natural anticancer pharmacy. Let their healing flavors explode in your mouth. As you look at their vibrant colors, remind yourself that each color is actually a potent natural medicine. Feel the nourishment of these foods gently flooding your body. Give thanks for the bounty of divine healing that Nature provides. Give thanks for the farmers who have devoted themselves to growing this food, devoid of toxic chemicals, and with consciousness of and respect for the Earth and the mind/body.

Before you can prepare your first meal of organic vegetables and fruits (be sure to feature a cruciferous vegetable—see page 51 for a list), you must first find a good source for organic produce. A great place to find organic produce is at your local health food store or at a larger chain store catering to organic products, such as Sprouts or Whole Foods (see the Resources section). If you don't have any of these stores nearby, find out if there's a local farmers' market or an individual farmer who sells seasonal organic fruits and vegetables. If there isn't such a market or farmer close to where you live, don't despair. There are many other creative ways to keep your kitchen filled with affordable organic produce.

For instance, you could start a community-sponsored agriculture (CSA) group (see the Resources section), which is simply a group of friends or neighbors who hire a farmer to grow organic foods for them on a plot of his or her land. Everyone shares in the cost of growing the food. What you pay for CSA organically grown produce is usually less than what you would pay for the same food in a grocery store. Another wonderful benefit of participating in a CSA is that your food is locally grown. That means it will be fresher and richer in nutrients than the food in grocery stores. Plants start to lose nutrients as soon as they are picked, so the fresher they are, the more nutrients they have. Often the organic food in stores has traveled long distances, and by the time you buy it and eat it, it is several weeks old and has lost many of its nutrients.

If you enjoy gardening, consider growing your own food organically. There are many books on organic gardening, so you can easily learn how to do it. Companies that specialize in organic lawn and garden care, such as Garden's Alive! or Arbico Organics (see the Resources section), are also great resources for tips and supplies for organic gardening. These companies have very knowledgeable people on staff who can help you get started and answer your questions.

The Internet makes it possible for you to get organic foods no matter where you live. Several companies offer an organic food–delivery service if you simply order from them on their Internet site (see the Resources section).

Remember that how you eat is just as important as what you eat. Review the *Ayurvedic* recommendations for enhancing digestion (see The Top 12 Aids to Digestion on page 47), and try to follow them as much as possible. By optimizing your digestion, you can substantially improve the value you get from your food.

The first step binds one to the second.

—FRENCH PROVERB

CUSTOM #1—POINTS TO REMEMBER

• Organically grown produce is grown without harmful chemical pesticides, herbicides, fertilizers, or genetic modifications. Studies show that it has a higher nutritional value and is much more supportive of your health and the environment than conventionally grown food.

- Organic fruits and vegetables are low in fat and calories and high in fiber, antioxidants, and vitamins.

- Organic produce contains a virtual anticancer pharmacy that includes hundreds of phytochemicals, including carotenoids, which are potent cancer and disease fighters.

- Cruciferous vegetables are particularly adept at reducing the risk of breast cancer as a result of three beneficial substances: indole-3 carbinol, sulforaphane, and D-glucaric acid.

  - Indole-3-carbinol fights breast cancer by forcing estrogen to break down into a protective, non-cancer-promoting type of estrogen. It also activates a tumor-suppression gene.

  - Sulforaphane stimulates enzymes in the liver to deactivate carcinogens.

  - D-glucaric acid supports a process in the liver that eliminates toxins and estrogen from your body.

- Women who eat the most cruciferous vegetables have a 40 percent lower risk of breast cancer.

- Vegetarians have a 50 percent lower incidence of most chronic disorders, including breast cancer.

Life is either a daring adventure, or it is nothing.

—HELEN KELLER

CUSTOM #2

Eat organic whole grains and seeds every day.

In the last century, it became popular to process grains to produce an ostensibly desirable white color for bread and rice. But this misguided practice also strips grains of many of their nutrients, especially B vitamins and fiber. That's why *whole* grains are so much better than processed grains for supporting your health and helping you to resist cancer.

Because whole grains are conspicuously absent from the traditional American diet, most of us are unfamiliar with the marvelous diversity of delectable grains. Based on our customs, you might think that the only way to eat whole grains is in cereal or bread. But whole grains can also be used to make delicious appetizers, side dishes, main courses, and even desserts. Look through a few cookbooks to find recipes that include whole grains. I recommend the excellent cookbook *Heaven's Banquet: Vegetarian Cooking for Lifelong Health the Ayurveda Way* by Miriam Kasin Hospodar. Not only does this book have wonderful recipes, but it also includes detailed information about each food: what it is, how to measure and cook it, its history, its nutritional and medicinal benefits, and how *Ayurveda* uses it as a medicine—all interlaced with beautiful quotes and entertaining stories.

Be exotic and try highly nutritious seeds, such as amaranth and quinoa. Amaranth, an important food to the Aztec Indians of Mexico centuries ago, is a tiny seed that is high in protein and calcium. Quinoa, its South American cousin and former staple of the ancient Inca diet, is also very high in protein. In fact, quinoa is a complete protein, meaning that it contains all the essential amino acids. Other savory grains that you can find at most grocery stores are barley, brown rice, buckwheat (kasha), millet, oats, spelt, rye, and kamut (a type of high-protein, hypoallergenic wheat).

Remember that each plant contains its own blend of unique medicines. The larger the medicine chest that you give to your body, the greater its ability is to keep you healthy. Big medicine chests come from eating a wide diversity of foods. Don't let the thought of cooking with new and unfamiliar foods intimidate you. With the help of a good cookbook, you'll find that creating new dishes with these nourishing foods is easy and fun.

Most health food stores, or grocery stores specializing in organic foods, stock seeds and grains in bulk bins at discount prices. There's also a list of Internet sites in the Resources section that sell organic grains. If you have one of these stores in your area, go there to see what types of organic grains they carry. Purchase a small amount of several different types of grains, and give each one a try. If you find that you don't like the taste of a certain type of grain, try it in at least three different recipes before you pass judgment and cross it off your list. With the right spices or combination of other ingredients, you will more than likely find a way that you *do* enjoy it. Remember, the more diverse the foods that you eat are, the wider the spectrum of healing nutrients you make available to your body.

If you have formed a Warrior Goddess group, have each member choose a different grain, create a soup, salad, main course, side dish, or dessert with it, and bring it to the meeting. Again, be creative, and have fun. Find an unusual recipe in a cookbook or invent your own. Great recipes don't have to be complex or require a lot of time. For instance, some grains are extremely tasty simply boiled in water and then tossed with sautéed spices. If you find a recipe—or make one up—that turns out to be great, please share it on my website at www.drchristinehorner.com.

*The responsibility for change . . . lies within us. We must begin
with ourselves, teaching ourselves not to close our minds
prematurely to the novel, the surprising, the seemingly radical.*

—ALVIN TOEFFLER

CUSTOM #2—POINTS TO REMEMBER

• Whole grains and seeds are rich in antioxidants, vitamins, trace minerals, fiber, and lignans.

• Soluble fiber deactivates carcinogens in the colon.

• Insoluble fiber absorbs water, dilutes carcinogens, binds estrogen and eliminates it, regulates insulin and glucose, promotes weight loss, lowers blood fats (lipids), and adds bulk to the stool.

• Women who eat a high-fiber diet have a 54 percent lower risk of breast cancer.

CUSTOM #3

Avoid all health-destroying fats.
Consume health-promoting fats every day.

Remember that there are both poisonous and protective fats. To nurture your health, avoid "bad" fats and consume "good" fats. If you don't already read food labels, start now. If a food contains trans fats, hydrogenated fats, or partially hydrogenated fats, don't buy it and don't eat it. These are the most dangerous types of fat for your health. Check all the foods you already have at home. If you find anything that contains these disease-promoting fats, throw it out!

Use organic olive, coconut, or macadamia nut oil for sautéing and for any other recipe that requires cooking oil. They are considered three of the best oils for these purposes, because they tolerate heat so well. Heating any oil—even olive oil—on high heat can destroy its antioxidants and create trans fats. So, when you cook with these oils, always use lower temperatures.

The most health-preserving and cancer-hindering type of fats you can eat are omega-3 fatty acids found in organic flaxseeds. These are so beneficial for your health that you should make it a point to consume at least 1 tablespoon of fresh, organic flax oil every day. Some people have no problem at all swallowing flax oil without mixing it with something—I'm not one of them, and you may not be either. Fortunately, Barlean's Organic Oils has created a delicious line of products that contain healthy oils called Omega Swirl. For example, flax oil comes in a strawberry-banana flavor that tastes like a fruit smoothie. They also have a product that contains a combination of oils, including flax and evening primrose oil, called Essential Woman. It comes in a scrumptious chocolate-raspberry flavor. Regular flax oil or the Omega-Swirl products can be added to a smoothie or a protein shake. Flax oil also makes an excellent salad dressing. Keep in mind that you are on a fun adventure, so be imaginative and share your ingenuity with your friends.

If you have started a Warrior Goddess group, you can add to the fun by giving an award, such as a gift certificate for a massage or any other stress-reducing service, to the person who comes up with the tastiest recipe. There's only one rule you should remember about using flax oil: *Do not heat it.* Heat destroys many of its healing properties.

Conjugated linoleic acid (CLA) and gamma linolenic acid (GLA) are two other types of health-promoting fats that also thwart breast cancer. It's not possible to consume enough CLA or GLA from food, so you must take them as a supplement. CLA comes in soft-gel capsules and is found in health food stores or stores that specialize in supplements for bodybuilders. Research shows that taking about 3,000 milligrams (mg) a day is enough to lower your risk of breast cancer. CLA is best taken in divided doses, usually 1,000 mg with each meal. GLA also comes in soft gels, or in the tasty Barlean's Essential Woman Swirl. The dose recommendation varies based on the condition it is being used to treat. Between 1,000 and 2,000 mg a day is advised for your breast health. Do not take more than 3,000 mg a day. (See the Resources section for sources for organic flax oil, organic olive oil, and CLAs.)

We cannot do everything at once, but we can do something at once.

—CALVIN COOLIDGE

CUSTOM #3—POINTS TO REMEMBER

- Fat is important for the proper functioning of your body.

- Some types of fat support health, while others destroy it.

- High-fat diets may increase your risk of breast cancer by as much as 50 percent.

- Saturated animal fats increase insulin resistance and, therefore, insulin levels in the blood. Women with high insulin levels have a 283 percent greater risk of breast cancer.

- Saturated animal fats concentrate toxic chemicals, including pesticides that are known to increase the risk of breast cancer.

- Insulin-like growth factor-1 (IGF-1), the most potent stimulator of breast cancer known, is found in high amounts in nonorganic whole-fat dairy products.

- Trans fats, partially hydrogenated fats, and hydrogenated fats are chemically altered fats that are very dangerous to your health because they promote inflammation and oxygen free radicals.

- Women who have the highest amounts of trans fats in their body have a 40 percent increased risk of breast cancer.

- The best ratio of omega-6 fatty acids to omega-3 fatty acids to consume is between 1:1 and 4:1. Americans typically eat an extremely unhealthy ratio of these fats—about 20:1.

- Women with the highest amounts of omega-6 fatty acids in their bodies have a 69 percent increased risk of breast cancer.

- Omega-3 fatty acids are the healthiest types of fat you can eat.

- The best plant source of omega-3 fatty acids is flaxseeds.

- Women with breast cancer who have high levels of omega-3 fatty acids in their bodies have a 50 percent lower incidence of metastasis.

- Omega-9 fatty acids, which are abundant in olive oil, are powerful antioxidants that suppress HER2/neu and decrease mammographic breast density.

- GLA and CLAs are a unique mixture of omega-6 fatty acids that lower the risk of breast cancer.

CUSTOM #4

Eat 2–3 tablespoons of flaxseeds every day.

Shoot for the moon.
Even if you miss, you'll land among the stars.

—LES BROWN

Remember that when it comes to lowering your risk of breast cancer and improving your chances of surviving it, research shows that flaxseeds are one of the most powerful medicinal foods you can eat. These tiny seeds provide a fortress of protection of such magnitude that you will want to make sure you consume them in some form every day.

To eat fresh organically grown flaxseeds, grind a few tablespoons in a coffee grinder until they become the consistency of a fine powder. Then sprinkle the delicious nutty flax powder over fruit, add it to a vegetable dish, stir it into a smoothie, or if you make your own bread or muffins, simply mix some of it into the dough before baking. Just like soy, there are many ways to enjoy flaxseeds, so I recommend getting a cookbook that specializes in recipes using flax.

If you have formed a Warrior Goddess group, have each member bring a different dish that incorporates flaxseeds to this meeting. Depending on how innovative and industrious you want to be, your group could make up new recipes, vote on the best ones, write them down, and create your own cookbook. Please share your recipes with me on my website at www.drchristinehorner.com.

Eating ground flaxseeds every day can be difficult, especially if you travel. You can also get the powerful anticancer substances in flax, called lignans, by taking a supplement called Brevail. One capsule of Brevail contains the same amount of lignans as about 4 tablespoons of flaxseeds. Health food stores usually carry all these items. (Sources for flaxseeds and Brevail are listed in the Resources section.)

Sow a thought, and you reap an act;
sow an act, and you reap a habit;
sow a habit, and you reap a character;
sow a character, and you reap a destiny.

—CHARLES READE

CUSTOM #4—POINTS TO REMEMBER

• Flaxseeds are one of the most powerful foods known to protect against and fight breast cancer.

• The richest plant source of omega-3 fatty acids is the flaxseed.

• Flaxseeds are high in fiber.

• The seeds of the flax plant contain 100 times more lignans than any other known edible plant.

• Lignans are powerful anticancer substances that are able to arrest and deter the growth of breast cancer in at least a dozen different ways.

• You can also get the daily recommended amount of flax lignans by taking one capsule of a supplement called Brevail.

CUSTOM #5

Eat soy-based whole-food products several times a week.

A vision must be followed by the venture.
It is not enough to stare up the steps—we must step up the stairs.

—Vance Havner

Research shows that whole soy foods are highly protective against breast cancer. In fact, women who eat the largest amounts of soy foods have a much lower risk of breast cancer. Begin by making a vegetarian dish that features a delicious, organically produced, soy-based whole-foods product such as natto, tofu, tempeh, fresh cooked soybeans, or miso, and make it at least three to four times a week. It's particularly important to buy soy foods that have been organically produced because most soybeans grown in the United States are genetically altered. Since the long-term consequences of eating genetically modified foods aren't known, you definitely want to avoid them as much as possible.

I recommend getting a good tofu or soy cookbook. You'll be amazed at all the creative, diverse, and surprisingly tasty dishes you can create using soy. For instance, you can craft fabulous salad dressings, dips, drinks, main meals, and desserts with tofu. Don't forget that roasted soy nuts make a delicious and healthy snack food. They are low in fat and are one of the best sources of the protective qualities of soy.

Remember to avoid genistein supplements isolated from soy, because studies show that genistein, without all the other substances in whole soy foods to interact with it, may not be protective and, in fact, may be harmful.

If you have formed a Warrior Goddess group, have each member bring something made with soy to this meeting. You might want each person to choose a different course or a different form of soy so you get a good sampling of the many ways to enjoy this wonderful food. (You'll find a list of companies that offer a large variety of soy foods in the Resources section.)

CUSTOM #5—POINTS TO REMEMBER

• Soy contains phytoestrogens, which act as weak estrogens that block stronger estrogens from attaching to estrogen receptors in the breast.

• The three major phytoestrogens in soy are genistein, daidzein, and glycitein.

• Turmeric enhances the estrogen-blocking abilities of soy.

- Don't take isolated genistein supplements because they may stimulate the growth of breast cells.

- Eat a wide variety of whole soy foods, but don't make your diet all about soy. Remember that food diversity is important.

- Women who eat the most whole soy foods have a 30 to 50 percent lower risk of breast cancer than women who don't.

- Soy matures breast cells and makes them more resistant to environmental toxins.

- Girls who consume soy around puberty and during the teen years have up to a 50 percent lower risk of breast cancer as adults.

CUSTOM #6

Eat exotic Asian foods such as maitake mushrooms often.

Asian women have a much lower incidence of breast cancer than American women do, and a large part of the reason is the foods they eat and don't eat. Asian cuisine is high in soy, but soy foods aren't the only types of Asian foods that ward off breast cancer. There are many others. (See Chapter 11 for a reminder.)

One special type of mushroom, the maitake mushroom, has been part of Japanese medicine for thousands of years and contains an armory of therapeutic weapons against breast cancer. Maitake mushrooms are considered a gourmet food in America. They come fresh or dried and can be found in the gourmet section of some grocery stores and at Asian markets. They are also available as a supplement—either in

> Trying to eat all the beneficial foods that defend against breast cancer every day isn't realistic. Taking supplements is sometimes an excellent alternative. If you decide to go this route on occasion, be sure to purchase only quality supplements from reputable companies. To make supplementation more convenient and affordable for women and to ensure excellent quality, I collaborated with the highly reputable company Enzymatic Therapy to create a supplement called Protective Breast Formula (PBF). PBF contains a combination of seven different supplements, each with powerful effects against breast cancer. This formulation includes indolplex 25 percent DIM (derived from indole-3-carbinol), calcium-D-glucarate, turmeric, green tea extract, maitake mushroom D-fraction, grape seed extract, and vitamin D_3. (See the Resources section or visit www.protective breast.com for more information.)

capsules or in a liquid extract. You can order maitake mushrooms or supplements over the Internet (see the Resources section). The recommended daily dose is 3–5 grams, or 10–30 drops of the liquid extract, three times a day.

There are no shortcuts to any place worth going.

—BEVERLY SILLS

CUSTOM #6—POINTS TO REMEMBER

• Maitake mushrooms stop tumor growth, cause tumors to shrink, and prevent them from spreading to other areas of the body.

• Maitake mushrooms stimulate the immune system.

• Maitake mushrooms can kill 95 percent of prostate cancer cells in twenty-four hours.

• Of those women with stage-2 to stage-4 breast cancers who were given maitake mushrooms, 68.8 percent experienced a reduction in tumor size and an improvement in symptoms.

• AHCC (active hexose correlated compound) is a mushroom formula made from the roots of shiitake mushrooms that supports all the cells in your immune system, deters several different types of cancer including breast cancer, improves survival, and takes away the side effects of chemotherapy.

The road to success is dotted with
many tempting parking places.

—AUTHOR UNKNOWN

CUSTOM #7

Drink green tea every day.

Drinking eight to ten cups of green tea each day can significantly lower your risk of breast cancer, and if you already have breast cancer, it may extend your life. Eight to ten cups a day may seem like a lot of green tea, but it's easy to drink that much if you sip it throughout the day. However, if you try to drink this much and find that you simply can't do it, just drink as much as you comfortably can.

If you don't like the taste of traditional green tea, you may like one of the flavored varieties. I've found organic green teas in many tantalizing flavors such as strawberry rose, mint, mango, Mandarin orange, cinnamon apple, and jasmine. If drinking tea just isn't your cup of tea, you can get the benefits of green tea by taking supplements. Two 250-mg capsules a day is recommended. (See the Resources section for a list of companies that make organic green tea and green-tea supplements.) You can also get your suggested daily intake of green tea by taking Protective Breast Formula (see the Resources section).

If you've formed a Warrior Goddess group, have a tea party. Have everyone bring a different flavor of green tea and an appetizer that includes a medicinal food, such as maitake mushroom puffs, tofu dip, fresh broccoli and cauliflower, and flax muffins.

CUSTOM #7—POINTS TO REMEMBER

- Green tea is considered the number-one anticancer beverage.

- Green tea contains powerful anti-inflammatories and antioxidants.

- Women who drink the most green tea have a lower risk of breast cancer and live much longer if they develop breast cancer than women who don't drink it.

- Green tea stops tumors from growing back, inhibits the growth of breast cancer, and decreases the incidence of tumors metastasizing to the lung.

- Always buy organic green tea because some nonorganic brands have been found to contain the pesticide DDT.

CUSTOM #8

Consume turmeric every day.

Turmeric is so extraordinary at protecting against and fighting breast cancer, as well as many other types of cancer, that it's considered the number-one anticancer spice. Turmeric inhibits cancer in several ways, including blocking all the powerful cancer-promoting actions of the inflammatory COX-2 enzyme.

Turmeric is a traditional spice used in Indian cooking, but you can use it in any dish of any ethnic origin. It's responsible for the intense bright yellow-orange color in curry, so you can either cook with turmeric or with a curry that contains turmeric.

Cooking with turmeric or curry is easy. *Ayurveda* recommends adding turmeric near the end of cooking because its healing properties are most powerful if it's lightly cooked. About one-fourth teaspoon of dried powdered turmeric should be added for each serving.

Adding turmeric to soy foods produces an especially potent medicine. Remember that turmeric enhances the estrogen-blocking capabilities of the phytoestrogens in soy. Combining turmeric and green tea also creates a phenomenal anticancer alchemy. Turmeric makes green tea's anticancer ability eight times stronger, and green tea enhances turmeric's by three times. So, if you want to get the most potent medicinal effects from turmeric, add this remarkable spice to your soy dish and serve it with a cup of green tea!

Turmeric comes as a dried powder and can be found in the spice section of any grocery or health food store. Favor using organically grown turmeric to avoid pesticide residue. If you can't find organic turmeric in your store, you can order it on the Internet.

On the days you don't cook with turmeric, you can take it as a supplement. The recommended dose is at least one 1,000-mg capsule a day. (See the Resources section for a list of companies that make organic turmeric supplements.) You can also get the suggested daily dose of turmeric by taking Protective Breast Formula (see the Resources section).

If you've formed a Warrior Goddess group, have each member bring a dish made with turmeric or curry. Serve organic green tea as the beverage.

CUSTOM #8—POINTS TO REMEMBER

• Turmeric is considered the number-one anticancer spice.

• This beautiful spice is 300 times more powerful as an antioxidant than vitamin E.

• An extraordinary COX-2 inhibitor, turmeric also blocks the estrogenic effects of breast cancer-inducing pesticides.

• Turmeric and green tea enhance each other's anticancer effects.

• The estrogen-blocking capabilities of soy are increased when you add turmeric.

• Turmeric defends against breast cancer in a multitude of ways.

CUSTOM #9

Eat at least one clove of garlic several times a week.

A nickel will get you on the subway, but garlic will get you a seat.

—OLD NEW YORK PROVERB

Not only is garlic delicious, but it's also a powerful medicine against breast cancer. It is extremely high in antioxidants and selenium, boosts the immune system, lessens the formation of carcinogens in the breast, prevents toxins from binding to DNA, and stops breast tumors from growing and dividing. Research shows that eating just a few cloves of garlic a week can significantly lower your risk of breast cancer.

The healing powers of garlic are best if you eat it raw. Crush it, wait fifteen minutes for it to activate its enzymes, and then put it on your salad or vegetables. If you choose to cook garlic, make sure you don't overcook it because you will destroy most of its antioxidants. If you prefer not to eat garlic because you're concerned about the odor of garlic radiating from your body, you can take an aged, odorless garlic supplement instead—600–900 mg a day is recommended. (Check the Resources section for good brands.)

If you've formed a Warrior Goddess group, have each member bring a different garlic dish, for example, roasted elephant garlic with olive oil on fresh whole-grain bread, pickled garlic, or gazpacho soup with extra garlic.

Custom #9—Points to Remember

- Women who eat as little as one clove of garlic a week have a statistically significant lower incidence of breast cancer.

- Garlic has more antioxidants than any other vegetable.

- This fragrant herb boosts the immune system.

- Garlic decreases the formation of carcinogens in breast tissue by 50 to 70 percent.

- You can take odorless garlic as a supplement to avoid the odor.

CUSTOM #10

Include wakame or mekabu seaweed in your diet.

Wakame and mekabu seaweeds are high in the mineral iodine, and research shows that they are at least as effective at killing breast cancer cells as many common chemotherapeutic drugs. These seaweeds can be found in the Asian section of grocery stores, health food stores, or Asian markets, or they can be ordered from the Internet (see the Resources section). Chop the seaweed up and add it to stir-fried vegetables, soups, grains, stews, or marinated dishes. Cooking instructions are usually on the package.

If you've formed a Warrior Goddess group, have each member bring a food to this session that features one of these seaweeds. You might also want to call a Japanese or Asian restaurant in your area to see if these items are included on their regular menu. If not, ask if they would be willing to order wakame or mekabu seaweed and prepare several dishes with it for your group.

Custom #10—Points to Remember

• Wakame and mekabu seaweeds are high in iodine, which suppresses breast cancer growth by causing cancer cells to die.

• These seaweeds can kill breast cancer cells and stop the growth of breast cancer more effectively than some common chemotherapeutic drugs.

• Iodine is taken up by breast cancer cells but not by normal cells. Scientists think that it may be possible to treat breast cancer in the future with radioactive iodine—a substance that is harmless to the body (except for the thyroid).

CUSTOM #11

Take a whole-food vitamin every day.

Vitamins are micronutrients that are needed to assist many of the chemical reactions in your body. Your body can't make most vitamins, so you must get them from an outside source. It's difficult to get all the vitamins you need from your food because our soil is nutrient-depleted and because food loses many of its nutrients as it travels long distances to market, sits on the shelf, is processed, and is cooked. Research shows that supplemental amounts of certain vitamins—especially vitamin A, vitamin B_{12}, folate, vitamin D, and vitamin E—can lower your risk of breast cancer. Since we typically don't absorb synthetic vitamins very well, I recommend taking a vitamin supplement made from whole foods. (Check the Resources section for a list of companies that make them.)

Vitamin D is unique because, unlike other vitamins, you can make your own. Sunlight stimulates your body to produce vitamin D naturally, so you can simply take a walk in the sunshine for fifteen minutes a day to meet all your daily requirements for vitamin D. An early-morning or late-afternoon walk is ideal. If you live in a place with unusually inclement weather, especially during the cold winter months, you'll need to either eat foods fortified with vitamin D or take a supplement. Many multivitamin supplements contain vitamin D_3—usually 400 international units (IU). Protective Breast Formula and Brevail each have 400 IU of vitamin D_3. If you took all three of these supplements for example, your daily dose would total 1,200 IU. Check all your supplements to see if they contain D_3. Make sure that you're getting at least 1,000 to 2,000 IU of vitamin D_3 daily.

Custom #11 — Points to Remember

• Vitamins assist your body's enzymes.

• Folic acid is crucial for making proteins and for constructing and repairing DNA.

• Alcohol, birth control pills, and nonsteroidal anti-inflammatory drugs (NSAIDs) cause folic acid levels to drop.

• Women who drink at least 15 grams a day of alcohol and have low folate levels have a very high risk of breast cancer.

• Vitamin B_{12} works with folate to make and repair DNA.

• Women with low B_{12} levels have high rates of breast cancer.

• Vitamin B_{12} applied directly to breast cancer cells stops them from growing.

• Vitamin D makes your breast cells more resistant to toxins, decreases the ability of breast cancer cells to grow and divide, stops tumor cells from growing, and boosts the immune system.

• You can make your own vitamin D through a chemical reaction in your skin that occurs when it is exposed to ultraviolet light.

• Just fifteen to twenty minutes a day of sunlight in the summer months is all you need to make your daily requirement of vitamin D. The sun is not strong enough in the winter in most locations in the United States for you to manufacture enough, so you'll need to take a supplement to keep your levels optimal.

• Vitamin E is a powerful antioxidant.

• Vitamin E slows down tumor growth, promotes the death of tumor cells, and prevents new blood vessels from growing into tumors.

• You absorb vitamin E better from food than from supplemental vitamins—especially synthetic vitamins.

• Vitamin C and coenzyme Q_{10} (CoQ_{10}) make the antitumor effects of vitamin E even stronger.

• Vitamin A decreases tumor cell growth, causes tumor cell death, stops the aromatase enzyme from converting androgens into estrogen, and modifies genes that govern the function of the alpha-estrogen receptor.

• Vitamin A greatly enhances the tumor-killing capabilities of omega-3 fatty acid, melatonin, and the chemotherapeutic drugs Tamoxifen and Herceptin (used for HER2/neu tumors).

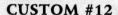

CUSTOM #12

Get adequate amounts of selenium every day.

Selenium is an essential part of one of your body's own powerful antioxidants, glutathione peroxidase. Remember that antioxidants eradicate excess oxygen free radicals—those tiny molecules of oxygen that ruthlessly attack your cells and DNA, causing damage that can lead to cancer, as well as a host of other serious diseases. Selenium gives a tremendous boost to your body's healing intelligence, so much so that research shows as little as 200 micrograms (mcg) a day lowers your risk of breast cancer—and most other types of cancer—by 50 percent.

Plants are our major source of selenium, but because our soil is now selenium-deficient and nutrient-poor, most of us don't get enough selenium. However, one food that is always packed full of large amounts of selenium is the delicious Brazil nut. Just a few organically grown Brazil nuts every day will give you more than enough selenium to fulfill your daily requirements.

If you don't like the taste of Brazil nuts or if you're allergic to them, begin taking 200 mcg a day of a good selenium supplement. (See the Resources section for a list of companies.)

CUSTOM #12—POINTS TO REMEMBER

• Selenium is an essential part of your body's own potent antioxidant, glutathione peroxidase.

• Women with breast cancer have much lower levels of selenium than women who don't have cancer.

• Selenium also helps to fight cancer by preventing cancer cells from growing, causing cancer cells to die, stopping blood-vessel growth into tumors, and enhancing the immune system.

• Iodine makes selenium more effective.

• Taking 200 mcg a day of selenium can lower your risk of breast cancer and most other cancers by 35 to 50 percent. If you have cancer, selenium can decrease your odds of dying from it by 52 percent.

• Selenium is found in garlic, onions, leafy green vegetables, mushrooms, and whole grains.

• Don't take too much selenium; if you do, you can develop a condition called selenosis, which is characterized by hair loss, gastrointestinal upset, white blotchy nails, and nerve damage.

CUSTOM #13

If you are over age thirty-five, take supplemental CoQ$_{10}$ every day.

CoQ$_{10}$ is a natural vitamin-like substance that is essential for the production of energy. It's also a powerful antioxidant. Researchers have found that supplemental CoQ$_{10}$ can stop the growth of breast cancer and dramatically shrink tumors.

CoQ$_{10}$ comes in many different strengths and varieties. The recommended amount depends on the type of CoQ$_{10}$ supplement. For instance, your body uses fermented CoQ$_{10}$ far more efficiently than synthetic CoQ$_{10}$. So, you need far less of the fermented CoQ$_{10}$ than the synthetic. About 22 mg of fermented CoQ$_{10}$ is equivalent to 400 mg of the synthetic variety. Ubiquinol is a more biologically active form of CoQ$_{10}$ recommended by some experts. (See the Resources section for a list of companies.)

CUSTOM #13—POINTS TO REMEMBER

- CoQ$_{10}$ is essential for the production of energy.
- CoQ$_{10}$ is a potent antioxidant.
- CoQ$_{10}$ appears to be very effective at shrinking tumors, including metastatic tumors.
- CoQ$_{10}$ prevents organ damage from chemotherapy.
- If you take medication for high blood pressure, cholesterol-lowering statin drugs, or red yeast rice, you should take supplemental CoQ$_{10}$.

Amrit Kalash—Another Powerful Antioxidant

When certain plants are combined, they form synergies that exponentially increase their antioxidant power. The *Ayurvedic* herbal preparation *Amrit Kalash* is a combination of forty-four herbs, spices, and fruits. This beneficial blend is at least 25,000 times more powerful than vitamin E as an antioxidant. In fact, it has been found to be the strongest antioxidant ever tested. This preparation can help to prevent the formation of tumors, slow tumor growth, shrink tumors, and help to alleviate the side effects of chemotherapy without interfering with its effectiveness (see page 150). Moreover, *Amrit Kalash* may slow the aging process and even reverse it. (If you wish to obtain this magnificent antioxidant, see the Resources section.)

CUSTOM #14

Take an herbal anti-inflammatory several times a week.

The so-called "secrets of success" will not work unless you do.
—AUTHOR UNKNOWN

Research shows that women who take an anti-inflammatory an average of three times a week, especially one that inhibits the COX-2 enzyme, have a 50 percent lower risk of breast cancer. Since pharmaceutical anti-inflammatories can have dangerous side effects, I recommend taking an herbal anti-inflammatory, particularly the potent herbal COX-2 inhibitor Zyflamend. This supplement is a combination of ten powerful herbs. Take two capsules of Zyflamend with a meal, several times a week. If you already have breast cancer, take two capsules every day.

CUSTOM #14—POINTS TO REMEMBER

• Chronic inflammation fuels the initiation and progression of many different types of cancer and chronic disorders.

• Chronic stress, some foods (such as refined carbohydrates and sugar), and certain fats (such as omega-6 fatty acids and trans fats) promote inflammation.

• The COX-2 enzyme, which is involved in the inflammatory process, also plays a key role in the initiation and progression of several types of cancer, including breast cancer.

• About 50 percent of all breast cancers overexpress the COX-2 enzyme.

• Research shows that taking a COX-2 anti-inflammatory at least three times a week can reduce the risk of breast cancer by 50 percent.

• Herbal COX-2 inhibitors may work just as well as the pharmaceutical ones, but without the potentially dangerous side effects.

• Cancer research is currently being conducted on the effectiveness of Zyflamend. So far, the results are impressive.

I'm a great believer in luck, and I find the harder I work,
the more I have of it.
—THOMAS JEFFERSON

Famous Vegetarians

Here's a list of a few famous people and historical figures who made the wise choice not to eat meat: Pythagoras, Leonardo da Vinci, Benjamin Franklin, Albert Einstein, Mahatma Gandhi, George Bernard Shaw, Robert Louis Stevenson, Henry David Thoreau, and Paul and Linda McCartney.

CUSTOM #15

Do not eat red meat.

Eating red meat, especially large amounts of well-done or grilled meats, significantly increases the risk of many diseases. These diseases include such common deadly diseases as breast cancer, prostate cancer, colon cancer, gallbladder disease, heart disease, high blood pressure, and stroke.

If you don't want to completely give up red meat, at least cut way back on the amount of it that you eat. Don't eat it more than once or twice a month, and eat only meat from animals that have been organically raised. Organically raised animals aren't fed toxic chemicals or growth hormones, which increase your risk of breast cancer even further. Also, by selecting organic, you are choosing not to support the conventional meat industry—an industry that pumps animals full of toxins and keeps them in horrific, abusive conditions. Never eat well-done or grilled meat because these cooking methods create excessive amounts of heterocyclic amines, dangerous carcinogens.

If slaughterhouses had glass walls,
everyone would be a vegetarian.

—PAUL MCCARTNEY

If you don't want to give up the flavor of red meat, the best choice you can make is to eat vegetable-based meat substitutes instead. For virtually any type of meat, there's a delicious alternative that closely mimics the flavor and texture of real meat without all the health hazards (see the Resources section for a list).

If you've formed a Warrior Goddess group, have each member bring a different type of meat substitute for everyone to sample.

Custom #15—Points to Remember

• Women who eat the most red meat have an 88 to 400 percent higher risk of breast cancer.

• Cooking animal protein creates dangerous carcinogens, especially when grilling or cooking meats at high temperatures.

• The saturated fat in animals stores cancer-causing toxins from the environment and growth hormones and increases other cancer promoters: insulin, inflammation, and oxygen free radicals.

• There are many delicious meat substitutes that can satisfy your desire for the taste and texture of meat without damaging your health.

CUSTOM #16

Avoid refined sugar. Use a natural sweetener such as stevia instead.

One half of knowing what you want
is knowing what you must give up before you get it.

—Sidney Howard

Cancer loves sugar. Refined sugar is the preferred food of tumors. Refined carbohydrates and sugars also cause insulin levels to go up, and excess insulin is a powerful promoter of diseases such as breast cancer, diabetes, and obesity. If you have a sweet tooth, satiate your yearnings with fresh organic fruit. For example, organic dates will satisfy even the most intense sweet-tooth attack. Instead of sprinkling sugar on your cereal or adding it to your favorite beverage, use a natural product such as stevia. The craving for sweets is actually an addiction that can be broken rather easily. Research shows that after only three weeks of avoiding sugar, you will lose your desire and taste for it. For instance, if you try a piece of candy after three weeks of consuming no sweets, it will taste so sweet to you that you won't like it.

If you've formed a Warrior Goddess group, have each member prepare a dessert or beverage sweetened with stevia. Cooking with stevia can be tricky, so I recommend getting a stevia cookbook (see the Recommended Reading section). There is a stevia product specifically made for baking made by NuNaturals called More Fiber Stevia Baking Blend. Some health food stores carry it. There are several websites that sell it, including Amazon.com. Support one another in breaking the sugar habit. Remember, all it usually takes is three weeks to lose your desire for sugar.

Bad habits are easier to abandon today than tomorrow.

—YIDDISH PROVERB

CUSTOM #16—POINTS TO REMEMBER

• Cancer loves sugar. The more you eat of this poison, the faster cancer will grow.

• Refined carbohydrates and sugars cause your pancreas to release high amounts of insulin.

• High insulin levels increase your risk of breast cancer by as much as 283 percent.

• Insulin causes cancer cells to divide and grow faster.

• Insulin lowers the number of protein binders in your blood and, thus, increases the amount of estrogen that can attach to your breast cells.

• After you eat sugar, your immune system becomes 50 to 94 percent less effective *for five hours.*

• Refined carbohydrates and sugars promote obesity.

• Stevia is a natural sweetener and a great sugar substitute with many health benefits.

• Artificial sweeteners may be damaging to your health, so avoid them.

CUSTOM #17

Keep your body-fat percentage low.

You cannot plough a field by turning it over in your mind.

—AUTHOR UNKNOWN

Keeping your body fat in check significantly lowers your risk of postmenopausal breast cancer. It also dramatically reduces your chances of developing diabetes, heart disease, and many other serious diseases. The Centers for Disease Control (CDC) and Prevention estimates that obesity-related health problems cause 300,000 deaths every year. If you have followed the program sequentially, you are already practicing many of the customs that will help you to lose and maintain a healthy weight—for example, eating fresh organic fruits, vegetables, and whole grains; avoiding red meat, processed foods, and sugar; taking flax oil or eating flaxseeds; and exercising every day.

If you find that you have frequent desires to snack, try this: Eat six small meals instead of three large meals, and plan what you're going to eat on a particular day the night before. Every three hours or so, eat a small portion of protein with a serving of vegetables. Include a serving of fresh fruit and whole grains in two of your meals. Eating planned, small, frequent meals will keep you from getting hungry, overeating, and having the compulsion to eat the wrong things.

If three meals a day works well for you, remember to eat your main meal at noon because that's when your digestion is strongest. In the evening when your digestion is much weaker, eat lightly. Make sure most of the foods you choose to eat are in alignment with the recommendations in this book; because what you eat and don't eat have a tremendous influence on your risk of breast cancer.

If you have a serious weight problem, joining a weight-loss program such as Weight Watchers can be very helpful. However, consult your doctor before starting a weight-loss program.

If you've formed a Warrior Goddess group, plan out how you are going to support each member to achieve and maintain a healthy weight. Perhaps you could go to a class together, help one another plan meals, exercise together, or create a buddy system for support.

> No diet will remove all the fat from your body because the brain is entirely fat. Without a brain, you might look good, but all you could do is run for public office.
>
> —GEORGE BERNARD SHAW

> I never worry about diets. The only "carrots" that interest me are the number you get in a diamond.
>
> —MAE WEST

CUSTOM #17—POINTS TO REMEMBER

• In the United States, 300,000 people die every year from obesity-related health problems.

• Obesity is thought to be responsible for 20 to 30 percent of all postmenopausal breast cancers.

- Fat cells manufacture estrogen, especially after menopause.

- Almost two-thirds of Americans are overweight or obese.

- Estimating your body-fat percentage is the best way to determine if you are overweight or obese.

- Toxins in the environment may contribute to obesity by disrupting our normal weight-control mechanisms; that's another reason to eat organic foods.

CUSTOM #18

Rarely, if ever, drink alcohol.

The best way out of a problem is through it.

—AUTHOR UNKNOWN

First you take a drink, then the drink takes a drink,
then the drink takes you.

—F. SCOTT FITZGERALD

Even one drink of alcohol a day increases your risk of breast cancer; however, taking a folic acid supplement appears to take away most of the damaging effects of one or two glasses a day. Do not regularly drink two or more glasses a day. If you find you don't have the self-control to limit how much you drink, it's best to avoid this potentially dangerous beverage completely. If you enjoy the taste of wine, there are several companies that make delicious and satisfying nonalcoholic wines.

If you have a serious drinking habit, now is the time to get help. You have taken the initiative to honor your body and mind by implementing many of the other customs, and this one is of utmost importance. Depending on the severity of your habit or addiction, you may need to enter an in-residence treatment program or participate in an excellent program such as Alcoholics Anonymous (AA). Alcohol can be very destructive to your health and your relationships, so make every effort to get it out of your life and keep it out. If it plays a big role in your life, now is the time to change that. Most people find that it's difficult or embarrassing to admit that they may have a drinking problem. But keep in mind that you're not alone. There are many wonderful programs and compassionate understanding people just waiting to help you.

If you've formed a Warrior Goddess group, have each member bring a non-alcoholic healthy beverage to this meeting. If you would like to try nonalcoholic wines, have each person bring a different brand and flavor to see if there is one you especially like. Remember that the potent antioxidant and cancer fighter resveratrol, which is responsible for many of the health benefits of red wine, is also found in grapes. So, try fresh grape juice made with a juicer or a blender such as Vitamix. (There's also a list of organic grape juices in the Resources section.) If you or any member of your group has a drinking problem, support one another by getting help.

You must do the thing you think you cannot do.

—ELEANOR ROOSEVELT

CUSTOM #18—POINTS TO REMEMBER

• Even one drink of alcohol a day increases the risk of breast cancer.

• The health detriments of alcohol far outweigh any health benefits.

• Alcohol increases estrogen and prolactin, both of which increase cell division in the breast.

• Grapes contain a substance called resveratrol, an antioxidant and COX-2 anti-inflammatory that research shows inhibits the formation and growth of breast cancer.

• Grape seeds also contain powerful antioxidants and can kill breast cancer cells and decrease the amount of estrogen your body produces.

• Overcoming a drinking problem can be difficult, so don't hesitate to seek help from one of the many excellent programs that are available.

CUSTOM #19

Never smoke tobacco products.

Smoking is one of the leading causes of statistics.

—AUTHOR UNKNOWN

Cigarettes are killers traveling in packs.

—AUTHOR UNKNOWN

Because of all the health problems caused by smoking tobacco products, including an increased risk of breast cancer, smoking is a bad habit that you never want to start. If you currently smoke, begin cutting back and choose a date when you will quit. Stopping this destructive habit is one of the most important things you can do for your health. As a fellow physician and former smoker said to me, "Smoking is a decision. You can decide not to smoke."

For some people, overcoming this addiction isn't that tough; but for others, it is extraordinarily difficult. Keep in mind that although breaking this habit may be very challenging, it's not impossible. You *can* do it. Most people need some support to be successful. Fortunately, there are many programs available to assist you. For example, research shows that the regular practice of Transcendental Meditation (TM) is one of the most successful approaches for helping you overcome any addiction. Make a plan, set goals and dates, find a program, enroll others to support you, and go for it.

If you've formed a Warrior Goddess group and any of your members smoke, everyone should offer their support to those members to help them stop. Be sure to let those who smoke tell you exactly what you can do to support them. Don't offer unrequested coaching or place unwanted demands on them. Allow them to direct and make choices for their own lives.

Men are made stronger on realization that the helping hand
they need is at the end of their own arm.

—SIDNEY PHILLIPS

Forget past mistakes. Forget failures. Forget everything
except what you're going to do now and do it.

—WILL DURANT

CUSTOM #19—POINTS TO REMEMBER

- Smoking during adolescence can increase the risk of breast cancer by 50 percent.

- Women who either smoke or inhale passive smoke may have as much as a 60 percent increased risk of breast cancer.

- For some people, breaking the cigarette habit is extremely difficult. If you are one of these people, seek help and support yourself in every way possible so that you can be successful.

CUSTOM #20

Don't take birth control pills or hormone replacement therapy (HRT),
except in rare circumstances determined by your doctor
and only for a brief time.

If you have been taking birth control pills or HRT for several years, schedule an appointment with your doctor to come up with a plan to get you off these medications. If your gynecologist or family physician won't work with you to get off these medications, find a physician who will. There are many doctors who specialize in natural or integrative medicine, and you may find one in your area.

Both birth control pills and HRT have been shown to significantly increase your risk of breast cancer, so you'll want to use alternative methods if you can. Sometimes, these medications are necessary for a short time, and when taken for brief periods, they will not have dire consequences to your health. If you find that you must take these medications, make sure that you're doing all the other steps in this program to minimize your risk. Remember that breast cancer isn't caused by one thing. It's the result of the balance of *everything* you do in your life. If you are doing enough to protect yourself, then the likelihood of one of these medications being able to tip the scale and cause breast cancer will be much lower.

In Chapter 20, I mentioned several very good books that provide excellent guidance on how to use natural approaches to restore balance to your body during menopause. These approaches, along with the use of a few herbs, may completely eliminate or significantly improve any uncomfortable symptoms you have during this natural transition of life. (These books are also listed in the Recommended Reading section.) You might find that the new customs that you're already practicing have created so much balance in your mind/body that your menopausal symptoms have gone away or have gotten much better.

If you are still of reproductive age, you don't have to rely on birth control pills to prevent pregnancy. There are many effective alternatives to choose from. If you are not monogamous, condoms are your best choice because they pro-

---

Be aware that certain heart medications and antidepressants can significantly increase the risk of breast cancer. If you are taking medication for depression or heart problems, find out what risks are associated with its use. If necessary, speak with your doctor about alternatives. Remember, both heart problems and depression have the potential to be extremely serious, so *never* discontinue medication without your doctor's approval and supervision.

vide protection from sexually transmitted diseases (STDs), including HIV (the virus that causes AIDS). If you are in a monogamous relationship, try different methods of birth control until you find the one that works best for you and your partner.

Anytime you make a change, it may seem uncomfortable at first just because it's new and different. But give it a chance. Usually, you can adjust in a short time, and it will no longer seem awkward. If you don't want any more children, seriously consider permanent sterilization. Surgical sterilization means either a vasectomy for a man or a tubal ligation for a woman. Surgical sterilization is usually easier for men, because the operation is done under local anesthesia, the recovery is short, and the complication rate is low.

If you've formed a Warrior Goddess group—and only if you feel comfortable doing so—share with one another what works for you, including your experience with different birth control methods or the names of gynecologists who have experience with natural approaches to menopause.

The greatest wealth is health.

—Virgil

Custom #20—Points to Remember

• Long-term use of birth control pills has been shown to increase the risk of breast cancer.

• Women who take the pill after age forty have a 50 percent higher risk of breast cancer.

• Women with a first-degree relative who has breast cancer and who take birth control pills long-term have a significantly higher risk of breast cancer.

• Menopause is not a disease. It is a natural transition of life that's best approached naturally, if possible.

• Menopausal symptoms arise from imbalances that, when corrected, usually improve or completely resolve.

• HRT increases the risk of heart disease, strokes, blood clots, gallbladder disease, invasive breast cancer, endometrial cancer, and ovarian cancer.

• HRT may increase the risk of breast cancer by as much as 66 to 100 percent and raise the risk of dying from breast cancer by as much as 22 percent.

• Taking a combination of estrogen and progestin contributes more to your risk of breast cancer than taking estrogen alone.

Never, never, never give up.

—WINSTON CHURCHILL

CUSTOM #21

Use only nontoxic cleaning products in your home and office.

We cannot direct the wind
but we can adjust the sails.

—AUTHOR UNKNOWN

Cleaning supplies are almost always filled with health-damaging toxins that you won't find listed on their labels. The federal government doesn't require that the ingredients in cleaning products be listed on the package. If a cleaning product isn't made by one of the companies that specifically make nontoxic cleaning products, you can bet it's got toxins in it. Throw it away. Buy only nontoxic cleaning products. (See the Resources section for a list of companies that make these products.) Most health food stores and some grocery stores carry nontoxic cleaning products. If your local store doesn't carry them, ask the manager to order them. These products are also available online and through certain catalogs, such as Harmony catalog sponsored by Gaiam.

If you've formed a Warrior Goddess group, have each member try a different nontoxic cleaning product, bring it to the meeting, and report what they liked or didn't like about it. There are many different companies that make nontoxic cleaning products, so if, for example, you don't like one company's glass cleaner, try another's. I have found good nontoxic products that work just as well as their toxic counterparts for *all* my cleaning needs. I'm sure you can, too.

CUSTOM #21 — POINTS TO REMEMBER

• Manufacturers are not required to list the harmful chemicals contained in their cleaning products on the product's label.

• Most cleaning products contain toxic chemicals.

• There is an effective nontoxic cleaning product to replace every toxic one you currently use.

Most of us can read the writing on the wall;
we just assume it's addressed to someone else.

—IVERN BALL

CUSTOM #22

Keep your home as toxin-free as possible.

In order to change, we must be sick and tired of being sick and tired.

—AUTHOR UNKNOWN

Cleaning products aren't the only sources of toxins in your home. They're everywhere! They are in your water, clothing, furnishings, construction materials, dry cleaning, personal-care products, lawn and garden products, insect repellant, flea collars, paints, wallpaper, carpet, tile, particleboard, and so on. Assume that everything is toxic. See Table 22.1 on page 228 for a reminder of the various sources of toxins in your home and their nontoxic alternatives.

Go through your house and find all the sources of possible toxins that you can easily do something about. For example, discard any pesticides or toxic lawn and garden products you have in your home, and research nontoxic ways to handle all your outdoor needs. Buy only chlorine-free paper products that are also labeled "tree-free," if possible. Use a water purifier, or buy purified drinking water (hard plastic bottles are safer than those that can be crushed easily). Purchase bed linens that are made of organic cotton when your old sheets are ready to be replaced. Likewise for your mattress. Whenever you do any home improvements, always choose nontoxic materials or use nontoxic sealers to prevent toxins from outgassing. (See the Resources section for companies that manufacture many of these products.)

If you live in an older home, the amount of toxins still outgassing from construction materials will be extremely low. However, if you live in a new home, it's a different story. If your house is fewer than two or three years old, the level of toxins in your home may be very high. Since heat causes the release of more toxins, keep your house on the cool side to keep the level of outgassing toxins lower. Keep your windows open as often as possible. It's also a good idea to buy a good air filter. Consider using a nontoxic sealer to trap the toxins. Certain houseplants, such as Boston ferns, English ivy, rubber plants, peace lilies, and bamboo, can absorb toxins from the air, so keep a few plants in each room.

Constantly be on the prowl to seek and avoid toxins. Develop an acute awareness of where toxins hide. Be aware of all the wonderful nontoxic alternatives, but don't feel that you must replace everything at once. For most, that's not practical or affordable. Don't stress over it. Move at a comfortable pace to gradually make your home as toxin-free as possible.

If you've formed a Warrior Goddess group, have each member investigate a nontoxic alternative for a common toxic item in the home and report what she discovers. If there's an organic lawn and garden service in your community, invite a representative to speak to your group.

Choices are the hinges of destiny.

—EDWIN MARKHAM

CUSTOM #22—POINTS TO REMEMBER

• Assume that everything is toxic unless specifically identified as nontoxic.

• Develop the habit of questioning the safety of a product and finding out if there's a nontoxic alternative.

• There are nontoxic alternatives to just about everything.

• You can prevent toxins from outgassing from particleboard, furniture, cabinets, and other construction materials in your home by using a nontoxic sealer.

• Organic lawn and garden companies have nontoxic solutions for all your needs, including pest problems.

• Don't stress over replacing everything in your home immediately. Make gradual changes.

• If you live in a new home, use an air filter, keep your house cool, and keep the windows open as often as possible.

CUSTOM #23

Purify your body several times a year.

If I'd known I was going to live so long, I'd have taken better care of myself.

—LEON ELDRED

No matter how pure your diet and lifestyle are, you're constantly being bombarded by unavoidable environmental toxins. Some of these toxins, such as organochlorine pesticides, significantly increase your risk of breast cancer. So, it's important to take a week or two, once or twice a year, to purify your body and get some of these toxins out. Research shows that the *Ayurvedic* purification procedures known as *panchakarma* are extremely effective at eliminating toxins. In fact, just one five-day series can cut your load of toxins in half.

There are many clinics throughout the world that specialize in *panchakarma* treatments. In the United States, there is an excellent clinic in Vedic City, Iowa. I've also located many other clinics in the United States that offer *panchakarma*, from Kauai, Hawaii, to Albuquerque and Taos, New Mexico, to Boulder, Colorado, to Coral Springs, Florida. If you'd prefer to go to Europe, where the cost is usually much less, there are several clinics in countries such as Switzerland and Germany, or you could go to India.

If getting away to a clinic for a week isn't possible, you can detoxify at home. However, there's been no research on home-detoxification programs, so it's impossible to say exactly what percentage of toxins you can get rid of this way. But, you'll almost certainly be able to reduce some of your toxin load. There are many programs for detoxifying at home. One simple way is to follow the home-prep program for *panchakarma* (see Chapter 23), stay on a purefoods diet for several weeks, and take herbs that help to purify your colon, liver, and kidneys. (Check the Resources section for websites that help with home detoxification.)

If you've formed a Warrior Goddess group, do something outlandish—go to a detox clinic together. Think outside the box; anything is possible. You could create a modified clinic at someone's home. For instance, invite massage therapists to come and give you sesame-oil massages or give them to one another. If someone has a sauna or has a membership at a gym that has one, you could all go there one day. Each member could volunteer to prepare vegetable juices or soups for everyone for one day of the week. Schedule colonics together—no kidding. Work together to create a detox program that everyone can do.

Limits exist only in your mind.

—Author unknown

Custom #23—Points to Remember

- Toxins can be eliminated from your body using purification techniques.

- Research shows that just one five-day *panchakarma* treatment can cut your toxin load in half.

- *Panchakarma* treatments also create profound balance, relieve depression, and improve many chronic conditions.

- If you can't go to a clinic, do a home-purification program.

- Although there's no research documenting the amount of toxins you may get rid of on a home-detoxification program, you *will* be able to get rid of some.

CUSTOM #24

Go to bed by 10:00 P.M., and get up before 6:00 A.M.

A good laugh and a long sleep are the best cures in the doctor's book.

—IRISH PROVERB

When you go to bed by 10:00 P.M. and get up before 6:00 A.M., you are following the natural rhythms of Nature and your body produces the highest surge of the astoundingly protective hormone, melatonin. Most people notice that when they begin to consistently sleep during these hours, they suddenly feel much better, have more energy, think more clearly, and are far more productive—wonderful side benefits to a habit that profoundly lowers your risk of breast cancer. Remember also that melatonin shuns light and loves the darkest of the dark. So, be sure to shut off all the lights and close the blinds in your bedroom.

If you have a habit of going to bed much later than 10:00 P.M., you may find that it's virtually impossible for you to fall asleep before 10:00 P.M. Experts recommend that, each week, you go to bed fifteen to thirty minutes earlier than you did the week before until you have adjusted to a 10:00 P.M. bedtime.

If you find you need some help getting to sleep while you are transitioning to an earlier bedtime, you might want to try supplemental melatonin. Research shows that melatonin supplements not only help you to sleep, but they may also provide additional protection against breast cancer. However, the safety of taking melatonin on a long-term basis hasn't been studied. Until there is research showing that long-term use of melatonin supplements is safe, limit your use of it to short periods. Be aware that if you use melatonin as a sleep aid every night for several weeks and then abruptly stop taking it, you may have difficulty falling asleep.

Studies show that supplemental melatonin usually produces a more restful sleep than pharmaceutical sleep aids, and it doesn't cause a "hangover." In my opinion, melatonin is safer than most pharmaceutical sleeping pills. So, if you occasionally have trouble sleeping and would like to take something to help, melatonin is an excellent option. However, if you frequently have trouble sleeping or know that you have a sleep disorder, see your physician.

If you've formed a Warrior Goddess group, discuss how each of you can complete your daily tasks and still get to bed by 10:00 P.M. Share your experiences with each other, especially concerning any emotional, physical, or spiritual changes you experience once you start this simple, yet powerful habit.

Some make it happen, some watch it happen,
and some say, "What happened?"

—AUTHOR UNKNOWN

CUSTOM #24—POINTS TO REMEMBER

• When you go to bed by 10:00 P.M. and get up before 6:00 A.M., you are following the natural rhythms of Nature. Hormonal fluctuations will be optimal, and the hormone melatonin will rise to its highest level.

• Melatonin is a powerful antioxidant and specifically arrests and deters breast cancer in many ways.

• Women who work the night shift produce far less melatonin and have a 50 percent higher risk of breast cancer.

• Melatonin supplements enhance the effectiveness of chemotherapy, protect against its damaging side effects, and improve your chances of survival from breast cancer.

• Melatonin is light sensitive. It needs complete darkness to rise to its highest level.

• Blind women have a 50 percent lower risk of breast cancer.

• Getting the proper amount of sleep at the right times is one of the most important things you can do to preserve and protect your health.

• Sleeping too many hours may actually increase your risk of illness.

• Alcohol and electromagnetic fields (EMFs) cause melatonin levels to drop.

CUSTOM #25

Minimize your exposure to electromagnetic fields (EMFs).

The impossible can always be broken down into possibilities.

—AUTHOR UNKNOWN

Electromagnetic fields (EMFs) emitted from common household appliances and wires have been shown to increase the risk of breast cancer. Go through your house and identify everything that might emit EMFs. Check your bedroom for electrical devices, such as clock radios, and move them at least several feet away from your head or consider replacing them with nonelectrical devices. For instance, change your clock radio to a battery-operated clock. The good news is that most of the EMF exposure you get from these devices becomes negligible when they are moved just a few feet away.

Microwave ovens produce significant EMFs. If you choose to use a microwave oven, avoid all the EMFs it emits simply by standing a few feet away or by going into another room while it's in use. (Incidentally, microwave cooking destroys most of the antioxidants in foods. Moreover, *Ayurvedic* physicians [*vaidyas*] say that microwave cooking changes the quality of the food so much that it creates imbalances in the body.)

Hair dryers produce more EMFs than any other appliance. If air-drying your hair isn't an option, purchase a low-EMF hair dryer (see the Resources section).

Be sure to apply cell chips made by GIA Wellness to all of your appliances and cell phones. It's also an excellent idea to wear the GIA Wellness pendant as much as possible. For more information on GIA Wellness products go to my website www.drchristinehorner.com.

If you've formed a Warrior Goddess group, make a game of identifying sources of EMFs in each member's home. Then, design a plan for keeping EMF exposure low in each of your homes.

CUSTOM #25—POINTS TO REMEMBER

- Research shows a definite link between EMF exposure and breast cancer.

- All electrical appliances and wires produce EMF.

- Hair dryers produce more EMFs than any other household appliance.

- EMF emissions drop very rapidly a short distance from an appliance. Just standing a few feet away from most electrical devices and appliances is all you need to do to avoid the EMFs they produce.

- Just 50 hertz (Hz) of EMFs causes breast cancer tumors to start growing and accelerates their growth.

- You can purchase EMF protection devices for your cell phone, computer, and other appliances.

- You can wear the GIA Wellness pendant.

CUSTOM #26

Embrace thirty minutes of aerobic activity every day.

Those who think they have not time for bodily exercise
will sooner or later have to find time for illness.

—EDWARD STANLEY

Movement is medicine for creating change
in a person's physical, emotional, and mental states.

—CAROL WELCH

This is the moment you've been waiting for. Now is the time you're going to begin an invigorating aerobic activity that raises your heart rate *every day*. First, check with your doctor before starting any exercise program. You must take your current state of health and aerobic condition into consideration when selecting the type of activity that best suits you. Usually, walking is an excellent choice for almost any beginner. If you haven't exercised in years, start walking at a comfortable pace, then gradually pick up the pace and increase your distance.

There's an endless list of activities that can improve and maintain your aerobic condition. Choose those that you enjoy because you are much more likely to continue doing something you like. Remember that exercising regularly is one of the most important things you can do to support your health. Not only does it lower your risk of breast cancer by 30 to 50 percent, but it also lowers your risk of many other diseases, including heart disease, colon cancer, diabetes, and obesity.

Review Chapter 25 for more suggestions about choosing an activity that elevates your heart rate. Remember to choose activities that bring you joy.

If you've formed a Warrior Goddess group, have one of the meetings at a fitness center and participate in an exercise class. Some members may buddy-up and take the class on a regular basis.

Don't say you don't have enough time. You have exactly the
same number of hours per day that were given to Helen Keller,
Pasteur, Michelangelo, Mother Teresa, Leonardo da Vinci,
Thomas Jefferson, and Albert Einstein.

—*LIFE'S LITTLE INSTRUCTION BOOK,*
COMPILED BY H. JACKSON BROWN, JR.

I have to exercise in the morning
before my brain figures out what I am doing.

—Marsha Doble

Custom #26—Points to Remember

• Regular aerobic exercise produces a cascade of health-promoting chemicals and hormones that significantly decrease your risk of many diseases including breast cancer.

• Just thirty minutes of aerobic activity three to five times a week can lower your risk of breast cancer by 30 to 50 percent.

• Teenagers who exercise regularly can lower their risk of breast cancer for the rest of their lives.

• Exercise can alleviate depression as effectively as many common antidepressant medications.

• The best time of day to exercise is in the morning.

• Regular invigorating movements also reduce your risk of heart disease; type 2 diabetes; cancers of the lung, ovary, uterus, and pancreas; lung diseases, such as asthma and emphysema; arthritis; glaucoma; and neurodegenerative diseases, such as Alzheimer's disease and dementia.

Stopping at third base adds no more runs than striking out.

—Author unknown

CUSTOM #27

Practice a stress-reducing meditation every day.

Too many people miss the silver lining
because they're expecting gold.

—Maurice Setter

Practicing a research-proven stress-reducing meditation every day is so balancing to your mind/body that it can lower your risk of all diseases by as much as

50 percent. The most effective form of meditation for relieving stress and promoting health is Transcendental Meditation (TM). To find a teacher near you, call 1-800-LEARN-TM (1-800-532-7686) or go to www.TM.org. Learning TM is relatively expensive, but its many health benefits make it worth the cost. If the cost is too much for your budget or there isn't a TM teacher in your area, begin another stress-reducing technique. Research shows that other techniques of meditation and relaxation may not be as effective as TM, but they are beneficial. Avoid techniques that require mental concentration because research shows they may actually increase stress.

You may find that listening to guided meditations or relaxing music on an audiotape or CD provides the stress reduction you need. There is a great device made by New Realities that has guided meditations programmed on an iPod-like device. Earbuds or headphones deliver the sound, which includes alternating subliminal beats called binaural beats. There are also goggles that you wear that look like sunglasses. The goggles produce light-emitting diode (LED) lights that are designed to stimulate your retinas while your eyes are closed. Both the sound and the lights help your brain to quickly go into a meditation state known as theta. You can find out more about this device on my website at www.drchristinehorner.com/transformationalguidedimagery.html.

If you're looking for more, yoga is a wonderful ancient practice you may want to consider. Research shows that it keeps the body supple, promotes balance, and reduces stress. There are many different types of yoga. Regardless of your physical condition, almost everyone can practice some form of yoga. Because of its wonderful health benefits, yoga has become very popular and is taught in most U.S. cities. You may want to purchase an instructional yoga videotape and practice it at home.

If you've formed a Warrior Goddess group, practice a relaxation technique at one of the meetings. Perhaps your group could sign up for yoga classes together, or you could create your own class with a few interested members.

CUSTOM #27—POINTS TO REMEMBER

• Stress plays a role in more than 90 percent of all illnesses, physical and mental.

• Women who have suffered a major stressful trauma have a twelve times greater risk of developing breast cancer within five years.

• Practicing a stress-reducing meditation every day can have profound beneficial effects on your mind, body, and spirit, and it can lower your risk of breast cancer.

• Research shows that TM is the most effective form of meditation in relieving stress and anxiety and in promoting health.

• People who practice this form of meditation have a 50 percent lower incidence of all diseases.

• Other stress-relieving techniques can have good health benefits, too; for example, *yoga* has been found to relieve stress and improve a variety of health conditions.

• Avoid meditation techniques that require mental concentration because they may actually increase anxiety.

• New Realities makes an excellent relaxation device with guided meditations, sounds, and lights (www.drchristinehorner.com/transformationalguidedimagery.html).

CUSTOM #28

Practice stress-reducing breathing techniques every day.

The time to relax is when you don't have time for it.
—Attributed to both Jim Goodwin and Sydney J. Harris

Stress has been found to contribute to about 90 percent of all illnesses, including breast cancer. So, practicing a daily stress-reducing technique, such as the simple breathing exercise called *pranayama*, can profoundly influence and support your health.

To perform *pranayama*, sit quietly where you won't be disturbed and begin breathing through alternating nostrils, as described under *Pranayama—Using Your Breath* on page 283. Notice how relaxed you feel afterward. The wonderful thing about *pranayama* is that it requires no equipment, special location, or expense. So, anyone can engage in this health-promoting technique anytime, anywhere. To achieve the greatest benefits from *pranayama*, practice it at least twice a day for five to ten minutes each time.

There are also many other techniques of *pranayama* that you could learn. The method I have described is one of the simpler, more basic ones. But if you're interested in learning other forms of *pranayama*, find out if there are any nearby classes available or research the other techniques (see the Resources section).

If you've formed a Warrior Goddess group, take a class together or have each member research a technique of *pranayama* and teach it to the other members. Practice each technique for five to ten minutes.

How beautiful it is to do nothing, and then rest afterward.
—Spanish proverb

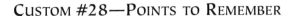

CUSTOM #28—POINTS TO REMEMBER

• *Pranayama* is a simple ancient practice of regulating the breath. It has profound health benefits.

• Research shows that the regular practice of *pranayama* increases the depth of your breath and your breath-holding capacity. It also improves stress-hormone balance, blood pressure, and heart rate, and it lowers cholesterol.

• Practicing *pranayama* is simple. It can be done anywhere, and it costs nothing.

CUSTOM #29

Take an herbal adaptogen every day to lower your body's response to stress.

Herbal adaptogens have been found to lower your body's response to stress and protect against its damaging effects in a multitude of ways. Some of the best adaptogen herbs are ginseng and the *Ayurvedic* herbs *ashwagandha* and holy basil. These supplements are available from most health food stores, some grocery stores, and on the Internet. (Check the Resources section for listings.) The recommended daily dosage for *ashwagandha* is 1–2 tablespoons of root powder or 1–2 grams of root, or simply follow the direction on the supplement label. The recommended daily dosage for ginseng is 1–2 grams of root or 200–400 mg in standardized capsules. The recommended daily dosage for holy basil is 1–2 standardized capsules. I recommend holy basil by New Chapter.

> Following an ideal daily routine lowers stress and brings balance. See Ideal *Ayurvedic* Daily Routine on page 282.

CUSTOM #29—POINTS TO REMEMBER

• Herbal adaptogens are effective at lowering your physiological response to stress.

• Holy basil, for example, decreases cortisol and enhances stamina, endurance, and the body's effective use of oxygen under stress. It also protects and boosts the immune system during stress.

• Don't rely on an herb alone to protect you from stress; adopt as many stress-reducing habits and behaviors as possible.

CUSTOM #30

Take care of your needs.

There must be quite a few things
a hot bath won't cure,
but I don't know many of them.

—SYLVIA PLATH, *THE BELL JAR*

Research shows that women who develop breast cancer are more likely to give too much at the expense of their own needs. Since our culture trains women to do this, we need to break this habit. Instead, we need to practice asking ourselves what serves us best and then do it. For instance, you may decide that a massage on a regular basis is something that supports you. Many women think that massages or other nurturing treatments are just frivolous pampering; they're wrong. Research shows that human touch is powerful medicine. Massage not only lessens muscular tension and discomfort, but it also stimulates the immune system and decreases depression—both of which have profound effects on keeping your body well and warding off disease. If you can't make it to a spa for a professional massage, request a massage from your significant other. Research shows that massage is beneficial to both the giver and the receiver. It's also a wonderful way to enhance intimacy with your partner. And nothing has been found to be more powerful in supporting health than the experience of love and intimacy. If you're not in an intimate relationship right now, massage yourself. In fact, self-massage contributes to good health so much that *Ayurveda* recommends daily sesame-oil self-massages as part of the ideal health routine.

Train yourself to listen to your needs. Nurture yourself like you would your children. As one of my good friends, a professional life coach, says, "The best way to take care of other people is to take care of you." You can't fully help others if you are stressed, exhausted, and emotionally spent. But if you keep yourself balanced, rested, and sourced, you can support those you love so much better. Nature gave each of us a miraculous mind/body and with it, the responsibility of taking care of it. No one else has been assigned to take care of your mind/body except you. It's your primary responsibility. If you don't accept this responsibility, you will become sick and then you won't be able to help those you love.

It is one of the most beautiful compensations of this life that
no man can sincerely try to help another without helping himself.

—RALPH WALDO EMERSON

The more you take care of yourself, the more likely you are to reach your full potential and *that* is the purpose of your life. You are here on a journey to experience the highest version of yourself and to contribute your unique gifts to the world. With few exceptions, you can only do that fully if you are healthy.

If you've formed a Warrior Goddess group, have each member reflect and share with the group a new practice she could start that takes care of her needs. Think about ways to support one another. For example, one member could babysit for another member's kids once a week for an hour or two. This will free up time for the other member to get a massage, go for a hike, read a book, or do whatever it is that takes care of her needs. Or, you could even free up time for *everyone* in the group by starting a dinner co-op. Each member takes a turn preparing large meals and sharing them with the other group members.

CUSTOM #30—POINTS TO REMEMBER

• Every emotion you feel creates a biochemical reaction in your body that affects your health.

• Negative emotions take a toll on your health, while positive emotions such as laughing stimulate your immune system and help to keep you healthy.

• It's important to feel all your emotions, but it's best to learn how to process your negative emotions so that they don't linger.

• Women with breast cancer tend to give too much at the expense of their own needs, stay in loveless relationships, have issues with hope and trust, and suffer from hurt, sorrow, and unfinished business.

When health is absent, wisdom cannot reveal itself,
art cannot become manifest, strength cannot be exerted,
wealth is useless, and reason is powerless.

—HEROPHILIES, 300 B.C.E.

The best way to predict your future is to create it.

—AUTHOR UNKNOWN

MISSION ACCOMPLISHED

That's it. You're now doing most everything we know of that will substantially lower your risk of breast cancer. If you haven't noticed her yet, look in the mirror. Look closely at your reflection. You should be able to see the Warrior Goddess within you shining in radiant health. Your new health-creating and health-preserving choices are contributing to making the enlightened culture of the next century a reality today. You can play an even larger role in making this

Grocery List

I recommend that you use the following list as a guide when you go to the health food store or the natural food section of your grocery store. These are all items that I've covered in this book, and if you can't find them locally, check the Internet. Remember to buy only organic, if you can!

- ❑ *Cruciferous vegetables: broccoli, cauliflower, kale, bok choy, or Brussels sprouts*
- ❑ *Brazil nuts*
- ❑ *Flaxseeds and flax oil*
- ❑ *Fruits: apples, apricots, oranges, berries, grapes, melon, and so on*
- ❑ *Garlic*
- ❑ *Green tea*
- ❑ *Olive oil*
- ❑ *Sesame oil*
- ❑ *Soy products: tofu, tempeh, miso, soy milk, or soy meat substitute*
- ❑ *Stevia*
- ❑ *Turmeric*
- ❑ *Vegetables: asparagus, beets, artichokes, garlic, spinach, and so on*
- ❑ *Wakame or mekabu seaweed*
- ❑ *Whole grains: brown rice, quinoa, amaranth, or barley*

Basic Supplement List

I recommended products made by Enzymatic Therapy, New Chapter, and Maharishi *Ayurvedic* Products International. These companies are highly reputable and put extremely careful thought into every step of creating each product. They principally use organically grown herbs or herbs grown and collected in the wild. They use no chemicals, pesticides, or harsh processing practices that could destroy the quality of the herbs. Generally, all the products are created from whole foods and are not synthetic. These companies make the highest quality products on the market, products that work in a manner most in harmony with your body. For your convenience most of the supplements I recommend throughout my book are available on my website www.drchristinehorner.com.

- ❏ *Multivitamin*
- ❏ *AHCC*
- ❏ *Amrit Kalash*
- ❏ *Brevail*
- ❏ *CoQ$_{10}$*
- ❏ *Holy basil*
- ❏ *Protective Breast Formula*
- ❏ *Resveratrol*
- ❏ *Zyflamend*

visionary culture real by sharing these new customs with your friends. The more of us there are who adopt these customs, the faster our world will change to one where good health is normal and chronic diseases such as cancer are rare.

Remember that the health benefits of all these customs or practices don't just add up, they multiply. So, the difference you're making in decreasing your risk of breast cancer is *huge*! Doing all these things won't give you a 100-percent guarantee that you'll never develop breast cancer. But your likelihood of getting this terrible disease will be very small. If you do get it, your chances of having a less aggressive tumor and surviving it are much greater. If you already have breast cancer, remember, all these things can help you, too.

Keep up the good work. It's important to keep all the customs you've adopted. Just doing a few things every once in a while won't give you the protection you really want. I do all these things. They can be done, and it's not hard. You just need to adjust to the changes, and you will. You should be feeling a lot better by now, too. Feeling better is good motivation. You will undoubtedly continue to feel better and better. Your energy levels should go up, and you will probably get sick less often. If you have other chronic disorders, you may notice an improvement in them, as well.

Nothing is more important than your health. Without it, you have nothing. Congratulations on completing the program!

I'd love to hear from you to see what differences it has made in your life already. Please contact me through my website at www.drchristinehorner.com.

 May you live with perfect health and fulfillment
all the days you walk this earth.

Thank you for allowing me to contribute to you.

Namasté

Resources

CONTENT GUIDE

Contact information is subject to change.

AHCC SUPPLEMENT

Quality of Life Labs, Inc.
2975 Westchester Avenue
Suite G-01
Purchase, NY 10577
Phone: 877-937-2422
Website: www.qualityoflife.net *or*
www.drchristinehorner.com

AIR-FILTRATION SYSTEMS

Gaiam, Inc.
Website: www.gaiam.com
Blueair HEPA Air Filter 501 and 402;
Healthmate HEPA Air Filter; SilentAir
4000; Desktop Air Filters; UV Air Purifier
(uses HEPA, carbon, UV light, and
ionization); Car Ionizer

AMRIT KALASH

Maharishi Ayurveda Products Int'l
1680 Highway 1 North, Suite 2200
Fairfield, IA 52556
Phone: 800-255-8332
Fax: 719-260-7400
E-mail: info@mapi.com
Website: www.mapi.com

ANTIOXIDANT SUPPLEMENTS

Maharishi Ayurveda Products Int'l
1680 Highway 1 North, Suite 2200
Fairfield, IA 52556
Phone: 800-255-8332
Fax: 719-260-7400
E-mail: info@mapi.com
Websites: www.mapi.com or
www.drchristinehorner.com

New Chapter
90 Technology Drive
Brattleboro, VT 05301
Phone: 800-543-7279
Fax: 800-470-0247
E-mail: info@newchapter.com
Websites: www.new-chapter.com,
www.newchapter.info, *or*
www.drchristinehorner.com

AYURVEDIC HEALTH SPAS

AuroMesa, LLC
101 Coyote Loop
P.O. Box 567
Arroyo-Hondo, NM 87571
Phone: 575-776-2212
E-mail: Tizia@auromesa.com
Website: www.auromesa.com

The Ayurvedic Institutes
11311 Menaul Boulevard, N.E.
Albuquerque, NM 87112
Phone: 505-291-9698
Website: www.ayurveda.com

Ayurvedic Natural Health Center
1342 North Fairfield Road, Suite B
Beavercreek (Dayton), OH 45432
Phone: 937-429-WELL (9355)
E-mail: ayurveda429WELL@sbcglobal.net
Website: www.midwestayurveda.com

Dr. John Douillard's LifeSpa
6662 Gunpark Drive East, Suite 102
Boulder, CO 80301
Phone: 303-516-4848 *or* 866-227-9843
E-mail: info@lifespa.com
Website: http://lifespa.com

The Raj
1734 Jasmine Avenue
Fairfield, IA 52556
Phone: 800-248-9050 *or* 641-472-9580
(in IA)
E-mail: theraj@lisco.com
Websites: www.theraj.com

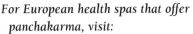

For European health spas that offer panchakarma, visit:

www.ayurveda.de/mag_forsch.htm

www.ayurvedabadems.de/
  english/haus/index.php

www.maharishi-european-
  sidhaland.org.uk

BEDS, BEDDING, FURNITURE

Amenity Home
4548 Ambrose Avenue
Los Angeles, CA 90027
Phone: 213-624-7309
E-mail: contact@amenityhome.com
Website: www.amenityhome.com

Coyuchi, Inc.
2501 Ninth Street, Suite 102
Berkeley, CA 94710
Phone: 510-903-0407 *or* 888-418-8847
E-mail: info@coyuchi.com
Website: www.coyuchi.com

Earthsake
1425 4th Street
Berkeley, CA 94710
Phone: 510-848-5023
Website: www.earthsake.com

Ecobaby Organics
7550 Miramar Road, Suite 220
San Diego, CA 92126
Phone: 800-596-7450
Website: www.purerest.com *or*
  www.ecobaby.com

Gaiam, Inc.
833 W. South Boulder Road
P.O. Box 3095
Boulder, CO 80307
Phone: 877-989-6321 *or* 800-254-8464
  (in Canada)
Website: www.gaiam.com

Tomorrow's World
9647 First View Street
Norfolk, VA 23503
Phone: 800-229-7571
Website: www.tomorrowsworld.com

BREVAIL SUPPLEMENTS

Barlean's Organic Oils
3660 Slater Road
Ferndale, WA 98248
Phone: 800-445-3529 *or* 360-384-0485
Fax: 360-384-1746
Websites: www.barleans.com *or*
  www.drchristinehorner.com

BUILDING CONSULTANTS AND PRODUCTS

Building for Health Materials Center
Website: www.buildingforhealth.com

Natural House Company
Website: www.naturalhouseco.com

CABINETS

Building for Health Materials Center
Website: www.buildingforhealth.com

Nirvana Safe Haven
Website: www.nontoxic.com

CALCIUM D-GLUCARATE SUPPLEMENTS

Enzymatic Therapy
825 Challenger Drive
Green Bay, WI 54311
Phone: 800-783-2286
Fax: 920-469-4444
Website: www.eticonsumer.com *or*
  www.drchristinehorner.com
Available in Protective Breast Formula

CARPETS AND FLOORING

Nature's Carpet
494 Railway Street
Vancouver, BC V6A 1B1
Canada
Phone: 800-667-5001
E-mail: myra@naturescarpet.com
Website: www.naturescarpet.com

EcoChoices
P.O. Box 1491
Glendora, CA 91740
Phone: 626-969-3707
Website: www.ecochoices.com/ecobydesign

Grown Green
1338 S. Foothill Drive, Suite 201
Salt Lake City, UT 84108
Phone: 877-233-7036
E-mail: info@growngreenrugs.com
Website: www.growngreenrugs.com

CLOTHING

Blue Canoe
1900 Oakdale Avenue
San Francisco, CA 94124
Phone: 888-923-1373
E-mail: info@bluecanoe.com
Website: www.bluecanoe.com

Blue Fish Clothing
58 S. Main Street
Fairfield, IA 52556
Phone: 800-395-4566
Website: www.bluefishclothing.com

Esperanza Threads
1370 West 69th Street
Cleveland, OH 44102
Phone: 800-397-0045
Website: www.esperanzathreads.com
Organic apparel and goods

Green Babies, Inc.
28 Spring Street
Tarrytown, NY 10591
Phone: 800-603-7508
Website: www.greenbabies.com

Maggie's Functional Organics
306 West Cross Street
Ypsilanti, MI 48197
Phone: 800-609-8593
Fax: 734-482-4175
E-mail: maggies@organicclothes.com
Website: www.organicclothes.com

Synergy Organic Clothing
Phone: 888-466-0411 (ext. 2) *or* 831-331-4015
E-mail: websales@synergyclothing.com
Website: www.synergyclothing.com

COENZYME Q$_{10}$/UBIQUINOL SUPPLEMENTS

Enzymatic Therapy
825 Challenger Drive
Green Bay, WI 54311
Phone:800-783-2286
Fax: 920-469-4444
Website: www.eticonsumer.com

New Chapter
90 Technology Drive
Brattleboro, VT 05301
Phone: 800-543-7279
E-mail: info@new-chapter.com
Websites: www.new-chapter.com *or* www.newchapter.info

COMMUNITY-SPONSORED AGRICULTURE (CSA)

Alternative Farming Systems Information Center (AFSIC)
Website: www.nal.usda.gov/afsic/csa

CONJUGATED LINOLEIC ACID (CLA)

NOW Foods
Website: www.nowfoods.com

DIGESTIVE FORMULAS
Enzymatic Therapy
825 Challenger Drive
Green Bay, WI 54311
Phone: 800-783-2286
Fax: 920-469-4444
Website: www.eticonsumer.com

New Chapter
90 Technology Drive
Brattleboro, VT 05301
Phone: 800-543-7279
Fax: 800-470-0247
E-mail: info@new-chapter.com
Websites: www.new-chapter.com *or*
   www.newchapter.info

Maharishi Ayurveda Products Int'l
1680 Highway 1 North, Suite 2200
Fairfield, IA 52556
Phone: 800-255-8332
Fax: 719-260-7400
E-mail: info@mapi.com
Website: www.mapi.com

EDAMAME (SOYBEANS)
SeaPoint Farms
2183 Fairview Road
Costa Mesa, CA 92627
Phone: 888-722-7098
E-mail: info@seapointfarms.com
Website: www.seapointfarms.com

Small Planet Foods (makers of Cascadian Farms)
P.O. Box 9452
Minneapolis, MN 55440
Phone: 800-624-4123
Website: www.cascadianfarm.com

EMOTIONAL RELEASE PRACTITIONERS

Body Memory Recall (BMR)
Jonathan Tripodi
www.freedomfrombodymemory.com

Telehealing with Gail Raborn
Transformational hypnosis and mind,
   body, spirit counselor
Phone: 707-0937-2271
Website: www.telehealing.com
*"My passion is to help people grow, heal,
   and transform their lives into ones of
   harmony, high health, and creativity."*

ENVIRONMENTAL TOXINS (INFORMATION)

Environmental Working Group
1436 U Street, NW, Suite 100
Washington, DC 20009 |
Phone: 202667-6982
Website: www.ewg.org

Scorecard (Environmental Defense)
Website: www.scorecard.org

U.S. Environmental Protection Agency
Website: www.epa.gov

FLAXSEEDS AND FLAX OIL

Barlean's Organic Oils
3660 Slater Road
Ferndale, WA 98248
Phone: 800-445-3529 *or* 360-384-0485
Fax: 360-384-1746
Websites: www.barleans.com *or*
   www.drchristinehorner.com

FOODS, ORGANIC

Amy's Kitchen, Inc.
P.O. Box 449
Petaluma, CA 94953
Phone: 707-781-7535
E-mail: amy@amyskitchen.net
Website: www.amyskitchen.com

Small Planet Foods (makers of Cascadian Farms)
P.O. Box 9452
Minneapolis, MN 55440
Phone: 800-624-4123
Website: www.cascadianfarm.com
Organic foods, including frozen fruits and vegetables

Earthbound Farm
1721 San Juan Highway
San Juan Bautista, CA 95045
Phone: 800-690-3200
Website: www.ebfarm.com
Organic fruits and vegetables

Eden Foods
701 Tecumseh Road
Clinton, MI 49236
Phone: 517-456-7424, 888-424-EDEN
Fax: 517-456-7854
Website: www.edenfoods.com
Variety of organic foods

Horizon Organic
12002 Airport Way
Broomfield, CO 80021
Phone: 888-494-3020
Fax: 503-652-1371
Website: www.horizonorganic.com
Organic dairy

Lotus Foods
c/o WorldPantry.com, Inc.
1192 Illinois Street
San Francisco, CA 94107
Phone: 866-972-6879
Fax: 510-525-4226
Website: www.lotusfoods.com
Organic grains

Lundberg Family Farms
P.O. Box 369
Richvale, CA 95974
Phone: 530-538-3500
Fax: 530-882-4500
Website: www.lundberg.com
Organic grains

Melissa's/World Variety Produce Inc.
P.O. Box 21127
Los Angeles, CA 90021
Phone: 800-588-0151
Fax: 323-584-7385
E-mail: hotline@melissas.com
Website: www.melissas.com
Organic foods and many recipes

Organic Kingdom
192 West 1480 South
Orem, UT 84058
Phone: 866-699-4950
Fax: 801-426-7627
Website: www.organickingdom.com

Organic Valley Family of Farms/CROPP Cooperative
One Organic Way
LaFarge, WI 54639
Phone: 888-444-6455
Fax: 608-625-3025
Website: www.organicvalley.com
Organic dairy

Purely Organic, Ltd.
P.O. Box 847
Fairfield, IA 52556
Phone: 877-201-0710
Fax: 641-472-1754
Website: www.purelyorganic.com
Imported organic condiments, grape juice from Italy

Seeds of Change
P.O. Box 4908
Rancho Dominguez, CA 90220
Phone: 888-762-7333
Website: www.seedsofchange.com

ShopOrganic
3450 S. Broadmont Drive, Suite 114
Tucson, AZ 85713
Phone: 520-792-0804
Website: www.shoporganic.com
Online organic food and products store

South Pacific Trading Company
15052 Ronnie Drive, Suite 100
Dade City, FL 33523
Phone: 888-505-4439 *or* 352-567-2200
Fax: 352-567-2257
Website: www.southpacifictrading.com

Sprouts Farmers Market
Corporate Office
11811 N. Tatum Blvd., Suite 2400
Phoenix, AZ 85028
Phone: 480-814-8016 *or*
  888-5-SPROUT (888-577-7688)
Fax: 480-814-8017
Website: http://sprouts.com

Stonyfield Farms
10 Burton Drive
Londonderry, NH 03053
Phone: 800-776-2697
Fax: 603-437-7594
Website: www.stonyfield.com
Organic dairy

SunOrganic Farm
411 S. Las Posas Road
San Marcos, CA 92078
Phone: 888-269-9888
Fax: 760-510-9996
Website: www.sunorganic.com
Online organic foods, free catalog

Whole Foods Market, Inc.
World Headquarters

550 Bowie Street
Austin, TX 78703
Phone: 512-477-4455
Fax: 512-482-7000
Website: www.wholefoodsmarket.com

GARLIC SUPPLEMENTS

Enzymatic Therapy
825 Challenger Drive
Green Bay, WI 54311
Phone: 800-783-2286
Fax: 920-469-4444
Website: www.eticonsumer.com

New Chapter
90 Technology Drive
Brattleboro, VT 05301
Phone: 800- 543-7279
Fax: 800-470-0247
E-mail: info@newchapter.com
Websites: www.newchapter.com *or*
  www.newchapter.info

Kyolic
23501 Madero
Mission Viejo, CA 92691
Phone: 949-855-2776 *or* 800-421-2998
Fax: 949-458-2764
E-mail: info@wakunaga.com
Website: www.kyolic.com

GRAPE SEED EXTRACT
Enzymatic Therapy
825 Challenger Drive
Green Bay, WI 54311
Phone: 800-783-2286
Fax: 920-469-4444
Websites: www.eticonsumer.com *or*
  www.drchristinehorner.com
Available in Protective Breast Formula

GREEN DRINKS

All Day Energy Greens
Institute for Vibrant Living
P.O. Box 3840

Camp Verda, AZ 86322
Phone: 800-218-1379
Website: www.IVLProducts.com

GREEN TEA

Blue Moon Tea
Website: www.bluemoontea.com

Celestial Seasonings
Website: www.celestialseasonings.com

Choice Organic Teas
Website: www.choiceorganicteas.com

Numi Teas and Teasans
Website: www.numitea.com

Stash Tea
Website: www.stashtea.com

Traditional Medicinals
Website: www.traditionalmedicinals.com
/products

Yogi Tea
Website: www.yogiproducts.com

GREEN TEA SUPPLEMENTS

Enzymatic Therapy
825 Challenger Drive
Green Bay, WI 54311
Phone: 800-783-2286
Fax: 920-469-4444
Websites: www.eticonsumer.com *or*
   www.drchristinehorner.com
Available in Protective Breast Formula

New Chapter
90 Technology Drive
Brattleboro, VT 05301
Phone: 800-543-7279
Fax: 800-470-0247
E-mail: info@newchapter.com
Websites: www.newchapter.com *or*
   www.newchapter.info

HERBAL ANTI-INFLAMMATORY (ZYFLAMEND)

New Chapter
90 Technology Drive
Brattleboro, VT 05301
Phone: 800-543-7279
Fax: 800-470-0247
E-mail: info@newchapter.com
Websites: www.newchapter.com,
   www.newchapter.info, *or*
   www.drchristinehorner.com

HERBS

Frontier Natural Products Co-op
P.O. Box 299
3021 78th Street
Norway, IA 52318
Phone: 800-669-3275
Fax: 800-717-4372
Website: www.frontiercoop.com
*World's largest supplier of organic herbs
   and spices—available in many stores
   including online stores.*

HOME DETOX PROGRAMS

**Enzymatic Therapy Natural
   Medicines**
Website: www.eticonsumer.com
Whole Body Cleanse Kit

HealthWorld Online
Website: www.healthy.net
*The Internet's leading resource on
   alternative medicine, wellness, and
   mind/body health, featuring the Wellness
   Inventory whole person assessment.*

Maharishi Ayurveda
Website: www.mapi.com
*Type in "home detox" into search engine to
   find several articles from past newsletters
   with instructions and recipes for home
   detox programs.*

HOUSEHOLD CLEANING PRODUCTS

Country Save
19704 60th Avenue NE
Arlington, WA 98223
Phone: 360-435-9868
Fax: 360-435-0896
E-mail: info@countrysave.com
Website:
   www.countrysave.com/prods.php

Earth Friendly Products
111 S. Rohlwing Road
Addison, IL 60101
Phone: 800-335-3267
Fax: 847-446-4437
Website: www.ecos.com

Ecover
P.O. Box 9111058
Commerce, CA 90091
Phone: 800-449-4925
Fax: 323-720-5732
Website: www.ecover.com

Planet, Inc.
2676 Wilfert Road, Suite 201
Victoria, BC V9B 5ZE
Canada
Phone: 250-478-8171 *or* 800-858-8449
Fax: 250-478-3238
Website: www.planetinc.com

INDOLE-3-CARBINOL SUPPLEMENTS

Enzymatic Therapy
825 Challenger Drive
Green Bay, WI 54311
Phone: 800-783-2286
Fax: 920-469-4444
Websites: www.eticonsumer.com *or*
   www.drchristinehorner.com
Available in Protective Breast Formula

INSECT REPELLENT

All Terrain
P.O. Box 840
920 Route 11
Sunapee, NH 03782
Phone: 800-246-7328
Website: www.allterrainco.com

Burt's Bees
Attn: Consumer Care
P.O. Box 3900
Peoria, IL 61612
Phone: 800-849-7112
Fax: 800-429-7487
Website: www.burtsbees.com

INSULATION

Building for Health Materials Center
Website: www.buildingforhealth.com

Cellulose
Website: www.cellulose.org

Icynene
Website: www.icynene.com

Nirvana Safe Haven
Website: www.nontoxic.com

LIGNAN SUPPLEMENTS

Brevail
Barlean's Organic Oils
3660 Slater Road
Ferndale, WA 98248
Phone: 800-445-3529 *or* 360-384-0485
Fax: 360-384-1746
Websites: www.barleans.com/brevail.asp
   or www.drchristinehorner.com

LOW-EMF HAIR DRYER

CHI Pro Low-EMF Hairdryer
*This hairdryer is sold on many different
   websites and retail stores—search the
   Internet to find the best price.*

MAHARISHI VEDIC ORGANIC AGRICULTURE

Maharishi Vedic Organic Agriculture Institute
P.O. Box 2006
Fairfield, IA 52556
Phone: 641-469-5477
Fax: 641-472-7873
E-mail: MVOAI@Maharishi.net
Website: www.mvoai.org

MAITAKE MUSHROOM SUPPLEMENTS

Enzymatic Therapy
825 Challenger Drive
Green Bay, WI 54311
Phone: 800-783-2286
Fax: 920-469-4444
Websites: www.eticonsumer.com *or*
  www.drchristinehorner.com
Available in Protective Breast Formula

Fungi Perfecti, LLC
P.O. Box 7634
Olympia, WA 98507
Order Line: 800-780-9126
Phone: 360-426-9292
Fax: 360-426-9377
E-mail: mycomedia@aol.com
Website: www.fungi.com

MycoLogical Natural Products, Ltd.
P.O. Box 24940
Eugene, OR 97402
Phone: 888-465-3247
Website: www.mycological.com
Organic dried maitake mushrooms

New Chapter
90 Technology Drive
Brattleboro, VT 05301
Phone: 800-543-7279
Fax: 800-470-0247
E-mail: info@newchapter.com

Websites: www.newchapter.com *or*
www.newchapter.info

MEAT SUBSTITUTES

Amy's Kitchen
P.O. Box 449
Petaluma, CA 94953
Phone: 707-781-7535 *or* 707-568-4500
Website: www.amys.com

BOCA Foods Company
P.O. Box 8995
Madison, WI 53708
Phone: 877-966-8769
Website: www.bocaburger.com

Light Life
53 Industrial Boulevard
Turners Falls, MA 10376
Phone: 800-SOYEASY (769-3279)
Website: www.lightlife.com

Morningstar Farms
Kellogg's Consumer Affairs
P.O. Box CAMB
Battle Creek, MI 49016
Phone: 800-962-1413
Websites: www.morningstarfarms.com *or*
  www.gardenburger.com

Yves Veggie Cuisine
Customer Care
Hain Celestial Group, Inc.
4600 Sleepytime Drive
Boulder, CO 80301
Phone: 800-434-4246
Website: www.yvesveggie.com/products
  /detail.php/good-dog
Made with organic ingredients

Tofurkey
Turtle Island Foods
P.O. Box 176
Hood River, OR 97031
Phone: 800-508-8100 (ext. 19)
Fax: 541-386-7754
Website: www.tofurkey.com/
  tofurkyproducts/holiday_products.html

MUSHROOMS, DRIED

Life Gourmet Shop, LLC
2814 Ashbury Heights Road
Decatur, GA 30030
Phone: 800-910-0849
E-mail: info@lifegourmetshop.com
Website: www.lifegourmetshop.com
/dried-mushrooms.html

MycoLogical Natural Products, Ltd.
P.O. Box 24940
Eugene, OR 97402
Phone: 888-465-3247
Website: www.mycological.com

NONALCOHOLIC WINES AND JUICES

Purely Organic, Ltd.
P.O. Box 847
Fairfield, IA 52556
Phone: 877-201-0710
Website: www.purelyorganic.com
Imported organic condiments, grape juice from Italy

Ariel
860 Napa Valley Corporate Way, Suite C
Napa, CA 94558
Phone: 800456-9472
E-mail: info@arielvineyards.com
Website: www.arielvineyards.com
Nonalcoholic wines

Walnut Acres
Customer Care
4600 Sleepytime Drive
Boulder, CO 80301
Phone: 800-434-4246
Website: www.walnutacres.com
Organic fruit and vegetable juices

Santa Cruz
Phone: 888-569-6994
E-mail: info@scojuice.com
Website: www.scojuice.com
Organic fruit and vegetable juices

PAINTS, STAINS, WALL COVERINGS, AND CLEANERS

American Formulating and Manufacturing
Phone: 800-239-0321
Website: www.afmsafecoat.com

Auro Natural Paints
Auro UK
Cheltenham Road
Bisley
Stroud
Gloucestershire, GL6 7BX
United Kingdom
Phone: 011 (44) 01452 772020 *or* 011 (44) 01452 772024
Website: www.auro.co.uk

Bioshield Paint Company
Plaza Entrada
3005 S. St. Francis, Suite 2A
Santa Fe, NM 87505
Phone: 505438-3448 *or* 800-621-2591
Fax: 505438-0199
E-mail: info@bioshieldpaint.com
Website: www.bioshieldpaint.com

Maya Romanoff
The Maya Romanoff Corporation
3435 Madison Street
Skokie, IL 60076
Phone: 773-465-6909
Fax: 773-465-7089
E-mail:
customerservice@mayaromanoff.com

Murco Wall Products, Inc.
2032 N. Commerce Drive
Fort Worth, TX 76164
Phone: 800-446-7124 *or* 817-626-1987
Fax: 817-626-0821
Website: http://murcowall.com

PAPER—TREE-FREE AND RECYCLED

Greenline Paper Company
631 South Pine Street
York, PA 17403
Phone: 800-641-1117
Website: www.greenlinepaper.com

New Leaf
116 New Montgomery Street, Suite 830
San Francisco, CA 94105
Phone: 888-989-5323
Website: www.newleafpaper.com

Living Tree Paper Company
1430 Willamette Street, Suite 367
Eugene, OR 97401
Phone: 800-309-2974
Website: www.livingtreepaper.com

PERSONAL-CARE PRODUCTS

Aubrey Organics
5046 W. Linebaugh Avenue
Tampa, FL 33624
Phone: 800-282-7394
Fax: 813-876-8166
Website: www.aubrey-organics.com

Burt's Bees
Attn: Consumer Care
P.O. Box 3900
Peoria, IL 61612
Phone: 800-849-7112
Fax: 800-429-7487
Website: www.burtsbees.com

Natracare, LLC
3620 West 10th Street, Unit B, #406
Greeley, CO 80634
Phone: 970-304-0076
Website: www.natracare.com
Chlorine-free feminine hygiene products

Tom's of Maine
P.O. Box 710
302 Lafayette Center
Kennebunk, ME 04043
Phone: 800-FOR-TOMS (800-367-8667)
Fax: 207-985-2196
Website: www.tomsofmaine.com

PEST CONTROL— LAWN AND GARDEN

Arbico Organics
P.O. Box 8910
Tucson, AZ 85738
Phone: 800-827-2847
Fax: 502-825-2038
E-mail: info@arbico.com
Website: www.arbico.com

Garden's Alive! Inc.
5100 Schenley Place, Dept. 4680
Lawrenceburg, IN 47025
Phone: 513-354-1482
Website: www.gardensalive.com

Peaceful Valley Farm Supply
P.O. Box 2209, #NGP
Grass Valley, CA 95945
Phone: 888-784-1722
Website: www.groworganic.com

PRANAYAMA

The Pranayama Institute
P.O. Box 660
Columbus, NM 88029
Website: www.pranayama.org

For instructions on how to perform pranayama, visit:
- www.yogajournal.com/practice/219
- www.integralyogastudio.com/basicpranayama.php
- www.yogawiz.com/breathing-exercises.html

PRODUCTS FOR THE HOME

Gaiam, Inc.
833 W. South Boulder Road
P.O. Box 3095
Boulder, CO 80307
Phone: 877-989-6321 *or*
  800-254-8464 (in Canada)
Website: www.gaiam.com
Free catalog: Harmony

ShopOrganic
3450 S. Broadmont Drive, Suite 114
Tucson, AZ 85713
Phone: 520-792-0804
Website: www.shoporganic.com
Online organic food and products store

PROTECTIVE BREAST FORMULA

Enzymatic Therapy
825 Challenger Drive
Green Bay, WI 54311
Phone: 800-783-2286
Fax: 920-469-4444
Website: www.eticonsumer.com *or*
  www.drchristinehorner.com

RAW-FOODS BLENDER

NutriBullet, LLC
Phone: 855-346-8874
Website: www.nutribullet.com

Vitamix Corporation
8615 Usher Road
Cleveland, OH 44138
Phone: 887-848-2649
Fax: 440-235-7155
Website: www.ultimateblender.com

RELAXATION DEVICES

Life Vessel Arizona
33747 North Scottsdale Road, Suite 115
Scottsdale, AZ 85266

Phone: 480-488-7780
Website: www.lifevesselarizona.com

Life Vessel Boulder
1625 Folsom Street
Boulder, CO 80302
Phone: 303-442-0122
Website: www.lightvesselboulder.com

Life Vessel California
20311 Birch Street, Suite 150
Newport Beach, CA 92660
Phone: 949-222-9991
Fax: 949-222-0630
E-mail: info@lvawusa.com
Website: www.lifevesselcalifornia.com

Life Vessel of the Rockies
1020 West 124th Avenue, Suite 100
Westminster, CO 80234
Phone: 303-630-9218
Website: www.lifevesseloftherockies.com

Life Vessel Santa Fe
66 Avenida Aldea Avenue
Santa Fe, NM 87507
Phone: 505-473-1200
Website:
  www.lightvesselsantafe.com/about-
  light-vessel

New Realities
Transformational Guided Imagery
Website: www.drchristinehorner.com/
  transformationalguidedimagery.html

RESOURCE ORGANIZATIONS

National Green Pages
Co-op America Business Network
1612 K Street NW, Suite 600
Washington, DC 20006
Phone: 800-58-GREEN
Website: www.greenpages.org
Directory to socially and environmentally
  responsible businesses

Natural Products Association
2112 East 4th Street, Suite 200
Santa Ana, CA 92705
Phone: 800-966-6632
Fax: 714-460-7444
Website: www.npainfo.org

Organic Consumers Association
6771 South Silver Hill Drive
Finland, MN 55603
Phone: 218-226-4164
Website: www.organicconsumers.org

Organic Trade Association
28 Vernon Street, Suite 413
Brattleboro, VT 05301
Phone: 802-275-3800
Fax: 802-275-3801
Website: www.ota.com

U.S. Green Building Council
2101 L Street NW, Suite 500
Washington, DC 20037
Phone: 800-795-1747
E-mail: info@usgbc.org
Website: www.usgbc.org

Vegetarian Resource Group
P.O. Box 1463
Baltimore, MD 21203
Phone: 410-366-8343
Website: www.vrg.org

RESVERATROL SUPPLEMENTS

Enzymatic Therapy
825 Challenger Drive
Green Bay, WI 54311
Phone: 800-783-2286
Fax: 920-469-4444
Websites: www.eticonsumer.com *or*
  www.drchristinehorner.com

ROSEMARY PRODUCTS

Frontier Natural Products Co-op
3021 78th Street

Norway, IA 52318
Phone: 800-669-3275
Website: www.frontiercoop.com

SELENIUM SUPPLEMENTS

New Chapter
90 Technology Drive
Brattleboro, VT 05301
Phone: 800-543-7279
Fax: 800-470-0247
E-mail: info@newchapter.com
Websites: www.newchapter.com *or*
  www.newchapter.info

SOCIALLY RESPONSIBLE INVESTING

Calvert Group, Ltd.
Phone: 800-368-2745
Website: www.calvert.com
Domini Social Investments
Phone: 800-762-6814
Website: www.domini.com

Domini Social Investments
Phone: 800-762-6814
Website: www.domini.com

Green Century Funds
Phone: 800-93-GREEN
Website: www.greencentury.com

Neuberger Berman Socially Responsible Fund
Phone: 800-223-6448
Website: www.nbfunds.com

Pax World Funds
Phone: 800-767-1729
Website: www.paxworld.com

Trillium Asset Management
Phone: 617-532-6665
Website: www.Trilliuminvest.com

SOY FOODS

Go Veggie Cheese
Galaxy Nutritional Foods
E-mail: www.galaxyfoods.com/about-us/contact-us
Website: www.galaxyfoods.com/galaxy-products/veggie

Light Life
153 Industrial Boulevard
Turners Falls, MA 10376
Phone: 800-SOYEASY (769-3279)
Website: www.lightlife.com
Tempeh and variety of soy meat substitutes

Morinaga Nutritional Foods, Inc.
3838 Del Amo Blvd., Suite 201
Torrance, CA 90503
Phone: 310-787-0200
Fax: 310-787-2727
E-mail: healthfoods@morinu.com
Website: www.morinu.com

Sensible Food Organic Roasted Soy Nuts
Website: www.amazon.com/Sensible-Foods-Organic-Roasted-1-5-Ounce/dp/B000EYLK2Y
Website: www.healthysnackstore.com

Vitasoy USA, Inc.
One New England Way
Ayer, MA 01432
Phone: 800-VITASOY (848-2769)
E-mail: info@vitasoy-usa.com
Website: www.nasoya.com

STEVIA PRODUCTS

Body Ecology/Stevia.Net
Website: www.stevia.net

HealthWorld Online
Website: www.healthy.net
Wisdom Natural Brands
1203 West San Pedro

Gilbert, AZ 85233
Phone: 800-899-9908
E-mail: wisdom@wisdomnaturalbrands.com
Website: www.wisdomherbs.com

STHAPATYAVEDA (VEDIC ARCHITECTURE)

Maharishi Sthapatya Veda
Website: www.maharishivastu.org

TRANSCENDENTAL MEDITATION (TM)

Maharishi Foundation USA
1100 N. 4th Street, Suite 128
Fairfield, IA 52556
Phone: 888-LEARN TM (888-532-7686)
Website: www.TM.org

TURMERIC PRODUCTS

Enzymatic Therapy
825 Challenger Drive
Green Bay, WI 54311
Phone: 800-783-2286
Fax: 920-469-4444
Websites: www.eticonsumer.com *or* www.drchristinehorner.com
Available in Protective Breast Formula

Frontier Natural Products Co-op
P.O. Box 299
3021 78th Street
Norway, IA 52318
Phone: 800-669-3275
Fax: 800-717-4372
Website: www.frontiercoop.com
World's largest supplier of organic herbs and spices—available in many stores including online stores.

New Chapter
90 Technology Drive
Brattleboro, VT 05301
Phone: 800-543-7279

Fax: 800-470-0247
E-mail: info@newchapter.com
Websites: www.newchapter.com,
www.newchapter.info, *or*
www.drchristinehorner.com

VITAMIN SUPPLEMENTS

Enzymatic Therapy
825 Challenger Drive
Green Bay, WI 54311
Phone: 800-783-2286
Fax: 920-469-4444
Website: www.eticonsumer.com

New Chapter
90 Technology Drive
Brattleboro, VT 05301
Phone: 800-543-7279
Fax: 800-470-0247
E-mail:info@newchapter.com
Websites: www.newchapter.com,
www.newchapter.info, *or*
www.drchristinehorner.com

WAKAME AND MEKABU SEAWEEDS

Eden Foods
701 Tecumseh Road
Clinton, MI 49236
Phone: 517-456-7424, 888-424-EDEN
Fax: 517-456-7854
Website: www.edenfoods.com

WATER-FILTRATION SYSTEMS

Building for Health Materials Center
Website: www.buildingforhealth.com

Nirvana Safe Haven
Website: www.nontoxic.com

WEDDING PLANNER, ORGANIC

Organic Weddings
Website:
www.greenbrideguide.com/learn/green-wedding-faq

Recommended Reading

AYURVEDA

Chopra, Deepak, M.D. *Perfect Health*. New York, NY: Harmony Books, 1991.

Dreyer, Ronnie. *Vedic Astrology*. York Beach, ME: Samuel Weiser, 1997.

Hagelin, John, Ph.D. *Manual for a Perfect Government*. Fairfield, IA: Maharishi University Management Press, 1998.

Levacy, William. *Beneath the Vedic Sky*. Carlsbad, CA: Hay House, 1999.

Lonsdorf, Nancy, M.D. *A Women's Best Medicine for Menopause*. New York, NY: Contemporary Books, 2002.

Lonsdorf, Nancy, M.D., Veronica Butler, M.D., and Melaine Brown, Ph.D. *A Woman's Best Medicine*. New York, NY: Putnam, 1995.

O'Connell, David, Ph.D., and Charles Alexander, Ph.D. *Self Recovery: Treating Addictions Using Transcendental Meditation and Maharishi Ayur-Veda*. Binghamton, NY: Harrington Park Press, 1994.

Roth, Robert. *Transcendental Meditation*. New York, NY: Donald Fine, 1994.

Sharma, Hari, M.D. *Freedom from Disease*. Toronto, Canada: Veda Publishing, 1993.

Sharma, Hari, M.D., and Christopher Clark, M.D. *Contemporary Ayurveda*. New York, NY: Churchill Livingstone, 1998.

Tirtha, Swami Sada Shiva. *The Ayurvedic Encyclopedia*. Bayville, NY: Ayurveda Holistic Center Press, 1998.

Wallace, Robert, Ph.D. *The Neurophysiology of Enlightenment*. Fairfield, IA: Maharishi International University Press, 1991.

Wallace, Robert, Ph.D. *The Physiology of Consciousness*. Fairfield, IA: Maharishi International University Press, 1993.

BREAST CANCER

Arnot, Bob, M.D. *The Breast Cancer Prevention Diet*. Boston, MA: Little, Brown & Co., 1998.

Epstein, Samuel, M.D., and David Steinman. *The Breast Cancer Prevention Program*. New York, NY: MacMillan, 1997.

Gaynor, Mitchell, M.D. *Dr. Gaynor's Cancer Prevention Program*. New York, NY: Kensington, 1999.

Gaynor, Mitchell, M.D. *Sounds of Healing*. New York, NY: Broadway Books, 1999.

Keuneke, Robin. *Total Breast Health*. New York, NY: Kensington, 1998.

Lee, John, M.D. *What Your Doctor May Not Tell You About Breast Cancer*. New York, NY: Warner Books, 2002.

Tagliaferri, M., M.D., Isaac Cohen, O.M.D., L.Ac., and Dubu Tripathy, M.D. *Breast Cancer: Beyond Convention*. New York, NY: Atria Books, 2002.

www.annieappleseedproject.org/ The Annie Appleseed Project, a 501 (c)3 non profit corporation, provides information, education, advocacy, and awareness for people with cancer, and family and friends interested in complementary alternative medicine (CAM)—natural therapies from the patient perspective.

EMOTIONAL AND SPIRITUAL HEALTH

Moorjani, Anita. *Dying to Be Me: My Journey from Cancer, to Near Death, to True Healing.* New York: Hay House, 2012.

Myss, Carolyn, Ph.D. *Anatomy of the Spirit: The Seven States of Power and Healing.* New York, NY: Harmony Books, 1996.

Myss, Carolyn, Ph.D. *Sacred Contracts.* New York, NY: Three Rivers Press, 2002.

Myss, Carolyn, Ph.D. *Why People Don't Heal and How They Can.* New York, NY: Three Rivers Press, 1997.

Ornish, Dean, M.D. *Love and Survival.* New York, NY: Harper Collins, 1995.

Tipping, Colin. *Radical Forgiveness.* Marietta, GA: Global 13, 2002.

Tolle, Eckhart. *The Power of Now.* Novato, CA: New World Library, 1999.

Tripodi, Jonathan. *Freedom from Body Memory.* 3rd ed. Virginia Beach, VA: Three Feet Publications, 2012.

FLAX COOKBOOKS

Beutler, Jade. *Flax for Life: 101 Delicious Recipes and Tips Featuring Fabulous Flax Oil.* Encinitas, CA: Progressive Health Publishing, 1996.

Magee, Elaine. *The Flax Cookbook: Recipes and Strategies for Getting the Most from the Most Powerful Plant on the Planet.* New York: Marlowe & Co., 2003.

Reinhardt-Martin. *Flax Your Way to Better Health.* Moline, IL: Jane Reinhardt-Martin, 2001.

FOOD AND NUTRITION

Boyens, Ingeborg. *Unnatural Harvest.* Toronto, Canada: Doubleday Canada, 1999.

Cummins, Ronnie, and Ben Lilliston. *Genetically Engineered Food.* New York, NY: Marlowe and Company, 2000.

Garrett, Howard. *J. Howard Garrett's Organic Manual.* Fort Worth, TX: The Summit Group, 1993.

Gastelu, Daniel, and Fred Hatfield, Ph.D. *Dynamic Nutrition for Maximum Performance.* Garden City Park, NY: Avery Publishing Group, 1997.

Hospodar, Miriam. *Heaven's Banquet: Vegetarian Cooking for Life Long Health the Ayurveda Way.* New York, NY: Dutton, 1999.

Johari, Harish. *The Healing Cuisine: India's Art of Ayurvedic Cooking.* Rochester, VT: Healing Arts Press, 1994.

Richard, David, and Dorie Byers. *Taste Of Life! The Organic Choice.* Bloominton, IL: Vital Health Publishing, 1998.

Robbins, John. *The Food Revolution.* Berkeley, CA: Conari Press, 2001.

Schlosser, Eric. *Fast Food Nation.* New York, NY: Houghton Mifflin, 2001.

Smith, Jeffrey. *Genetic Roulette: The Documented Health Risks of Genetically Engineered Foods* (4th edition). White River Junction, VT: Chelsea Green, 2007.

Smith, Jeffrey. *Genetic Roulette: The Gambles of Our Lives.* DVD. Fairfield, IA: Institute for Responsible Technology, 2012.

Steinman, David. *Diet for a Poisoned Planet.* New York, NY: Harmony, 1990.

HERBS AND SUPPLEMENTS

Murray, Michael, N.D. *Encyclopedia of Nutritional Supplements.* Roseville, CA: Prima Publishing, 1996.

Newmark, Thomas M., and Paul Schulick. *Beyond Aspirin: Nature's Challenge to Arthritis, Cancer & Alzheimer's Disease.* Prescott, AZ: Hohm Press, 2000.

NONTOXIC HOME

Harwood, Barbara. *The Healing House.* Carlsbad, CA: Hay House, 1997.

Marinelli, Janet, and Paul Beirman-Lytle. *Your Natural Home.* Boston, MA: Little, Brown & Co., 1995.

Pearson, David. *The Natural House Catalog.* New York, NY: Fireside, 1996.

Pearson, David. *The New Natural House Book.* New York, NY: Fireside, 1998.

QUANTUM PHYSICS

Greene, Brian. *The Elegant Universe.* New York, NY: Vintage Books, 1999.

TOFU COOKBOOKS

Ecookbooks.com. static.ecookbooks.com/categories/h/healthycookingsoyandtofu/

Greenberg, Patricia. *The Whole Soy Cookbook, 175 Delicious, Nutritious, Easy-to-Prepare Recipes Featuring Tofu, Tempeh, and Various Forms of Nature's Healthiest Bean.* New York: Three Rivers Press, 1998.

Hagler, Louise. *Tofu Cookery.* Summertown, TN: The Book Publishing Co., 1991.

Hagler, Louise. *Tofu Quick and Easy.* Summertown, TN: The Book Publishing Co., 1992.

Landgrebe, Gary. *Everyday Tofu: From Pancakes to Pizza.* Santa Cruz, CA: Crossing Press, 1999.

Madison, Deborah. *This Can't Be Tofu: 75 Recipes to Cook Something You Never Thought You Would—and Love Every Bite.* New York: Broadway Books, 2001.

WOMEN'S HEALTH

Love, Susan, M.D. *Dr. Susan Love's Breast Book.* Reading, MA: Addison-Wesley, 1990.

Love, Susan, M.D. *Dr. Susan Love's Hormone Book.* New York, NY: Times Books, 1998.

Northrup, Christiane, M.D. *Women's Bodies, Women's Wisdom.* Revised edition. New York, NY: Bantam Books, 1998.

Northrup, Christiane, M.D. *The Wisdom of Menopause.* New York, NY: Bantam Books, 2001.

References

Chapter 1: Breast Cancer Epidemic

www.bloomberg.com. "Breast Cancer Rate in US Dropped 7 percent in 2003." Presented at the Breast Cancer Symposium, San Antonia, TX (Dec 14, 2006). www.cancer.org

Calderon-Margalit, R., and O. Patiel. "Prevention of breast cancer in women who carry BRCA1 or BRCA2 mutations: a critical review of the literature." *International Journal of Cancer* Vol. 112. (Nov 2004): 356–364.

Dziaman, T.. T. Huzarski, D. Gackowski, et al. "Selenium supplementation reduced oxidative DNA damage in adnexectomized BRCA1 mutation carriers." *Cancer Epidemiology, Biomarkers & Prevention* Vol. 18. (Nov 2009): 2923–2928.

Elmore, J.G., P.A. Carney, L.A. Abraham, et al. "The association between obesity and screening mammography accuracy." *Archives of Internal Medicine* Vol.164. (May 24, 2004): 1140–1147.

Evans, D., A. Shelton, E. Woodward, et al. "Penetrance estimates for BRCA1 and BRCA2 based on genetic testing in the Clinical Cancer Genetics service setting: risks of breast/ovarian cancer quoted should reflect the cancer burden in the family." *BMC Cancer* Vol. 8. (May 2008): 155.

Gigert, R., V. Hanf, G. Emons, et al. "Membrane-bound melatonin receptor MT1 down-regulates estrogen responsive genes in breast cancer cells." *Journal of Pineal Research* Vol. 47. (Aug 2009): 23–31.

Hill, S., T. Frasch, S. Xiang, et al. "Molecular mechanisms of melatonin anticancer effects." *Integrative Cancer Therapies* Vol. 8. (Dec 2009): 337–346.

Jiang, W., W. Qiu, Y. Wang, et al. "Ginkgo may prevent genetic-associated ovarian cancer risk: mmultiple biomarkers and anticancer pathways induced by ginkgolide B in BRCA1-mutant ovarian epithelial cells." *European Journal of Cancer Prevention* Vol. 20. (Nov 2011): 508–517.

Jourdan, M., K. Maheo, A. Barascu, et al. "Increased BRCA1 protein in mammary tumours of rats fed marine omega-3 fatty acids." *Oncology Reports* Vol. 17. (Apr 2007): 713–719.

Keyserlink, J.R., P.D. Ahlgren, E. Yu, et al. "Functional infrared imaging of the breast." Journal of IEEE, *Engineering in Medicine & Biology Magazine* Vol. 19. (May/June 2000): 30–41.

Liort, G., M. Peris, I. Blanco. "[Hereditary breast and ovarian cancer: primary and secondary *prevention for BRCA1 and BRCA2 mutation carriers]." Medicina Clínica* Vol. 128. (Mar 2007): 468–476.

Mettlin, C. "Global breast cancer mortality statistics." CA: *A Cancer Journal for Clinicians* Vol. 49. (May/ June 1999): 138–144.

Parisky, Y.R., A. Sardi, R. Hamm, et al. "Efficacy of computerized infrared imaging analysis to evaluate mammographically suspicious lesions." *American Journal of Roentgenology* Vol. 180. (Jan 2003): 263– 269.

Pijpe, A., N. Andrieu, D. Easton, et al. "Exposure to diagnostic radiation and risk of breast cancer among carriers of BRCA1/2 mutations: retrospective cohort study (GENE-RAD-RISK). *British Medical Journal* Vol. 345. (2112): e5660.

Tomasz, H., B. Tomasz, J. Gronwald, et al. " A lowering of breast and ovarian cancer risk in women with the BRCA 1 mutation by selenium supplementation of diet." *Hereditary Cancer in Clinical Practice* Vol. 4. (Jan 2006): 58.

Chapter 2: Rediscovering Ancient Healing

Chopra, Deepak, M.D. *Perfect Health.* New York. NY: Harmony Books, 1991.

Sharma, Hari, M.D., and Christopher Clark, M.D. *Contemporary Ayurveda.* New York, NY: Churchill Livingstone, 1998.

Chapter 3: The Birth of the Beast

Arnot, B. *The Breast Cancer Prevention Diet.* Boston, MA: Little, Brown & Co., 1998.

Almada, A. "Brevail: SDG precision standardized flaxseed extract." *Scientific Research Monograph.* San Diego, CA: Lignan Research, 2003.

Lee, J. *What Your Doctor May Not Tell You About Breast Cancer.* New York, NY: Warner Books, 2002.

Love, Susan, M.D. *Dr. Susan Love's Breast Book.* Reading, MA: Addison-Wesley, 1990.

Chapter 4: Your Inner Healing Intelligence

Sharma, Hari, M.D., and Christopher Clark, M.D. *Contemporary Ayurveda.* New York, NY: Churchill Livingstone, 1998.

Chapter 5: The Intelligence of Plants

Arnot, B. *The Breast Cancer Prevention Diet.* Boston, MA: Little, Brown & Co., 1998.

About organic. Organic Farming Research Foundation www.ofrf.org/about_organic/index.html 1998.

Brandi, G., G.F. Schiavano, N. Zaffaroni, et al. "Mechanisms of action and antiproliferative properties of Bassica oleracea juice in human breast cancer cell lines." *The Journal of Nutrition* Vol. 135. (June 2005): 1503–1509.

Chang, X., J.C. Tou, C. Hong, et al. "3,3'-diindolylmethane inhibits angiogenesis and the growth of transplantable human breast carcinoma in athymic mice." *Carcinogenesis* Vol. 26. (April 2005): 771–778.

Dalessandri, K.M., G.L. Firestone., M.D. Fitch, et al. "Pilot study: effect of 3,3'-diindolylmethane supplements on urinary hormone metabolites in postmenopausal women with a history of early-stage breast cancer." *Nutrition and Cancer* Vol. 50. (2004):161–167.

De Santos, Silva I., P. Mangtani, V. McCormack, et al. "Lifelong vegetarianism and risk of breast cancer: a population-based case-control study among South Asian migrant women living in England." *International Journal of Cancer* Vol. 99. (May 10, 2002): 238–244.

Garcia, H.H., G.A. Brar, D.H. Nguyen, et al. "Indole-3-carbinol (I3C) inhibits cyclin-dependent kinase-2 function in human breast cancer cells by regulating the size distribution, associated cyclin E forms, and subcellular localization of the CDK2 protein complex." *The Journal of Biological Chemistry* Vol. 280. (March 11, 2005): 8756–8764.

Howe, G.R., T. Hirohata, T.G. Hislop, et al. "Dietary factors and risk of breast cancer: combines analysis of 12 case-control studies." *Journal of the National Cancer Institute* Vol. 82. (April 4, 1990): 561–569.

Hulten, K., A.L. Van Kappel, A. Winkvist, et al. "Carotenoids, alpha-tocopherols, and retinol in plasma and breast cancer in northern Sweden." *Cancer Causes Control* Vol. 12. (August 2001): 529–537.

La Marchand, L. "Cancer preventative effects of flavonoids—a review." *Biomedical Pharmacotherapy* Vol. 56. (Aug 2002): 296–301.

Le Vecchia, C., A. Altieri, and A. Tavani. "Vegetables, fruits, antioxidants and cancer: a review of Italian studies." *European Journal of Nutrition* Vol. 40. (Dec 2001): 261–267.

Levi, F., C. Pasche, F. Lucchini, et al. "Dietary intake of selected micronutrients and breast cancer risk." *International Journal of Cancer* Vol. 91. (Jan 15, 2001): 260–263.

McCarty, M.F. "Vegan proteins may reduce risk of cancer, obesity, and cardiovascular disease by promoting increased glucagon activity." *Medical Hypotheses* Vol. 53. (Dec 1999): 459–485.

McGuire, K.P., N. Ngoubilly, M. Neavyn et al. "3,3'-diindolylmethane and paclitaxel act synergistically to promote apoptosis in HER2/Neu human breast cancer cells." *The Journal of Surgical Research* Vol. 132. (May 15, 2006): 208–213.

Peterson, J., P. Lagiou, E. Samoli, et al. "Flavonoid intake and breast cancer risk: a case-controlled study in Greece." *British Journal of Cancer* Vol. 89. (Oct 6, 2003): 1255–1259.

Piernick, E. "The color of health." www.organicfrog.com/pub.article2.asp The Organic Frog Inc., 2002.

Rahman, K.W., and F.H. Sarkar. "Inhibition of nuclear translocation of nuclear factor-(kappa)B contributes to 3,3'-diindolylmethane-induced apoptosis in breast cancer cells." *Cancer Research* Vol.65. (Jan 1, 2005): 364–371.

Riby, J.E., L. Xue, U. Chatterji, et al. "Activation and potentiation of interferon-gamma signaling by 3,3'-diindolylmethane in MCF-7 breast cancer cells." *Molecular Pharmacology* Vol. 69. (Feb 2006): 430–439.

Ronco, A., E. De Stefani, P. Boffetta, et al. "Vegetables, fruits, and related nutrients and risk of breast cancer: a case control study in Uruguay." *Nutrition & Cancer* Vol. 35. (Issue 2, 1999): 111–119.

Segasothy, M., and P.A. Phillips. "Vegetarian diet: panacea for modern lifestyle diseases?" *QJM: An International Journal of Medicine* QJM: monthly journal of the Association of Physicians Vol. 92. (Sept 1999): 531–544.

Smith-Warner, S., D. Spiegelman, and S.S. Yaun. "Intake of fruits and vegetables and risk of breast cancer." *Journal of the American Medical Association* (*JAMA*) Vol. 285. (Feb 14, 2001): 769–776.

Toniolo, P., A.L. Van Kappel, A. Akhmedkhanov, et al. "Serum carotenoids and breast cancer." *Ameri-*

can Journal of Epidemiology Vol. 153. (Jun 15, 2001): 1142–1147.

Wang, T.T., M.J. Milner, J.A. Milner, et al. "Estrogen receptor alpha as a target for indole-3-carbinol." Journal of Nutritional Biochemistry Vol. 17. (Oct 2006): 659–664.

Worthington, V. "Nutritional quality of organic verses conventional fruits, vegetables, and grains." Journal of Alternative & Complementary Medicine Vol. 7. (Issue 2, 2001): 161–173.

Cruciferous Vegetables

Ashok, B.T., Y. Chen, X. Liu, et al. "Abrogation of estrogen-mediated cellular and biochemical effects by indole-3 carbinol." Nutrition & Cancer Vol. 41. (Issue 1-2, 2001): 180–187.

Ahmad, A., S. Ali, A. Ahmed, et al. "3, 3-diindolylmethane enhances the effectiveness of herceptin against her-2/neu-expressing breast cancer cells." PloS One Vol. 8. (Jan 2013): e54657.

Ahmad, A., S. Ali, Z. Wang, et al. "3, 3-diindolylmethane enhances taxotere-induced growth inhibition of breast cancer cells through downregulation of FoxM1." International Journal of Cancer Vol. 129. (Oct 2011): 1781–1791.

Ashok, B.T., Y. Chen, X. Liu, et al. "Multiple molecular targets of indole-3 carbinol, a chemopreventative anti-estrogen in breast cancer." European Journal of Cancer Prevention Vol. 11. (Aug 2002; Suppl 2): S86–S93.

Degner, S., A. Papoutsis, O. Selmin, et al. "Targeting of aryl hydrocarbon receptor-mediated activation of cyclooxygenase-2 expression by the indole-3-carbinol metabolite 3, 3-diindolylmethane in breast cancer cells." The Journal of Nutrition Vol. 139. (Jan 2009): 26–32.

Fahey, J.W., Y. Zhang, and P. Talalay. "Broccoli sprouts: an exceptionally rich source of inducers of enzymes that protect against chemical carcinogens." Proceedings of the National Academy of Science USA Vol. 94. (Sept 16, 1997): 10367–10372.

Higdon, J., B. Delage, D. Dashwood. "Cruciferous vegetables and human cancer risk: epidemiologic evidence and mechanistic basis." Pharmacological Research: The Official Journal of the Italian Pharmacological Society Vol. 55. (Mar 2007): 224–236.

Jin, Y. "3, 3-diindolylmethane inhibits breast cancer cell growth via miR-21-mediated Cdc25A degradation." Molecular and Cellular Biochemistry Vol. 358. (Dec 2011): 345–354.

Kim, E., M. Shin, H. Park, et al. "Oral administra-

tion of 3, 3-diindolylmethane inhibits lung metastasis of 4T1 murine mammary carcinoma cells in BALB/c mice." The Journal of Nutrition Vol. 139. (Dec 2009): 2373–2379.

Laidlaw, M., C. Cockerline, D. Sepkovic. "Effects of a breast-health herbal formula supplement on estrogen metabolism in pre-and post-menopausal women not taking hormonal contraceptives or supplements: a randomized controlled trial." Breast Cancer: Basic and Clinical Research Vol. 4. (Dec 2010): 85–95.

Li, Y., T. Zhang, H. Korkaya, et al. "Sulforaphane, a dietary component of broccoli/broccoli sprouts, inhibits breast cancer stem cells." Clinical Cancer Research Vol. 16. (May 2010): 2580–2590.

Lord, R.S., B. Bongiovanni, and J.A. Bralley. "Estrogen metabolism and the diet-cancer connection: rationale for assessing the ratio of urinary hydroxylated estrogen metabolites." Alternative Medicine Review Vol. 7. (Apr 2002): 112–129.

Meng, Q., I.D. Goldberg, E.M. Rosen, et al. "Inhibitory effects of indole-3-carbinol on invasion and migration in human breast cancer cells." Breast Cancer Research & Treatment Vol. 63. (Sept 2000): 147–152.

Meng, Q., M. Qi, D.Z. Chen, et al. "Suppression of breast cancer invasion and migration by indole-3 carbinol: associated with up-regulation of the BRCA1 and E-cadherin/catenin complexes." Journal of Molecular Medicine Vol. 78. (Issue 3, 2000): 155–165.

Meng, Q., F. Yuan, I.D. Goldberg, et al. "Indole-3 carbinol is a negative regulator of estrogen receptor-alpha signaling in human tumor cells." Journal of Nutrition Vol. 12. (Dec 2000): 2927–2931.

Nguyen, H., I. Aronchik, G. Brar, et al. "The dietary phytochemical indole-3-carbinol is a natural elastase enzymatic inhibitor that disrupts cyclin E protein processing." Proceedings of the National Academy of Sciences Vol. 105. (Dec 2008): 19750–19755.

Oganesian, A., J.D. Hendricks, and D.E. Williams. "Long term dietary indole-3 carbinol inhibits diethylnitrosamine-initiated hepatocarcinogenesis in the infant mouse." Cancer Letters Vol. 18. (Sept 16, 1997): 87–94.

Rahimi, M., K. Huang, C. Tang. "3, 3-diindolylmethane (DIM) inhibits the growth and invasion of drug-resistant human cancer cells expressing EGFR mutants." Cancer Letters Vol. 295. (Sept 2010): 59–68.

Rahman, K.M., O. Aranha, A. Glazyrin, et al.

"Translocation of Bax to mitochondria induces apoptotic cell death in indol-3 carbinol (I3C) treated breast cancer cells." *Oncogene* Vol. 19. (Nov 23, 2000): 5764–5771.

Rahman, K.M., O. Aranha, and F.H. Sarkar. "Indole-3 carbinol induces apoptosis in tumorigenic but not in nontumorigenic breast epithelial cells." *Nutrition & Cancer* Vol. 45. (Issue 1, 2003): 101–112.

Riby, J.E., G.H. Chang, G.L. Firestone, et al. "Ligand-independent activation of estrogen receptor function by 3,3' diindolylmethane in human breast cancer cells." *Biochemical Pharmacology* Vol. 60. (Jul 15, 2000): 167–177.

Riby, J.E., C. Feng, Y.C. Chang, et al. "The major cyclic trimeric product of indole-3 carbinol is a strong agonist of the estrogen receptor signaling pathway." *Biochemistry* Vol. 39. (Feb 8, 2000): 910–918.

Saati, G., and M. Archer. "Inhibition of fatty acid synthase and Sp1 expression by 3, 3-diindolylmethane in human breast cancer cells." *Nutrition and Cancer* Vol. 63. (June 2011): 790–794.

Sepkovic, D.W., H.L. Bradlow, and M. Bell. "Quantitative determination of 3, 3' diindolylmethane in urine of individuals receiving indole-3 carbinol." *Nutrition & Cancer* Vol. 41. (Issue 1-2, 2001): 57–63.

Stoner, G., B. Casto, S. Ralston, et al. "Development of a multi-organ rat model for evaluation chemoprotective agents: efficacy of indole-3 carbinol." *Carcinogenisis* Vol. 23. (Feb 2002): 265–272.

Szaefer, H., B. Licznerska, V. Krajka-Kuzniak, et al. "Modulation of CYP1A1, CYP1A2 and CYP1B1 expression by cabbage juices and indoles in human breast cell lines." *Nutrition and Cancer* Vol. 64. (Aug 2012): 879–888.

Telang, N.T., H.L. Bradlow, and M.P. Osborne. "Molecular and endocrine biomarkers in non-involved breast: relevance to cancer chemoprevention." *Journal of Cellular Biochemistry.* (16G, 1992): 161–169.

"Calcium-D-Gluterate." *Alternative Medicine Review: A Journal of Clinical Therapeutic* Vol. 7. (Aug 2002): 336–339.

Xue, L., J. Pestka, M. Li, et al. "3, 3-diindolylmethane stimulates murine immune function in vitro and in vivo." *The Journal of Nutritional Biochemistry* Vol. 19. (May 2008): 336–344.

Chapter 6: Mother Nature Knows Best

Aubé, M., C. Larochelle, and P. Ayotte. "Differential effects of a complex organochlorine mixture on the proliferation of breast cancer cell lines." *Environmental Research* Vol. 111. (Apr 2011): 337–347.

Bernstein, I.L., J. A. Bernstein, M. Miller, et al. "Immune Responses in farm workers after exposure to Bacillus thuringiensis pesticides." *Environmental Health Perspectives* Vol. 107. (July 1999): 575–582.

Bradlow, H.L., D.L. Davis, G. Lin, et al. "Effects of pesticides on the ratio of 16 alpha/2-hydroxyestrone: a biologic marker of breast cancer risk." *Environmental Health Perspectives* Vol. 103 Supplement. (Oct 1995): 147–150.

Bratton, M., D. Frigo, H. Segar, et al. "The organochlorine o, p'-DDT plays a role in coactivator-mediated MAPK crosstalk in MCF-7 breast cancer cells." *Environmental Health Perspectives* Vol. 120. (Sept 2012): 1291–1296.

Cabello, G., A. Juarranz, L.M. Botella, et al. "Organophosphorous pesticides in breast cancer progression." *Journal of Submicroscopic Cytology & Pathology* Vol. 35. (Jan 2003): 1–9.

Canales-Aguirre, A., E. Padilla-Camberos, U. Gómez-Pinedo, et al. "Genotoxic effect of chronic exposure to DDT on lymphocytes, oral mucosa and breast cells of female rats." *International Journal of Environmental Research and Public Health* Vol. 8. (Feb 2011): 540–553.

Canales-Aguirre, A., E. Padilla-Camberos, U. Gómez-Pinedo, et al. "Genotoxic effect of chronic exposure to DDT on lymphocytes, oral mucosa and breast cells of female rats." *International Journal of Environmental Research and Public Health* Vol. 8. (Feb 2011): 540–553.

Coco, P., N. Kazerouni, and S.H. Zahm. "Cancer mortality and environmental exposure to DDE in the United States." *Environmental Health Perspectives* Vol. 108. (Jan 2000): 1–4.

Cohn, Barbara A. "Developmental and environmental origins of breast cancer: DDT as a case study." *Reproductive Toxicology* Vol. 31. (Apr 2011): 302–311.

Cohn, B., M. Wolff, P. Cirillo, et al. "DDT and breast cancer in young women: new data on the significance of age at exposure." *Environmental Health Perspectives* Vol. 115. (Oct 2007): 1406–1414.

Davis, J. "Alleviating political violence through enhancing coherence in collective consciousness: impact assessment amlusis of the Lebanon war." *Dis-*

sertations & Abstracts International Vol. 49. (Issue 8, 1988): 2381A.

Demers, A., P. Ayotte, J. Brisson, et al. "Risk and aggressiveness of breast cancer in relation to plasma organochlorine concentrations." Cancer Epidemiology, Biomarkers & Prevention Vol. 9. (Feb 2000): 161–166.

"Environmental estrogens and other hormones." Tulane University website: www.tmc.tulane.edu/ecme/eehome/basics/

Epstein, S. "Pesticides and Cancer." Transcript of lecture given in 1993.

Guttes, S., K. Failing, K. Neumann, et al. "Chlororganic pesticides and polychlorinated biphenyls in breast tissue of women with benign and malignant breast disease." Archives of Environmental Contamination and Toxicology Vol. 35. (Jul 1998): 140–147.

Holloway, A.C., K.A. Stys, W.G. Foster, "DDE-induced changes in aromatase activity in endometrial stromal cells in culture." Endocrine Vol. 27. (June 2005): 45–50.

Horner, C., M.D. "Organic means pure food." Channelcincinnati.com. June 9, 2001.

Horner, C., M.D. "GE food questioned." Channelcincinnati.com. May 15, 2001.

Horner, C., M.D. "Genetically engineered foods." Channelcincinnati.com. May 17, 2001.

Hoyer, A., T. Jorgensen, P. Grandjean, et al. "Repeated measurements of organochlorine exposure and breast cancer risk (Denmark)." Cancer Causes and Control Vol. 11. (Feb 2000): 177–184.

Hoyer, A.P., P. Grandjean, T. Jorgensen, et al. "Organochlorine compounds and breast cancer— is there a connection between environmental pollution and breast cancer." Ugeskr Laeger Vol. 162. (Feb 14, 2000): 922–926.

Hoyer, A.P., T. Jorgensen, J.W. Brock, et al. "Organochlorine exposure and breast cancer survival." Journal of Clinical Epidemiology Vol. 53. (Mar 2000): 323–330.

Jaga, K., and D. Brosius. "Pesticide exposure: human cancers on the horizon." Reviews on Environmental Health Vol. 14. (Jan-Mar 1999): 39–50.

Jaga, K., and H. Duvvi. "Risk reduction for DDT toxicity and carcinogenesis through dietary modifications." Journal of the Royal Society of Health Vol. 121. (Jun 2001): 107–113.

Johnson, N., A. Ho, J. Cline, et al. "Accelerated mammary tumor onset in a HER2/Neu mouse model exposed to DDT metabolites locally delivered to the mammary gland." Environmental Health Perspectives Vol. 120. (Aug 2012): 1170–1176.

Mathur, V., P. Bhatnagar, R.G. Sharma, et al. "Breast cancer incidence and exposure to pesticides among women originating from Jaipur." Environment International Vol. 28. (Nov 2002): 331–336.

Moysich, K.B., C.B. Ambrosone, P. Mendola, et al. "Exposures associated with serum organochlorine levels among postmenopausal women from western New York State." American Journal of Industrial Medicine Vol. 41. (Feb 2002): 102–110.

Northwest Coalition for Alternatives to Pesticides (NCAP). "Are pesticides hazardous to our health." Journal of Pesticide Reform Vol. 19. (Issue 2, 1999): 2–3.

Ociepa-Zawal, M., B. Rubis, D. Wawrzynczak, et al. "Accumulation of environmental estrogens in adipose tissue of breast cancer patients." Journal of Environmental Science and Health Part A Vol. 45. (Jan 2010): 305–312.

Organic trade association website for new organic standards, www.ota.com.

Orme-Johnson, D.W., C.N. Alexander, J.L. Davies, et al. "International peace project in the Middle East: the effects of Maharishi Technology of the Unified Field." Journal of Conflict Resolution Vol. 32. (1988): 776–812.

Tarone, R. "DDT and breast cancer trends." Environmental Health Perspectives Vol. 116. (Sept 2008): A374.

Valerón, P., J. Pestano, O. Luzardo, et al. "Differential affects exerted on human mammary epithelial cells by environmentally relevant organochlorine pesticides either individually or in combination." Chemico-Biological Interactions Vol. 180. (Aug 2009): 485–491.

Worthington, V. "Effects of agriculture methods on nutritional quality: a comparison of organic and conventional crops." Alternative Therapies in Health & Medicine Vol. 4. (Jan 1998): 58–69.

Chapter 7: Fields of Gold

Arts, C.J., C.A. Govers, H. Van den berg, et al. "Effect of wheat bran on excretion of radioactively labeled estradiol-17 beta and estrone-glucuronide injected intravenously in male rats." Journal of Steroid Biochemistry & Molecular Biology Vol. 42. (Mar 1992): 103–111.

Arts, C.J., and J.H. Thijssen. "Effects of wheat bran on blood and tissue hormone levels in adult female

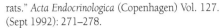

rats." *Acta Endocrinologica* (Copenhagen) Vol. 127. (Sept 1992): 271–278.

Aune, D., D. Chan, D. Greenwood, et al. "Dietary fiber and breast cancer risk: a systematic review and meta-analysis of prospective studies." *Annals of Oncology* Vol. 23. (June 2012): 1394–1402.

Belle, F., E. Kampman, A. McTiernan, et al. "Dietary fiber, carbohydrates, glycemic index, and glycemic load in relation to breast cancer prognosis in the HEAL cohort." *Cancer Epidemiology Biomarkers & Prevention* Vol. 20. (May 2011): 890–899.

Buck, K., A.K. Zaineddin, A. Vrieling, et al "Estimated enterolignans, lignan-rich foods, and fibre in relation to survival after postmenopausal breast cancer." *British Journal of Cancer* Vol. 105. (Oct 2011): 1151–1157.

Cade, J.E., Burley, V.J., Greenwood, D.C. "Dietary fibre and risk of breast cancer in the UK Women's Cohort Study." *International Journal of Epidemiology* Vol. 36. (2007): 431–438.

Challier, B., J.M. Perarnau, and J.F. Viel. "Garlic, onion, and cereal fiber as protective factors for breast cancer: French case control study." *European Journal of Epidemiology* Vol. 14. (Dec 1998): 737–747.

Daniells, S. "Fibre could halve young women's breast cancer risk, says study." *NutraIngredients.com.* (Jan 2007). Accessed May 19 2013.

Ferrari, P., S. Rinaldi, M. Jenab, et al. "Dietary fiber intake and risk of hormonal receptor–defined breast cancer in the European Prospective Investigation into Cancer and Nutrition study." *The American Journal of Clinical Nutrition* Vol. 97. (Feb 2013): 344–353.

Kolodziejczyk, J., S. Flatt, L. Natarajan, et al. "Associations of soluble fiber, whole fruits/vegetables, and juice with plasma beta-carotene concentrations in a free-living population of breast cancer survivors." *Women & Health* Vol. 52. (Nov 2012): 731–743.

Park, Y., L. Brinton, A. Subar, et al. "Dietary fiber intake and risk of breast cancer in postmenopausal women: the National Institutes of Health–AARP Diet and Health Study." *The American Journal of Clinical Nutrition* Vol. 90. (Sept 2009): 664–671.

Pena-Rosas, J.P., S. Rickard, and S. Cho. "Wheat bran and breast cancer: revisiting the estrogen hypothesis." *Archivos Latinoamericanos de Nutricion* Vol. 49. (Dec 1999): 309–317.

Slavin, J. "Why whole grains are protective: biolog-ical mechanisms." *Proceedings of the Nutrition Society* Vol. 62. (Feb 2003): 129–134.

Suzuki, R., T. Rylander-Rudqvist, W. Ye, et al. "Dietary fiber intake and risk of postmenopausal breast cancer defined by estrogen and progesterone receptor status—a prospective cohort study among Swedish women." *International Journal of Cancer* Vol.122. (Jan 2008): 403–412.

Weisenburger, J.H., B.S. Reddy, D.P. Rose, et al. "Protective mechanisms of dietary fibers in nutritional carcinogenesis." *Basic Life Sciences* Vol. 61. (1993): 45–63.

Zhang, C.X., S.C. Ho, S.Z. Cheng, Et Al. "Effect of Dietary Fiber Intake on Breast Cancer Risk According to Estrogen and Progesterone Receptor Status." *European Journal of Clinical Nutrition* Vol. 65. (Aug 2011): 929–936.

Chapter 8: Fats—The Good and the Bad

Arnot, B. *The Breast Cancer Prevention Diet.* Boston, MA: Little, Brown & Co., 1998.

Bagga, D. "Dietary modulation of Omega-3/Omega-6 poly-unsaturated fatty acids ratios in patients with breast cancer." *Journal of the National Cancer Institute* Vol. 89. (Issue 15, 1997): 1123–1131.

Barrett-Conner, E., and N.J. Friedlander. "Dietary fat, calories, and the risk of breast cancer in postmenopausal women: a prospective population based study." *Journal of the American College of Nutrition* Vol 12. (Aug 1993): 390–399.

Beasley, J., P. Newcomb, A. Trentham-Dietz, et al. "Post-diagnosis dietary factors and survival after invasive breast cancer." *Breast Cancer Research and Treatment* Vol. 128. (July 2011): 229–236.

Chajès, V., A. Thiébaut, M. Rotival, et al. "Association between serum trans-monounsaturated fatty acids and breast cancer risk in the E3N-EPIC Study." *American Journal of Epidemiology* Vol. 117. (June 2008): 1312-1320.

Cho, E., et al. "Premenopausal fat intake and the risk of breast cancer." Journal of the National Cancer Institute Vol. 95. (Jul 2003): 1079–1085.

de Lorgeril, M., and P. Salen. "New insights into the health effects of dietary saturated and omega-6 and omega-3 polyunsaturated fatty acids." *BMC Medicine* Vol. 21. (May 2012): 50.

Horvitz, B. "McDonald's tinkers with beloved fries." *USA Today* (Jan 2007).

Hu, J., C. La Vecchia, M. de Groh, et al. "Dietary transfatty acids and cancer risk." *European Journal of Cancer Prevention* Vol. 20. (Nov 2011): 530–538.

Kallianpur, A., S. Lee, Y. Gao, et al. "Dietary animal-derived iron and fat intake and breast cancer risk in the Shanghai Breast Cancer Study." *Breast Cancer Research and Treatment* Vol. 107. (Jan 2008): 123–132.

Laake, I., M. Carlsen, J. Pedersen, et al. "Intake of trans fatty acids from partially hydrogenated vegetable and fish oils and ruminant fat in relation to cancer risk." *International Journal of Cancer* Vol. 132. (Mar 2013): 1389–1403.

Medvedovic, M., R. Gear, J. Freudenberg, et al. "Influence of fatty acid diets on gene expression in rat mammary epithelial cells." *Physiological Genomics* Vol. 38. (June 2009): 80–88.

Nettleton, J. "Omega-3s shine at international fatty acid conference." *Holistic Primary Care.* (Oct 15, 2002).

Simopoulos, A.P. "The importance of the ratio of omega-6/omega-3 essential fatty acids." *Biomedicine & Pharmacotherapy* Vol. 56. (Oct 2002): 365–379.

Stannard, E. "Depression, brain cells, and essential fatty acids." *Well Being Journal.* (Issue 7, 2000): 8–9.

Stoll, A.L. "The omega-3 solution fatty acids fight heart disease, arthritis, obesity and more." *Bottom Line Health.* (June 2001).

Stoll, A.L., W.E. Severus, M.P. Freeman, et al. "Omega-3 fatty acids in bipolar disorder: a preliminary double-blind, placebo-controlled trial." *Archive of General Psychiatry* Vol. 56. (May 1999): 407–412.

Thiébaut, A., V. Kipnis, S. Chang, et al. "Dietary fat and postmenopausal invasive breast cancer in the National Institutes of Health–AARP Diet and Health Study cohort." *Journal of the National Cancer Institute* Vol. 99. (Mar 2007): 451–462.

Turner, L. "A meta-analysis of fat intake, reproduction, and breast cancer risk: an evolutionary perspective." *American Journal of Human Biology* Vol. 23. (Oct 2011): 601–608.

Conjugated Linoleic Acid (CLA)

Aro, A., S. Mannisto, and I. Salminen. "Inverse association between dietary and serum conjugated linoleic acid and the risk of breast cancer in postmenopausal women." *Nutrition & Cancer* Vol. 38. (Issue 2, 2000): 151–157.

Chajes, V., F. Lavillonniere, and V. Maillard. "Conjugated linoleic acid content in breast adipose tissue of breast cancer patients and the risk of metastasis." *Nutrition & Cancer* Vol. 45. (Issue 1, 2003): 17–23.

Cunningham, D.C., L.Y. Harrison, and T.D. Shultz. "Proliferative response of normal mammary and MCF-& breast cancer cells to linoleic acid, conjugated linoleic acid, and eicosanoid synthesis inhibitors in culture." *Anticancer Research* Vol. 17. (Jan-Feb 1997): 197–203.

Durgan, V.R. "The growth inhibitory effects of conjugated linoleic aid on MCF-7 cells related to estrogen response system." *Cancer Letters* Vol. 116. (Jun 24, 1997): 121–130.

Ip, C., and J.A. Scimeca. "Conjugated linoleic acid and linoleic acid are distinctive modulators of mammary carcinogenesis." *Nutrition & Cancer* Vol. 27. (Issue 2, 1997): 131–135.

Ip, C., S.F. Chin, J.A. Scimeca, et al. "Mammary cancer prevention by conjugated deinoic derivative of linoleic acid." *Cancer Research* Vol 51. (Nov 15, 1991): 6118–6124.

Ip, C., J.A. Scimeca, and H.J. Thompson. "Conjugated linoleic acid. A powerful anticarcinogen from animal fat sources." *Cancer* Vol. 74. (Aug 1, 1994; 3 Suppl): 1050–1054.

Mjumder, B., K.W. Wahle, and S. Moir. "Conjugated linoleic acids (CLAs) regulate the expression of key apoptotic genes in human breast cancer cells." *The FASEB Journal* Vol. 16. (Sept 2002): 1447–1449.

Thompson, H., Z. Zhu, and S. Banni. "Morphological and biochemical status of the mammary gland as influenced by conjugated linoleic acid: implications for a reduction in mammary cancer risk." *Cancer Research* Vol. 15. (Nov 1997): 5067–5072.

Visonneau, S., A. Cesano, S.A. Tepper, et al. "Conjugated linoleic acid suppresses the growth of human breast adenocarcinoma cells in SCID mice." *Anticancer Research* Vol. 17. (Mar-Apr 1997): 969–973.

Evening Primrose Oil

Menendez, J.A., Vellon, L., Colomer, R., et al. "Effects of gamma-linolenic acid on the transcriptional activity of the Her-2/neu (erbB-2) oncogene." *Journal of the National Cancer Institute* Vol. 98. (May 17, 2006): 718–720.

Zaugg, J., Potterat, O., Plescher, A., et al. "Quantitative analysis of anti-inflammatory and radical scavenging triterpenoid esters in evening primrose seeds." *Journal of Agriculture and Food Chemistry* Vol. 54. (Sept 6, 2006): 6623–6628.

Fats

Brenna, T., N. Salem Jr, A. Sinclair, et al. "Alpha-linolenic acid supplementation and conversion to n-3 long-chain polyunsaturated fatty acids in humans." *Prostaglandins, Leukotrienes, and Essential Fatty Acids* Vol. 80. (Feb-Mar 2009): 85–91.

Cui, P., T. Rawling, K. Bourget, et al. "Antiproliferative and antimigratory actions of synthetic long chain n-3 monounsaturated fatty acids in breast cancer cells that overexpress cyclooxygenase-2." *Journal of Medicinal Chemistry* Vol. 55. (Aug 2012): 7163–7172.

Ghoreishi, Z., A. Esfahani, A. Djazayeri, et al. "Omega-3 fatty acids are protective against paclitaxel-induced peripheral neuropathy: a randomized double-blind placebo controlled trial." *BMC Cancer* Vol. 12. (Aug 2012): 355.

Hardman, W.E., C.P. Avula, G. Fernandes, et al. "Three percent dietary fish oils concentrate increased efficacy of doxorubicin against MDA-MB 231 cancer xenografts." *Clinical Cancer Research* Vol. 7. (July 2001): 2041–2049.

Isbilen, B., S.P. Fraser, M.B. Djamgoz. "Docosahexaenoic acid (omega-3) blocks voltage-gated sodium channel activity and migration of MDA-MB-231 human breast cancer cells." *The International Journal of Biochemistry and Cell Biology* Vol. 38. (July 16, 2006): 2173–2182.

Jin, F., D. Nieman, W. Sha, et al. "Supplementation of milled chia seeds increases plasma ALA and EPA in postmenopausal women." *Plant Foods for Human Nutrition* Vol. 67. (June 2012): 105–110.

Larsson, S.C., Kumlin, M., Ingelman-Sundberg, M., et al. "Dietary long chain n-3 fatty acids for the prevention of cancer: a review of potential mechanisms." *American Journal of Clinical Nutrition* Vol. 79. (June 2004): 935–945.

Menéndez, J., A. Vázquez-Martín, S. Ropero, et al. "HER2 (erbB-2)-targeted effects of the omega-3 polyunsaturated fatty acid, alpha-linolenic acid (ALA; 18: 3n-3) in breast cancer cells: the fat features of the 'Mediterranean diet' as an 'anti-HER2 cocktail'." *Clinical and Translational Oncology* Vol. 11. (Nov 2006): 812–820.

Menendez, J.A., R. Lupu, and R. Colomer. "Exogenous supplementation with omega-3 polyunsaturated fatty acid docosahexaenoic acid (DHA; 22:6n-3) synergistically enhances taxane cytotoxicity and downregulates Her-2/neu (c-erbB-2) oncogene expressions in human breast cancer cells." *European Journal of Cancer Prevention* Vol. 14. (June 2005): 263–270.

Moore, N.G., F. Wang-Johanning, P.L. Chang, et al. "Omega-3 fatty acids decrease protein kinase expression in human breast cancer cells." *Breast Cancer Research and Treatment* Vol. 67. (June 2001): 279–283.

Oh, D., S. Talukdar, E. Bae, et al. "GPR120 is an omega-3 fatty acid receptor mediating potent anti-inflammatory and insulin-sensitizing effects." *Cell* Vol.142. (Sept 2010): 687–698.

Rose, D.P., Connolly, J.M. "Regulation of tumor angiogenesis by dietary fatty acids and eicosanoids." *Nutrition and Cancer* Vol. 37. (2000): 119–127.

Saggar, J., J. Chen, P. Corey, et al. "Dietary flaxseed lignan or oil combined with tamoxifen treatment affects MCF 7 tumor growth through estrogen receptor and growth factor signaling pathways." *Molecular Nutrition & Food Research* Vol. 54. (Mar 2010): 415–425.

Saldeen, P., and T. Saldeen. "Women and omega-3 fatty acids." *Obstetrical and Gynecological Survey* Vol. 59. (Oct 2004): 722–730.

Siddiqui, R.A., M. Zerouga, M. Wu, et al. "Anticancer properties of propofol-docosahexaenoate and propofol-eicosapentaenoate on breast cancer cells." *Breast Cancer Research* Vol. 7. (July 7, 2005): R645–654.

Signori, C., C. DuBrock, J.P. Richie, et al. "Administration of omega-3 fatty acids and raloxifene to women at high risk of breast cancer: interim feasibility and biomarkers analysis from a clinical trial." *European Journal of Clinical Nutrition* Vol. 66. (Aug 2012): 878–884.

Simon, J., Y. Chen, and S. Bent. "The relation of -linolenic acid to the risk of prostate cancer: a systematic review and meta-analysis." *The American Journal of Clinical Nutrition* Vol. 89. (May 2009): 1558S–1564S.

Sun, H., I.M. Berquin, and I.J. Edwards. "Omega-3 polyunsaturated fatty acids regulate syndecan-1 expression in human breast cancer cells." *Cancer Research* Vol. 65. (May 15, 2005): 4442–4447.

Truan, J., J. Chen, and L. Thompson. "Flaxseed oil reduces the growth of human breast tumors (MCF 7) at high levels of circulating estrogen." *Molecular Nutrition & Food Research* Vol. 54. (Oct 2010): 1414–1421.

Ulbricht, C., W. Chao, K. Nummy, et al. "Chia (Salvia hispanica): a systematic review by the Natural Standard Research Collaboration." *Reviews on Recent Clinical Trials* Vol. 4. (Sept 2009): 168–174.

Olive Oil

Alarcon de la Lastra, C., M.D. Barranco, V. Motila, et al. "Mediterranean diet and health: biological importance of olive oil." *Current Pharmaceutical Design* Vol. 7. (July 2001): 933–950.

Aguas, F., A. Martins, T.P. Gomes, et al. "Prophylaxis approach to a-symptomatic post-menopausal women: breast cancer." *Maturitas* Vol. 52. (Nov 15, 2005): S23–31.

Buckland, G., N. Travier, A. Agudo, et al. "Olive oil intake and breast cancer risk in the Mediterranean countries of the European Prospective Investigation into Cancer and Nutrition sStudy." *International Journal of Cancer* Vol. 131. (Nov 2012): 2465–2469.

Busnena, B., A. Foudah, T. Melancon, et al. "Olive secoiridoids and semisynthetic bioisostere analogues for the control of metastatic breast cancer." *Bioorganic & Medicinal Chemistry* Vol. 21. (Apr 2013): 2117–2127.

Casaburi, I., F. Puoci, A. Chimento, et al. "Potential of olive oil phenols as chemopreventive and therapeutic agents against cancer: a review of in vitro studies." *Molecular Nutrition & Food Research* Vol. 57. (Jan 2013): 71–83.

Colomer, R., Menendez, J.A. "Mediterranean diet, olive oil and cancer." *Clinical and Translational Oncology* Vol. 8. (Jan 2006): 15–21.

Colomer, R., R. Lupu, A. Papadimitropoulou, et al. "Giacomo Castelvetro's salads. Anti-HER2 oncogene nutraceuticals since the 17th century?" *Clinical and Translational Oncology* Vol. 10. (Jan 2008): 30–34.

Costa, I., R. Moral, M. Solanas, et al. "High-fat corn oil diet promotes the development of high histologic grade DMBA-induced mammary adenocarcinomas, while olive oil diet does not." *Breast Cancer Research and Treatment* Vol. 86. (Aug 2004): 225–235.

Elamin, M., M. Daghestani, S. Omer, et al. "Olive oil oleuropein has anti-breast cancer properties with higher efficiency on ER-negative cells." *Food and Chemical Toxicology* Vol. 53. (Mar 2013): 310–316.

Escrich, E., M. Solanas, R. Moral, et al. "Modulatory effects and molecular mechanisms of olive oil and other dietary lipids in breast cancer." *Current Pharmaceutical Design* Vol. 17. (Mar 2011): 813–830.

Escrich, E., R. Moral, and M. Solanas. "Olive oil, an essential component of the Mediterranean diet, and breast cancer." *Public Health Nutrition* Vol. 14. (Dec 2011): 2323–2332.

Fistoni , I., M. Šitum, V. Bulat, et al. "Olive oil biophenols and women's health." *Medicinski Glasnik* Vol. 9. (Feb 2012): 1–9.

Garcia-Segovia, P., A. Sanchez-Villegas, J. Doreste, et al. "Olive oil consumption and risk of breast cancer in the Canary Islands: a population-based case-control study." *Public Health Nutrition* Vol. 9. (Feb 2006): 163–167.

Hassan, Z., M. Elamin, M. Daghestani, et al. "Oleuropein induces anti-metastatic effects in breast cancer." *Asian Pacific Journal of Cancer Prevention* Vol. 13. (Jan 2012): 4555–4559.

Masala, G., Ambrogetti, D., Assedi, M., et al. "Dietary and lifestyle determinants of mammographic breast density. A longitudinal study in a Mediterranean population." *International Journal of Cancer* Vol. 118. (April 1, 2006): 1782–1789.

Menendez, J.A., A. Papadimitropoulou, L. Vellon, et al. "A genomic explanation connecting 'Mediterranean diet,' olive oil and cancer: Oleic oleic acid, the main monounsaturated fatty acid of olive oil, induces formation of inhibitory 'PEA3 transcription factor-PEA3 DNA binding site' complexes at the Her-2/neu (erbB-2) oncogene promoter in breast, ovarian and stomach cancer cells." *European Journal of Cancer* Vol. 42. (Jan, 4, Oct 2006): 2425–2432.

Menendez, J., A. Vazquez-Martin, R. Colomer, et al. "Olive oil's bitter principle reverses acquired autoresistance to trastuzumab (Herceptin) in HER2-overexpressing breast cancer cells." *BMC Cancer* Vol. 7. (May 2007): 80.

Menendez, J.A., L. Vellon, R. Colomer, et al. "Oleic acid, the main monounsaturated fatty acid of olive oil, suppresses Her-2/neu (erbB-2) expression and synergistically enhances the growth inhibitory effects of trastuzumab (Herceptin) in breast cancer cells with Her-2/neu oncogene amplification." *Annals of Oncology* Vol. 16. (Mar 2005): 339–371.

Menendez, J.A., L. Vellon, R. Colomer, et al. "Oleic acid, the main monounsaturated fatty acid of olive oil, suppresses Her-2/neu (erbB-2) expression and synergistically enhances the growth inhibitory effects of trastuzumab (Herceptin) in breast cancer cells with Her-2/neu oncogene amplification." *Annals of Oncology* Vol. 16. (Oct 2005): 359–371.

Moral, R., Solanas, M., Garcia, G., et al. "Modulation of EGFR and neu expression by n-6 and n-9 high-fat diets in experimental mammary adenocarcinomas." *Oncology Reports* Vol. 10. (Sept-Oct 2003): 1417–1424.

Oliveras-Ferraros, C., S. Fernández-Arroyo, A. Vazquez-Martin, et al. "Crude phenolic extracts from extra virgin olive oil circumvent de novo breast cancer resistance to HER1/HER2-targeting drugs by inducing GADD45-sensed cellular stress, G2/M arrest and hyperacetylation of Histone H3." *International Journal of Oncology* Vol. 38. (June 2011): 1533–1547.

Owen, R.W., Giacosa, A., Hull, W.E., et al. "The antioxidant/anticancer potential of phenolic compounds isolated from olive oil." *European Journal of Cancer* Vol. 36. (June 2000): 1235–1247.

Pelucchi, C., C. Bosetti, E. Negri, et al. "Olive oil and cancer risk: an update of epidemiological findings through 2010." *Current Pharmaceutical Design* Vol. 17. (Mar 2011): 805–812.

Perez-Jimenez F, G. Alvarez de Cienfuegos , L. Badimon, et al. "International Conference on the Healthy Effect of Virgin Olive Oil." *European Journal of Clinical Investigation* Vol. 35. (July 2005): 421–424.

Psaltopoulou, T., R. Kosti, D. Haidopoulos, et al. "Olive oil intake is inversely related to cancer prevalence: a systematic review and a meta-analysis of 13800 patients and 23340 controls in 19 observational studies." *Lipids Health* Vol. 30. (July 2011): 127.

rBGH/IGF1

Chen, J., P.M. Starvo, and L.U. Thompson. "Dietary flaxseed inhibits human breast cancer growth and metastasis and down regulates expression of insulin-like growth factor and epidermal growth factor receptor." *Nutrition & Cancer* Vol. 43. (Issue 2, 2002): 187–192.

Dong, Y., L. Zhang, K. He, et al. "Dairy consumption and risk of breast cancer: a meta-analysis of prospective cohort studies." *Breast Cancer Research and Treatment* Vol. 127. (May 2011): 23–31.

Epstein, S. "Monsanto's hormonal milk poses serious risks of breast cancer." *PRNewswire*. (Jun 22, 1998).

Kahan, Z., J. Gardi, T. Nyari, et al. "Elevated levels of circulating insulin-like growth factor-1, IGF-binding globulin-3 and testosterone predict hormone-dependent breast cancer in postmenopausal women: a case-control study." *International Journal of Oncology* Vol. 29. (July 2006): 193–200.

Krajcik, R.A., N.D. Borofsky, S. Massardo, et al. "Insulin-like growth factor I (IGF-1), IGF-binding proteins, and breast cancer." *Cancer Epidemiology, Biomarkers & Prevention* Vol. 11. (Dec 2002): 1566–1573.

Larsen, Hans. "Milk and the cancer connection." *International Health News*. (April 1998).

Lukanova, A., P. Toniolo, A. Zeleniuch-Jacquotte, et al. "Insulin-like growth factor 1 in pregnancy and maternal risk of breast cancer." *Cancer, Epidemiology, Biomarkers and Prevention* Vol. 15. (Dec 2006): 2489–2493.

Martin, M.B., and A. Stoica. "Insulin-like growth

factor-1 and estrogen interactions in breast cancer." *Journal of Nutrition* Vol. 132. (Dec 2002): 3799S–3801S.

Outwater, J.L., A. Nicholson, and N. Barnard. "Dairy products and breast cancer: the IGF-1, estrogen, and rBGH hypothesis." *Medical Hypotheses* Vol. 48. (Jun 1997): 453–461.

Schmitz, K.H., R.L. Ahmed, and D. Yee. "Effects of a 9-month strength training intervention on insulin, insulin-like growth factor (IGF-1), IGF-binding protein (IGFBP)-1, and IGFBP-3 in 30–50 year old women." *Cancer Epidemiology, Biomarkers & Prevention* Vol. 11. (Dec 2002): 1597–1604.

Silva, J., A. Beckedorf, and E. Bieberich. "Osteoblast-derived oxysterol is a migration-inducing factor for human breast cancer cells." *Journal of Biology & Chemistry* (May 6, 2003). www.ncbi.nlm.nih.gov/entrez/query.fcgi?cmd=Retrieve&db=journals&list_uids=4559&dopt=full.

CLA

Białek, A., A. Tokarz. "Conjugated linoleic acid as a potential protective factor in prevention of breast cancer." *Postepy Higieny i Medycyny Doswiadczalnej* (Online) Vol. 67. (Jan 2012): 6–14.

Chen, J. "Src may be involved in the anti-cancer effect of conjugated linoleic acid. Comment on: CLA reduces breast cancer cell growth and invasion through ER and PI3K/Akt pathways." *Chemico-biological Interactions* Vol. 186. (July 2010): 250–251.

El R., J. M. Bard, J. M. Huvelin, et al. "The anti-proliferative and pro-apoptotic effects of the trans9, trans11 conjugated linoleic acid isomer on MCF-7 breast cancer cells are associated with LXR activation." *Prostaglandins, Leukotrienes and Essential Fatty Acids* Vol. 88. (Apr 2013): 265–272.

Flowers, M., J. Schroeder, A. Borowsky, et al. "Pilot study on the effects of dietary conjugated linoleic acid on tumorigenesis and gene expression in PyMT transgenic mice." *Carcinogenesis* Vol. 31. (Sept 2010): 1642–1649.

Heinze, V., and A. Actis. "Dietary conjugated linoleic acid and long-chain n-3 fatty acids in mammary and prostate cancer protection: a review." *International Journal of Food Sciences and Nutrition* Vol. 63. (Feb 2012): 66–78.

Kelley, N., N. Hubbard, and K. Erickson. "Conjugated linoleic acid isomers and cancer." *The Journal of Nutrition* Vol. 137. (Dec 2007): 2599-2607.

McGowan, M., B. Eisenberg, L. Lewis, et al. "A proof of principle clinical trial to determine whether conjugated linoleic acid modulates the lipogenic pathway in human breast cancer tissue."

Breast Cancer Research and Treatment Vol. 138. (Feb 2013): 175–183.

Song, H-J., A. A. Sneddon, S. D. Heys, and K. W. J. Wahle. "Regulation of fatty acid synthase (FAS) and apoptosis in estrogen-receptor positive and negative breast cancer cells by conjugated linoleic acids." *Prostaglandins, Leukotrienes and Essential Fatty Acids* Vol. 87. (Dec 2012): 197–203.

Tao, M., J. Wang, J. Wang, et al. "Enhanced anticancer activity of gemcitabine coupling with conjugated linoleic acid against human breast cancer in vitro and in vivo." *European Journal of Pharmaceutics and Biopharmaceutics* Vol. 82. (Oct 2012): 401–409.

Evening Primrose Oil/ GLA

Menendez, J., L. Vellon, R. Colomer, et al. "Effect of γ-linolenic acid on the transcriptional activity of the Her-2/neu (erbB-2) oncogene." *Journal of the National Cancer Institute* Vol. 97. (Sept 2005): 1611–1615.

Menendez, J., S. Ropero, I. Mehmi, et al. "Overexpression and hyperactivity of breast cancer-associated fatty acid synthase (oncogenic antigen-519) is insensitive to normal arachidonic fatty acid-induced suppression in lipogenic tissues but it is selectively inhibited by tumoricidal alpha-linolenic and gamma-linolenic fatty acids: a novel mechanism by which dietary fat can alter mammary tumorigenesis." *International Journal of Oncology* Vol. 24. (June 2004): 1369–1383.

Menendez, J., S. Ropero, R. Lupu, et al. "Omega-6 polyunsaturated fatty acid gamma-linolenic acid (18: 3n-6) enhances docetaxel (Taxotere) cytotoxicity in human breast carcinoma cells: Relationship to lipid peroxidation and HER-2/neu expression." *Oncology Reports* Vol. 11. (June 2004): 1241–1252.

Menendez, J., L. Vellon, R. Colomer, et al. "Effect of γ-linolenic acid on the transcriptional activity of the Her-2/neu (erbB-2) oncogene." *Journal of the National Cancer Institute* Vol. 97. (Nov 2005): 1161–1615.

Chapter 9: A Fortress Made of Seeds

Alexander, J.W. "Immunonutrition: the role of omega-3 fatty acids." *Nutrition* Vol. 14. (Jul-Aug 1998): 627–633.

Almada, A. "Brevail: SDG precision standardized flaxseed extract." *Scientific Research Monograph.* (2003).

Barlean's Organic Oils. "A very important message to women: Lignans reduce risk and spread of malignant disease." *The Breast Cancer Prevention Files:* *The Doctor's Prescription for Healthy Living* Vol. 4. (Issue 10).

Basch, E., S. Bent, J. Collins, et al. "Flax and flaxseed oil (Linum usitatissimum): a review by the Natural Standard Research Collaboration." *Journal of the Society for Integrative Oncology* Vol. 5. (June 2007): 92–105.

Bhathena, S.J., Velasquez, M.T. "Beneficial role of dietary phytoestrogens in obesity and diabetes." *American Journal of Clinical Nutrition* Vol. 76. (Dec 2002): 1191–1201.

Chajes, V., W. Sattler, A. Stranzl, et al. "Influence of n-3 fatty acids on the growth of human breast cancer cells in vitro: relationship to peroxides and vitamin E." *Breast Cancer Research & Treatment* Vol. 34. (Jun 1995): 199–212.

Chen, J., J. Saggar, P. Corey, et al. "Flaxseed and pure secoisolariciresinol diglucoside, but not flaxseed hull, reduce human breast tumor growth (MCF-7) in athymic mice." *The Journal of Nutrition* Vol. 139. (Nov 2009): 2061–2066.

Chen, J., J. Saggar, P. Corey, et al. "Flaxseed cotyledon fraction reduces tumour growth and sensitises tamoxifen treatment of human breast cancer xenograft (MCF-7) in athymic mice." *British Journal of Nutrition* Vol. 105. (Feb 2011): 339–347.

Chen, J., J. Saggar, W. Ward, et al. "Effects of flaxseed lignan and oil on bone health of breast-tumor-bearing mice treated with or without tamoxifen." *Journal of Toxicology and Environmental Health, Part A* Vol. 74. (May 2011): 757–768.

Chen, J., K. Power, J. Mann, et al. "Flaxseed alone or in combination with tamoxifen inhibits MCF-7 breast tumor growth in ovariectomized athymic mice with high circulating levels of estrogen." *Experimental Biology and Medicine* Vol. 232. (Sept 2007): 1071–1080.

Chen, J., P.M. Starvo, and L.U. Thompson. "Dietary Flaxseed inhibits human breast cancer growth and metastasis and down regulates expression of insulin-like growth factor and epidermal growth factor receptor." *Nutrition & Cancer* Vol. 43. (Issue 2, 2002): 187–192.

Cotterchio, M., B. Boucher, N. Kreiger, et al. "Dietary phytoestrogen intake—lignans and isoflavones —and breast cancer risk (Canada)." *Cancer Causes & Control* Vol. 19. (Apr 2008): 259–272.

Dabrosin, C., J. Chen, L. Wang, et al. "Flaxseed inhibits metastasis and decreases extracellular vascular endothelial growth factoring human breast cancer xenografts." *Cancer Letters* Vol. 185. (Nov 2002): 31–37.

Dai, Q., A.A. Franke, F. Jin, et al. "Urinary excretion of phytoestrogens and risk of breast cancer among Chinese women in Shanghai." *Cancer, Epidemiology, Biomarkers and Prevention* Vol. 11. (Sept 2002): 815– 821.

Fife, B. "The facts on flax" from the book *Saturated Fats May Save Your Life*. Website: www.Coconut-info.com/facts_on_ flax.htm.

Haggens, C.J., A.M. Hutchins, B.A. Olson, et al. "Effects of flaxseed consumption on urinary estrogen metabolites in postmenopausal women." *Nutrition & Cancer* Vol. 33. (Issue 2, 1999): 188–195.

Haggans, C.J., E.J. Travelli, W. Thomas, et al. "The effects of flaxseed and wheat bran consumption on urinary estrogen metabolites in premenopausal women." *Cancer Epidemiology, Biomarkers & Prevention* Vol. 9. (Jul 2000): 719–725.

Horner, C., M.D. "Flax: the food no home should be without." *Channelcincinnati.com*. (Mar 15, 2001).

Jungeström, B., L. Thompson, and C. Dabrosin. "Flaxseed and its lignans inhibit estradiol-induced growth, angiogenesis, and secretion of vascular endothelial growth factor in human breast cancer xenografts in vivo." *Clinical Cancer Research* Vol. 13. (Feb 2007): 1061–1067.

Kitts, D.D., Y.V. Yuan, A.N. Wijewickreme, et al. "Antioxidant activity of flaxseed lignan secoisolariciresinol diglycoside and its mammalian lignan metabolites enterolactone." *Molecular and Cellular Biochemistry* Vol. 202. (Dec 1999): 91–100.

Kurzer, M.S., J.W. Lampe, M.C. Martini, et al. "Fecal lignan and isoflavonoid excretion in premenopausal women consuming flaxseed powder." *Cancer Epidemiology*, Biomarkers & Prevention Vol. 4. (Jun 1995): 353–358.

McCann, S., K. Hootman, A. Weaver, et al. "Dietary intakes of total and specific lignans are associated with clinical breast tumor characteristics." *The Journal of Nutrition* Vol. 142. (Jan 2012): 91–98.

McCann, S., K.B. Moyisch, J.L. Freudenheim, et al. "The risk of breast cancer associated with dietary lignans differs by CYP17 genotype in women." *Journal of Nutrition* Vol. 132. (Oct 2002): 3035–3041.

McCann, S., L. Thompson, J. Nie, et al. "Dietary lignan intakes in relation to survival among women with breast cancer: the Western New York Exposures and Breast Cancer (WEB) Study." *Breast Cancer Research and Treatment* Vol. 122. (July 2010): 229–235.

Michaels, K.B., Solomon, C.G., Hu, F.B., et al. "Type 2 diabetes and subsequent incidence of breast cancer in the Nurses' Health Study." *Diabetes Care* Vol. 26. (June 2003): 1752–1758.

Nagel, G., Mack, U., von Fournier, D., et al. "Dietary phytoestrogens intake and mammographic density-results of a pilot study." *European Journal of Medical Research* Vol. 10. (Sept 12, 2005): 389–394.

Phippes, W.R., M.C. Martini, J.W. Lampe, et al. "Effects of flax seed ingestion on the menstrual cycle." *The Journal of Clinical Endocrinology & Metabolism* Vol. 77. (Nov 1993): 1215–1219.

Pietinen, P., Stumpf, K., Mannisto, S., et al. "Serum enterolactone and risk of breast cancer: a case-control study in eastern Finland." *Cancer Epidemiology, Biomarkers, and Prevention* Vol. 10. (April 2001): 339–344.

Saarinen, N., and L. Thompson. "Prolonged administration of secoisolariciresinol diglycoside increases lignan excretion and alters lignan tissue distribution in adult male and female rats." *British Journal of Nutrition* Vol. 104. (Sept 2010): 833–841.

Sacco, S., J. Jiang, L. Thompson, et al. "Flaxseed does not enhance the estrogenic effect of low-dose estrogen therapy on markers of uterine health in ovariectomized rats." *Journal of Medicinal Food* Vol. 15. (Sept 2012): 846–850.

Saggar, K., J. Chen, P. Corey, et al. "Dietary flaxseed lignan or oil combined with tamoxifen treatment affects MCF-7 tumor growth through estrogen receptor- and growth factor-signaling pathways." *Molecular Nutrition & Food Research* Vol. 54. (Mar 2010): 415–425.

Simopulos, A.P. "Essential fatty acids in health and chronic disease." *American Journal of Clinical Nutrition* Vol. 70. (Sept 1999; 3 Suppl): 560S–569S.

Stuedal, A., I.T. Gram, Y. Bremmes, et al. "Plasma levels of enterolactone and percentage mammographic density among postmenopausal women." *Cancer Epidemiology, Biomarkers, and Prevention* Vol. 14. (Sept 2005): 2154–2159.

Touillaud, M., A. Thiébaut, A. Fournier, et al. "Dietary lignan intake and postmenopausal breast cancer risk by estrogen and progesterone receptor status." Journal of the *National Cancer Institute* Vol. 99. (Jan 2007): 475–486.

Truan, J., J. Chen, and L. Thompson. "Comparative effects of sesame seed lignan and flaxseed lignan in reducing the growth of human breast tumors (MCF-7) at high levels of circulating estrogen in athymic mice." *Nutrition and Cancer* Vol. 64. (Dec 2012): 65–71.

Velasquez, M.T., Bhathena, S.J. "Dietary phytoestrogens: a possible role in renal disease protection." *American Journal of Kidney Disease* Vol. 37. (May 2001): 1056–1068.

Wang, L.Q. "Mammalian phytoestrogens: enterodiol and enterolactone." Journal of Chromatography. B, Analytical Technologies in the Biomedical and Life Sciences Vol. 25. (Sept 25, 2002): 289–309.

Ward, W.E., F.O. Jiang, and L.U. Thompson. "Exposure to flaxseed or purified lignan during lactation influences rat mammary gland structures." Nutrition & Cancer Vol. 37. (Issue 2, 2000): 187–192.

Zaineddin, A., K. Buck, A. Vrieling, et al. "The association between dietary lignans, phytoestrogen-rich foods, and fiber intake and postmenopausal breast cancer risk: a German case-control study." Nutrition and Cancer Vol. 64. (May 2012): 652–665.

Chapter 10: Asian Defense

Allred, C.D., K.F. Allred, H.J. Young, et al. "Soy processing influences growth of estrogen-dependent breast cancer tumors in mice." Carcinogenesis Vol. 25. (Sept 2004): 1649–1657.

Auborn, K.J., Fan, S., Rosen, E.M., et al. "Indole-3 carbinol is a negative regulator of estrogen." Journal of Nutrition Vol. 133. (July 2003): 2470S-2475S.

Boucher, B., M. Cotterchio, L. Anderson, et al. "Use of isoflavone supplements is associated with reduced postmenopausal breast cancer risk." International Journal of Cancer Vol. 132. (Mar 2013): 1439-1450.

Bouker, K.B., and L. Hilakivi-Clarke. "Genistein: does it prevent or promote breast cancer?" Environmental Health Perspectives Vol. 108. (Aug 2000): 701-708.

Dai, Q., A.A. Franke, F. Jin, et al. "Urinary excretion of phytoestrogens and risk of breast cancer among Chinese women in Shanghai." Cancer Epidemiology, Biomarkers & Prevention Vol. 11. (Issue 9, 2002): 815-821.

Dave, B., Eason, R.R., Till, S.R., et al. "The soy isoflavone genistein promotes apoptosis in mammary epithelial cells by inducing the tumor suppressor PTEN." Carcinogenesis Vol. 26. (Oct 2005): 1793- 1803.

Dong, Y., and L. Qin. "Soy isoflavones consumption and risk of breast cancer incidence or recurrence: a meta-analysis of prospective studies." Breast Cancer Research and Treatment Vol. 125. (Jan 2011): 315-323.

"Environmental estrogens and other hormones: phytoestrogens." 2001. Website: www.com.tulane.edu/ecme/eehome/basics/phytoestrogens/.

Fan, S., Q. Meng, K. Auburn, et al. "BRCA1 and BRCA2 as molecular targets for phytochemicals indole-3-carbinol and genistein in breast and prostate cancer cells." British Journal of Cancer Vol. 94. (Feb 13, 2006): 407–426.

Ghen, M. "Supplements and alternatives." International Journal of Integrative Medicine Vol. 3. (Issue 3, 2001): 37–38.

Hargreaves, D.F., C.S. Potten, C. Harding, et al. "Two-week dietary soy supplementation has an estrogenic effect on normal premenopausal breast." Journal of Clinical Endocrinology & Metabolism Vol. 84. (Nov 1999): 4017–4024.

Helferich, W. G., J. E. Andrade, and M. S. Hoagland. "Phytoestrogens and breast cancer: a complex story." Inflammopharmacology Vol. 16. (Oct 2008): 219–226.

Ingram, D., K. Sanders, M. Kolybaba, et al. "Case-control study of phyto-estrogens and breast cancer." The Lancet Vol. 350. (Issue 9083, 1997): 990–994.

Kang, B., Y. Zhang, J. Yang, and K. Lu. "Study on soy isoflavone consumption and risk of breast cancer and survival." Asian Pacific Journal of Cancer Prevention Vol. 13. (Mar 2012): 995–998.

Kim, H., H. Xia, L. Li, et al. "Attenuation of neurodegeneration-relevant modifications of brain proteins by dietary soy." Biofactors Vol. 12. (2000): 243–250.

Kim, M., J. Kim, S. Nam, et al. "Dietary intake of soy protein and tofu in association with breast cancer risk based on a case-control study." Nutrition and Cancer Vol. 60. (Sept 2008): 568–576.

Kishida, T., M. Beppu, et al. "Effects of dietary soy isoflavone aglycones on the urinary 16 alpha-to-22 hydroxyestrone ratio in C3H/HeJ mice." Nutrition & Cancer Vol. 38. (Issue 2, 2000): 209–214.

Lal, A., S. Warber, and A. Kirakosyan. "Upregulation of isoflavonoids and soluble proteins in edible legumes by light and fungal elicitor treatments." Journal of Alternative & Complementary Medicine Vol. 9. (Issue 3, 2003): 371–378.

Li, Y., F. Ahmed, S. Ali, et al. "Inactivation of nuclear factor kappB by soy isoflavone genistein contributes to increased apoptosis induced by chemotherapeutic agents in human cancer cells." Cancer Research Vol. 65. (Aug 1, 2005): 6934– 6942.

Low Dog, T., D. Riley, and T. Carter. "Traditional and alternative therapies for breast cancer." Alternative Therapies in Health & Medicine Vol. 7. (Issue 3, 2001): 36–47.

McCarty, M.F. "Isoflavones made simple-genistein's agonist activity for the beta-type estrogen receptor mediates their health benefits." Medical Hypotheses Vol. 66. (March 2, 2006): 1093–1114.

Magee, P., and I. Rowland. "Soy products in the management of breast cancer." Current Opinion in Clinical Nutrition & Metabolic Care Vol. 15. (Nov 2012): 586–591.

Maskarinec, G., N. Ollberding, S. Conroy, et al. "Estrogen levels in nipple aspirate fluid and serum during a randomized soy trial." *Cancer Epidemiology Biomarkers & Prevention* Vol. 20. (Sept 2011): 1815–1821.

Mercola, J. "The trouble with tofu: soy and the brain." Website: www.Mercolacom/2000/sept17/soy_brain. htm.

Messina, M., and C. Wood. "Soy isoflavones, estrogen therapy, and breast cancer risk: analysis and commentary." *Nutrition Journal* Vol. 7. (June 2008): 17–28.

Messina, M.J., and C.L. Loprinzi. "Soy for breast cancer survivors: a critical review of the literature." *Journal of Nutrition* Vol. 131. (Nov 2001): 3095S–3108S.

Montales, M., O. Rahal, J. Kang, et al. "Repression of mammosphere formation of human breast cancer cells by soy isoflavone genistein and blueberry polyphenolic acids suggests diet-mediated targeting of cancer stem-like/progenitor cells." *Carcinogenesis* Vol. 33. (Mar 2012): 652–660.

Morimoto, Y., S. Conroy, I. Pagano, et al. "Influence of diet on nipple aspirate fluid production and estrogen levels." *Food & Function* Vol. 2. (Nov 2011): 665–670.

Myung, S-K., W. Ju, H. J. Choi, et al. "Soy intake and risk of endocrine-related gynaecological cancer: a meta-analysis." *BJOG: An International Journal of Obstetrics & Gynaecology* Vol. 116. (Dec 2009): 1697–1705.

Nagata, C. "Factors to consider in the association between soy isoflavone intake and breast cancer risk." *Journal of Epidemiology* Vol. 20. (Feb 2010): 83–89. 11.

Nakagawa, H., Yamamoto, D., Kiyozuka, Y., et al. "Effects of genistein and synergistic action in combination with eicosapentaenoic acid on the growth of breast cancer cell lines." *Journal of Cancer Research and Clinical Oncology* Vol. 126. (Aug 2000): 448–454.

Nechuta, S., B. Caan, W. Chen, et al. "Soy food intake after diagnosis of breast cancer and survival: an in-depth analysis of combined evidence from cohort studies of US and Chinese women." *The American Journal of Clinical Nutrition* Vol. 96. (July 2012): 123–132.

Pabona, J., B. Dave, Y. Su, et al. "The soybean peptide lunasin promotes apoptosis of mammary epithelial cells via induction of tumor suppressor PTEN: similarities and distinct actions from soy isoflavone genistein." *Genes & Nutrition* Vol.8. (Jan 2013): 79–90.

Peeters, P.H., L. Keinan-Boker, et al. "Phytoestrogens and breast cancer risk. Review of the epidemiological evidence." *Breast Cancer Research & Treatment* Vol. 77. (Jan 2003): 171–183.

Petrakis, N.L., S. Barnes, E.B. King, et al. "Stimulatory influence of soy protein on breast secretion in pre- and postmenopausal women." *Cancer Epidemiology, Biomarkers & Prevention* Vol. 5. (Oct 1996): 785–794.

Salvo, V.A., Boue, S.M., Fonseca, J.P., et al. "Antiestrogenic glyceollins suppress human breast and ovarian carcinoma tumorigenesis." *Clinical Cancer Research* Vol. 12. (Dec 1, 2006): 7159–7164.

Satoh, H., K. Nishikawa, K. Suzuki, et al. "Genistein, a soy isoflavone, enhances necrotic-like cell death in a breast cancer cell treated with a chemotherapeutic agent." *Research Communications in Molecular Pathology and Pharmacology* Vol. 133–114. (2003): 149–158.

Schmidl, M. "Soybeans and nutraceuticals." 1999 lecture.

Setchell, K., N. Brown, X. Zhao, et al. "Soy isoflavone phase II metabolism differs between rodents and humans: implications for the effect on breast cancer risk." *The American Journal of Clinical Nutrition* Vol. 94. (Nov 2011): 1284–1294.

Stephens, F.O. "Breast cancer: Aetiological factors and associations (a possible protective role of phyto-estrogens)." *Australia and New Zealand Journal of Surgery* Vol. 67. (Nov 1997): 755–760.

"The Phytochemistry of Herbs Phytochemicals of the Month: November 2002." *Phytoestrogens.* Website: www.herbalchem.net/introductory.htm.

Tominaga, Y., A. Wang, R.H. Wang, et al. "Genistein inhibits BRCA1 mutant tumor growth through activation of DNA damage checkpoints, cell cycle arrest, and mitotic catastrophe." *Cell Death and Differentiation* Vol. 14. (Mar 2007): 472–479.

Trock, B.J., L. Hilakivi-Clarke, R. Clarke. "Meta-analysis of soy intake and breast cancer risk." *Journal of the National Cancer Institute* Vol. 98. (April 5, 2006): 430–431.

Valladares, L., A. Garrido, and W. Sierralta. "Soy isoflavones and human health: breast cancer and puberty timing." *Revista Médica de Chile* Vol. 140. (April 2012): 512–516.

van Duursen, M., S. M. Nijmeijer, E. S. de Morree, et al. "Genistein induces breast cancer-associated aromatase and stimulates estrogen-dependent tumor cell growth in in vitro breast cancer model." *Toxicology* Vol. 289. (Nov 2011): 67–73.

Wada, K., K. Nakamura, Y. Tamai, et al. "Soy isoflavone intake and breast cancer risk in Japan:

from the Takayama Study." *International Journal of Cancer* (Feb 2013): doi: 10.1002/ijc.28088.

Warri, A., N. M. Saarinen, S. Makela, et al. "The role of early life genistein exposures in modifying breast cancer risk." *British Journal of Cancer* Vol. 98. (May 2008): 1485-1493.

Weil, A. "CAM and continuing education: the future is now." *Alternative Therapies in Health & Medicine* Vol. 7. (Issue 3, 2001): 32–34.

Whitsett, T.G., Lamartiniere, C.A. "Genistein and resveratrol: Mammary cancer chemoprevention and mechanisms of action in the rat." *Expert Review of Anticancer Therapy* Vol. 6. (Dec 2006): 1699–1706.

Woo, D., K. Park, J. Ro, et al. "Differential influence of dietary soy intake on the risk of breast cancer recurrence related to HER2 status." *Nutrition and Cancer* Vol. 64. (Jan 2012): 198–205.

Wood, C.E., Register, T.C., Franke, A.A., et al. "Dietary soy isoflavones inhibit estrogen in the postmenopausal breast." *Cancer Research* Vol. 66. (Jan 15, 2006): 1241–1249.

Wu, A. H., M. C. Yu, C. C. Tseng, et al. "Epidemiology of soy exposures and breast cancer risk." *British Journal of Cancer* Vol. 98. (Jan 2008): 9–14.

Yamamoto, S., et al. "Soy, isoflavones, and breast cancer risk in Japan." *Journal of the National Cancer Institute* Vol. 95. (Jul 18, 2003): 906–913.

Zhang, F., H. Kang, B. Li, et al. "Positive effects of soy isoflavone food on survival of breast cancer patients in China." *Asian Pacific Journal of Cancer Prevention* Vol. 13. (Feb 2012): 479–482.

Zheng, W., Q. Dai, et al. "High isoflavone consumption can mean lower risk of breast cancer." *Cancer Epidemiology, Biomarkers & Prevention* Vol. 8. (Jan 1999): 35–40.

Zhong, X., and C. Zhang. "Soy food intake and breast cancer risk: a meta-analysis." *Journal of Hygiene Research* Vol. 41. (July 2012): 670–676.

Zhu, Y., L. Zhou, S. Jiao, et al. "Relationship between soy food intake and breast cancer in China." *Asian Pacific Journal of Cancer Prevention* Vol. 12. (July 2011): 2837–2840.

Chapter 11: Magic Mushrooms and More

Maitake Mushrooms

Berry, J. "Maitake." *Natural Health Magazine*. (Aug 2001).

Kidd, P.M. "The use of mushroom glucans and proteoglycans in cancer treatment." Alternative Medicine Review Vol. 5. (Feb 2000): 4–27. Kodama, N.,
K. Komuta, and H. Nanba. "Can maitake MD-fraction aid cancer patients?" *Alternative Medicine Review* Vol. 7. (Jun 2002): 236–239.

Soares, R., M. Meireles, A. Rocha, et al. "Maitake (D fraction) mushroom extract induces apoptosis in breast cancer cells by BAK-1 gene activation." *Journal of Medicinal Food* Vol. 14. (June 2011): 563–572.

Reishi Mushrooms

Hu, H., N.S. Ahn, X. Yang, et al. "Ganoderma lucidum extract induces cell cycle arrest and apoptosis in MCF-7 human breast cancer cells." *International Journal of Cancer* Vol. 102. (Nov 20, 2002): 250–253.

Jin, X., J. Beguerie, D. Man-yeun Sze, et al. "Ganoderma lucidum (reishi mushroom) for cancer treatment." *Cochrane Database Syst Rev* Vol. 6. (June 2012): CD007731. doi: 10.1002/14651858.CD007731.

Lu, Q.Y., M.R. Sartippour, M.N. Brooks, et al. "Ganoderma lucidum spore extract inhibits endothelial and breast cancer cells in vitro." *Oncology Report* Vol. 12. (Sept 2004): 659–662.

Sanodiya, B., G. Thakur, R. Baghel, et al. "Ganoderma lucidum: a potent pharmacological macrofungus." *Current Pharmaceutical Biotechnology* Vol. 10. (Dec 2009): 717–742.

Shang, D., Y. Li, C. Wang, etc. "A novel polysaccharide from Se-enriched Ganoderma lucidum induces apoptosis of human breast cancer cells." *Oncology Reports* Vol. 25. (Jan 2011): 267–272.

Sliva, D. "Ganoderma lucidum (Reishi) in cancer treatment." *Integrative Cancer Therapies* Vol. 2. (Dec 2003): 358–364.

Sliva, D., M. Sedlak, V. Slivova, et al. "Biologic activity of spores and dried powder from Ganoderma lucidum for inhibition of highly invasive human breast and prostate cancer cells." *Journal of Alternative & Complementary Medicine* Vol. 9. (Aug 2003): 491–497.

Sliva, D., C. Labarrere, V. Slivova, et al. "Ganoderma lucidum suppresses motility of highly invasive breast and prostate cancer cells." *Biochemical and Biophysical Research Communications* Vol. 298. (Nov 8, 2002): 603–612.

Weng, C., and G. Yen. "The in vitro and in vivo experimental evidences disclose the chemopreventive effects of Ganoderma lucidum on cancer invasion and metastasis." *Clinical & Experimental Metastasis* Vol. 27. (May 2010): 361–369.

Xu, Z., X. Chen, Z. Zhong, et al. "Ganoderma lucidum polysaccharides: immunomodulation and potential anti-tumor activities." *The American Journal of Chinese Medicine* Vol. 39. (Jan 2011): 15–27.

Other Mushrooms

Breau, M. "AHCC as an immunotherapy for breast cancer–new study is promising." *AHCC Research Blog*. Website: www.ahccresearch.com.

Chen, S., Oh, S.R., Phung, S., et al. "Anti-aromatase activity of phytochemicals in white button mushrooms (Agaricus bisporus)." *Cancer Research* Vol. 66. (Dec 2006): 12026–12034.

Dotan, N., S. Wasser, and J. Mahajna. "The culinary-medicinal mushroom Coprinus comatus as a natural antiandrogenic modulator." *Integrative Cancer Therapies* Vol. 10. (June 2011): 148–159.

Gu, Y.H., and J. Leonard. "In vitro effects on proliferation, apoptosis and colony inhibition in ER-dependent and ER-independent human breast cancer cells by selected mushroom species." *Oncology Reports* Vol. 15. (Feb 2006): 417–423.

Hong, S., K. Kim, S. Nam, et al. "A case–control study on the dietary intake of mushrooms and breast cancer risk among Korean women." *International Journal of Cancer* Vol. 122. (Feb 2008): 919–923.

Jeong, C., S. Koyyalamudi, Y. Jeong, et al. "Macrophage immunomodulating and antitumor activities of polysaccharides isolated from Agaricus bisporus white button mushrooms." *Journal of Medicinal Food* Vol.15. (Jan 2012): 58–65.

Jiang, J., and D. Sliva. "Novel medicinal mushroom blend suppresses growth and invasiveness of human breast cancer cells." *International Journal of Oncology* Vol. 37. (Dec 2010): 1529–1536.

Lee, M.L., N.H. Tan, S.Y. Fung, et al. "The antiproliferative activity of sclerotia of Lignosus rhinocerus (tiger milk mushroom)." *Evidence-Based Complementary and Alternative Medicine* 2012 (Feb 2012): 697603. doi: 10.1155/2012/697603.

Mansour, A., A. Daba, N. Baddour, et al. "Schizophyllan inhibits the development of mammary and hepatic carcinomas induced by 7, 12 dimethylbenz (α) anthracene and decreases cell proliferation: comparison with tamoxifen." *Journal of Cancer Research and Clinical Oncology* Vol. 138. (Sept 2012): 1579–1596.

Martin, K., and S. Brophy. "Commonly consumed and specialty dietary mushrooms reduce cellular proliferation in MCF-7 human breast cancer cells." *Experimental Biology and Medicine* Vol. 235. (Nov 2010): 1306–1314.

Novaes, M., F. Valadares, M. Reis, et al. "The effects of dietary supplementation with Agaricales mushrooms and other medicinal fungi on breast cancer: evidence-based medicine." *Clinics* Vol. 66. (July 2011): 2133–2139.

Wang, C., T. Ng, L. Jin Cen Fang, et al. "Isolation of a polysaccharide with antiproliferative, hypoglycemic, antioxidant and HIV-1 reverse transcriptase inhibitory activities from the fruiting bodies of the abalone mushroom Pleurotus abalonus." *Journal of Pharmacy and Pharmacology* Vol. 63. (June 2011): 825–832.

Zhang, M., J. Huang, X. Xie, et al. "Dietary intakes of mushrooms and green tea combine to reduce the risk of breast cancer in Chinese women." *International Journal of Cancer* Vol. 124. (Mar 2009): 1404–1408.

Green Tea

Boehm, K., F. Borrelli, E. Ernst, et al. "Green tea (Camellia sinensis) for the prevention of cancer." *Cochrane Database System Review* Vol. 3. (July 2009): CD005004. doi: 10.1002/14651858.CD005004.pub2.

Butt, M., and M. Sultan. "Green tea: nature's defense against malignancies." *Critical Reviews in Food Science and Nutrition* Vol. 49. (May 2009): 463-473.

Chen, D., S. Pamu, Q. Cui, et al. "Novel epigallocatechin gallate (EGCG) analogs activate AMP-activated protein kinase pathway and target cancer stem cells." *Bioorganic & Medicinal Chemistry* Vol. 20. (May 2012): 3031–3037.

Clement, Y., and E. Ernst. "Can green tea do that? A literature review of the clinical evidence." *Preventive Medicine* Vol. 49. (Aug-Sept 2009): 83–87.

De Amicis, F., A. Russo, P. Avena, et al. "In vitro mechanism for downregulation of ER-α expression by epigallocatechin gallate in ER+/PR+ human breast cancer cells." *Molecular Nutrition & Food Research* Vol. 57. (May 2013): 840–853.

Eddy, S., S. Kane, and G. Sonenshein. "Trastuzumab-resistant HER2-driven breast cancer cells are sensitive to epigallocatechin-3 gallate." *Cancer Research* Vol. 67. (Oct 2007): 9018–9023.

El-Beshbishy, H.A. "Hepatoprotective effect of green tea (Camellia sinensis) extract against Tamoxifen-induced liver injury in rats." *Journal of Biochemistry and Molecular Biology* Vol. 38. (Sept 30, 2005): 563–570.

Farabegoli, F., C. Barbi, E. Lambertini, et al. "(–)-Epigallocatechin-3-gallate downregulates estrogen receptor alpha function in MCF-7 breast carcinoma cells." *Cancer Detection and Prevention* Vol. 31. (Oct 2007): 499–504.

Ferrario, A., M. Luna, N. Rucker, et al. "Pro-apoptotic and anti-inflammatory properties of the green tea constituent epigallocatechin gallate increase photodynamic therapy responsiveness." *Lasers in Surgery and Medicine* Vol. 43. (Sept 2011): 644-650.

Fijiki, H., M. Suganuma, S. Okabe, et al. "Mechanistic findings of green tea as a cancer preventative for humans." *Proceedings of the Society for Experimental Biology and Medicine* Vol. 220. (Apr 1999): 225–228.

Guo, S., S. Yang, C. Taylor, et al. "Green tea polyphenols epigallocatechin-3 gallate (EGCG) affects gene expression of breast cancer cells transformed by the carcinogen 7, 12-dimethylbenz[a]anthracene." *Journal of Nutrition* Vol. 135. (Dec 2005): 2978S– 2986S.

Hirose, M., T. Hoshiya, K. Akagi, et al. "Inhibition of mammary gland carcinogenesis by green tea catechins and other naturally occurring antioxidants in female Sprague-Dawley rats pretreated with 7,12-dimethylbenz[alpha]anthracene." *Cancer Letters* Vol. 83. (Aug 15, 1994): 149–156.

Horner, C., M.D. "Green tea: a hot healing beverage." *Channelcincinnati.com.* (Jan 9, 2001).

Iwasaki, M., and S. Tsugane. "Risk factors for breast cancer: epidemiological evidence from Japanese studies." *Cancer Science* Vol. 102. (Sept 2011): 1607–1614.

Iwasaki, M., M. Inoue, S. Sasazuki, et al. "Green tea drinking and subsequent risk of breast cancer in a population to based cohort of Japanese women." *Breast Cancer Res* Vol. 12. (Oct 2010): R88.

Iwasaki, M., M. Inoue, S. Sasazuki, et al. "Plasma tea polyphenol levels and subsequent risk of breast cancer among Japanese women: a nested case–control study." *Breast Cancer Research and Treatment* Vol. 124. (Dec 2010): 827–834.

Johnson, R., S. Bryant, and A. Huntley. "Green tea and green tea catechin extracts: an overview of the clinical evidence." *Maturitas* Vol.73. (Dec 2012): 280–287.

Leong, H., P. Mathur, and G. Greene. "Green tea catechins inhibit angiogenesis through suppression of STAT3 activation." *Breast Cancer Research and Treatment* Vol. 117. (Oct 2009): 505–515.

Luo, T., J. Wang, Y. Yin, et al. "(-)-Epigallocatechin gallate sensitizes breast cancer cells to paclitaxel in a murine model of breast carcinoma." Vol. 12. (2010): R8. doi: 10.1186/bcr2473.

Meeran, S., S. Patel, Y. Li, et al. "Bioactive dietary supplements reactivate ER expression in ER-negative breast cancer cells by active chromatin modifications." *PloS One* Vol. 7. (May 2012): e37748.

Nagata, C., M. Kabuto, and H. Shimizu. "Associa-

tion of coffee, green tea, and caffeine intake with serum concentrations of estradiol and sex hormone-binding globulin in premenopausal Japanese women." *Nutrition & Cancer* Vol. 30. (Issue 1, 1998): 21–24.

Nagle, D., D. Ferreira, and Y. Zhou. "Epigallocatechin-3-gallate (EGCG): chemical and biomedical perspectives." *Phytochemistry* Vol. 67. (Sept 2006): 1849–1855.

Nakachi, K., K. Suemasu, K. Suga, et al. "Influence of drinking green tea on breast cancer malignancy among Japanese patients." *Japanese Journal of Cancer Research* Vol. 89. (Mar 1998): 254–261.

Ogunleye, A., F. Xue, and K. Michels. "Green tea consumption and breast cancer risk or recurrence: a meta-analysis." *Breast Cancer Research and Treatment* Vol. 119. (Jan 2010): 477–484.

Rathore, K., and H. Wang. "Green tea catechin extract in intervention of chronic breast cell carcinogenesis induced by environmental carcinogens." *Molecular Carcinogenesis* Vol. 51. (Mar 2012): 280–289.

Rathore, K., and H. Wang. "Mesenchymal and stem-like cell properties targeted in suppression of chronically-induced breast cell carcinogenesis." *Cancer Letters* Vol. 333. (June 2013): 113–123.

Sadzuka, Y., Y. Yamashita, and T. Sonobe. "Effect of dihydrokainate on the antitumor activity of doxorubicin." *Cancer Letters* Vol. 179. (May 28, 2002): 157–163.

Sadzuka, Y., T. Sugiyama, and T. Sonobe. "Efficacies of tea components on doxorubicin induced antitumor activity and reversal of multidrug resistance." *Toxicology Letters* Vol. 114. (Apr 3, 2000): 155–162.

Sadzuka, Y., T. Sugiyama, and S. Hirota. "Modulation of cancer chemotherapy by green tea." *Clinical Cancer Research* Vol. 4. (Jan 1998): 153–156.

Sadzuka, Y., T. Sugiyama, A. Miyagishima, et al. "The effects of theanine, as a novel biochemical modulator, on the antitumor activity of Adriamycin." *Cancer Letters* Vol. 105. (Aug 2, 1996): 203–209.

Sartippour, M.R., R. Pietras, D.C. Marquez-Garban, et al. "The combination of green tea and tamoxifen is effective against breast cancer." *Carcinogenesis* Vol. 27. (Dec 2006): 2424–2433.

Seely, D., E. Mills, P. Wu, et al. "The effects of green tea consumption on incidence of breast cancer and recurrence of breast cancer: a systematic review and meta-analysis." *Integrative Cancer Therapies* Vol. 4. (June 2005): 144–155.

Shimizu, M., S. Adachi, M. Masuda, et al. "Cancer

chemoprevention with green tea catechins by targeting receptor tyrosine kinases." *Molecular Nutrition & Food Research* Vol. 55. (June 2011): 832–843.

Shrubsole, M., W. Lu, Z. Chen, et al. "Drinking green tea modestly reduces breast cancer risk." *The Journal of Nutrition* Vol. 139. (Feb 2009): 310–316.

Sugiyama, T., and Y. Sadzuka. "Enhancing effects of green tea components on the antitumor activity of Adriamycin against M5076 ovarian sarcoma." *Cancer Letters* Vol. 133. (Nov 13, 1998): 19–26.

Sugiyama, T., and Y. Sadzuka, et al. "Inhibition of glutamate transporter by theanine enhances the therapeutic efficacy of doxorubicin." *Toxicology Letters* Vol. 121. (Apr 30, 2001): 89–96.

Sugiyama, T., and Y. Sadzuka. "Theanine and glutamate transporter inhibitor enhance the antitumor efficacy of chemotherapeutic agents." *Biochimica et Biophysica Acta* Vol. 1653. (Dec 5, 2003): 47–59.

Sun, C.L., Yuan, J.M., Koh, W.P., et al. "Green tea, black tea and breast cancer risk: a meta-analysis of epidemiological studies." *Carcinogenesis* Vol. 27. (July 2006): 1310–1315.

Tanaka, H., M. Hirose, M. Kawabe, et al. "Post-initiation inhibitory effects of green tea catechins on 7,12-dimethylbenz[alpha]anthracene-induced mammary gland carcinogenesis in female Sprague Dawley rats." *Cancer Letters* Vol. 116. (Jun 1997): 47–52.

Thangapazham, R., N. Passi, and R. Maheshwari. "Green tea polyphenol and epigallocatechin gallate induce apoptosis and inhibit invasion in human breast cancer cells." *Cancer Biology & Therapy* Vol. 6. (Dec 2007): 1938–1943.

Valcic, S., B.N. Timmermann, D.S. Alberts, et al. "Inhibitory effect of six green tea catechins and caffeine on the growth of four selected human tumor cell lines." *Anticancer Drugs* Vol. 7. (Jun 1996): 461–468.

Wu, A.H., Arakawa, K., Stanczyk, F.Z., et al. "Tea and circulating estrogen levels in postmenopausal Chinese women in Singapore." *Carcinogenesis* Vol. 26. (May 2005): 976–980.

Yuan, M., C. Sun, and L. Butler. "Tea and cancer prevention: epidemiological studies." *Pharmacological Research* Vol. 64. (Aug 2011): 123–135.

Zhang, M., C.D. Holman, J.P. Huang, et al. "Green tea and the prevention of breast cancer: a case-control study in southeast China." *Carcinogenesis* Vol. 28. (May 2007): 1074–1078.

Zhang, M., J. Huang, X. Xie, et al. "Dietary intakes of mushrooms and green tea combine to reduce the risk of breast cancer in Chinese women." *International Journal of Cancer* Vol. 124. (Mar 2009): 1404–1408.

Zhao, X., Tian, H., Ma, X., et al. "Epigallocatechin gallate, the main ingredient of green tea induces apoptosis in breast cancer cells." *Frontiers in Bioscience: A Journal and Virtual Library* Vol. 11. (Sept 1, 2006): 2428–2433.

Turmeric

Aggarwal, B., C. Sundaram, N. Malani, et al. "Curcumin: the Indian solid gold." *Advances in Experimental Medicine and Biology* Vol. 595. (Jan 2007):1–75.

Agrawal, K., and P. Mishra. "Curcumin and its analogues: potential anticancer agents." *Medicinal Research Reviews* Vol. 30. (Sept 2010): 818–860.

Alappat, L., and A. Awad. "Curcumin and obesity: evidence and mechanisms." *Nutrition Reviews* Vol. 68. (Dec 2010): 729–738.

Anand, P., A. Kunnumakkara, R. Newman, et al. "Bioavailability of curcumin: problems and promises." *Molecular Pharmaceutics* Vol. 4. (Nov 2007): 807–818.

Anand, P., C. Sundaram, S. Jhurani, et al. "Curcumin and cancer: an "old-age" disease with an "age-old" solution." *Cancer Letters* Vol. 267. (Aug 2008): 133–164.

Bachmeier, B., A. Nerlich, C. Iancu, et al. "The chemopreventive polyphenol Ccurcumin prevents hematogenous breast cancer metastases in immunodeficient mice." *Cellular Physiology and Biochemistry* Vol. 19. (Jan 2007): 137–152.

Bisht, S., and A. Maitra. "Systemic delivery of curcumin: 21st century solutions for an ancient conundrum." *Current Drug Discovery Technologies* Vol. 6. (Sept 2009): 192-199.

Boonrao, M., S. Yodkeeree, C. Ampasavate, et al. "The inhibitory effect of turmeric curcuminoids on matrix metalloproteinase-3 secretion in human invasive breast carcinoma cells." *Archives of Pharmacal Research* Vol. 33. (July 2010): 989–998.

De La, C., E. Saludables, and Y. De Los Curcuminoides. "Plant-derived health-the effects of turmeric and curcuminoids." *Nutrición hospitalaria : organo oficial de la Sociedad Española de Nutrición Parenteral y Enteral* Vol. 24. (May-June 2009): 273–281.

Goel, A., and B. Aggarwal. "Curcumin, the golden spice from Indian saffron, is a chemosensitizer and radiosensitizer for tumors and chemoprotector and radioprotector for normal organs." *Nutrition and Cancer* Vol. 62. (July 2010): 919–930.

Gupta, S.C., S. Patchva, W. Koh, et al. "Discovery

of curcumin, a component of golden spice, and its miraculous biological activities." *Clinical and Experimental Pharmacology and Physiology* Vol. 39. (Mar 2012): 283–299.

Hassan, Z., and M. Daghestani. "Curcumin effect on MMPs and TIMPs genes in a breast cancer cell line." *Asian Pacific Journal of Cancer Prevention* Vol. 13. (Jan 2012): 3259–3264.

Hedelin, M., M. Löf, M. Olsson, et al. "Dietary phytoestrogens are not associated with risk of overall breast cancer but diets rich in coumestrol are inversely associated with risk of estrogen receptor and progesterone receptor negative breast tumors in Swedish women." *The Journal of Nutrition* Vol. 138. (May 2008): 938–945.

Jagetia, C., and B. Aggarwal. "'Spicing up'" of the immune system by curcumin." *Journal of Clinical Immunology* Vol. 27. (Jan 2007): 19–35.

Jiang, M., O. Huang, X. Zhang, et al. "Curcumin induces cell death and restores tamoxifen sensitivity in the antiestrogen-resistant breast cancer cell lines MCF-7/LCC2 and MCF-7/LCC9." *Molecules* Vol. 18. (Jan 2013): 701–720.

Kim, H., H. Huang, S. Cheepala, et al. "Curcumin inhibition of integrin (6 4)-dependent breast cancer cell motility and invasion." *Cancer Prevention Research* Vol. 1. (Oct 2008): 385–391.

Kunnumakkara, A., P. Anand, and B. Aggarwal. "Curcumin inhibits proliferation, invasion, angiogenesis and metastasis of different cancers through interaction with multiple cell signaling proteins." *Cancer Letters* Vol. 269. (Oct 2008): 199–225.

Lee, H., T. Khor, L. Shu, et al. "Dietary phytochemicals and cancer prevention: Nrf2 signaling, epigenetics, and cell death mechanisms in blocking cancer initiation and progression." *Pharmacology & Therapeutics* Vol. 137. (Feb 2013): 153–171.

Liu, Q., W. Loo, S. C. W. Sze, et al. "Curcumin inhibits cell proliferation of MDA-MB-231 and BT-483 breast cancer cells mediated by down-regulation of NF B, cyclinD and MMP-1 transcription." *Phytomedicine* Vol. 16. (Oct 2009): 916–922.

Menon, V., and A. Sudheer. "Antioxidant and anti-inflammatory properties of curcumin." *Advances in Experimental Medicine and Biology.* Vol. 595. (2007): 105–125.

Palange, A., D. Di Mascolo, J. Singh, et al. "Modulating the vascular behavior of metastatic breast cancer cells by curcumin treatment." *Frontiers in Oncology* Vol. 2. (Nov 2012): 161.

Polasa, K., T.C. Raghuram, T. Krishna, et al. "Effect of turmeric on urinary mutagens in smokers." *Mutagenesis* Vol. 7. (Issue 2, 1992): 107–109.

Ramachandran, C., H. Fonseca, P. Jhabvala, et al. "Curcumin inhibits telomerase activity through human telomerase reverse transcritpase in MCF-7 breast cancer cell line." *Cancer Letters* Vol. 184. (Oct 2002): 1–6.

Ravindran, J., S. Prasad, and B. Aggarwal. "Curcumin and cancer cells: how many ways can curry kill tumor cells selectively?" *The AAPS Journal* Vol. 11. (Sept 2009): 495–510.

Singletary, K., C. MacDonald, M. Iovinelli, et al. "Effect of the beta-diketones diferuloylmethane (curcumin) and dibenzoylmethane on rat mammary DNA adducts and tumor induced by 7,12-dimethylbenz[alpha]anthracene." *Carcinogenesis* Vol. 19. (Jun 1998): 1039–1043.

Sun, X. D., X. E. Liu, and D. S. Huang. "Curcumin induces apoptosis of triple-negative breast cancer cells by inhibition of EGFR expression." *Molecular Medicine Reports* Vol. 6. (Dec 2012): 1267–1270.

Verna, S.P., B.R. Goldin, and P.S. Lin. "The inhibition of estrogenic effects of pesticides and environmental chemicals by curcumin and isoflavonoids." *Environmental Health Perspectives* Vol. 106. (Dec 1998): 807–812.

Verma, S.P., E. Salamone, and B. Goldin. "Curcumin and genistein, plant natural products, show synergistic inhibitory effects on the growth of human breast cancer MCF-7 cells induced by estrogenic pesticides." *Biochemical and Biophysical Research Communications* Vol. 233. (Apr 28, 1997): 692–696.

Garlic

Altonsy, M., T. Habib, and S. Andrews. "Diallyl disulfide-induced apoptosis in a breast-cancer cell line (MCF-7) may be caused by inhibition of histone deacetylation." *Nutrition and Cancer* Vol. 64. (Nov 2012): 1251–1260.

Amagase, H., and J. Milner. *The FASEB Journal* Vol. 6. (Issue 4, 1992): 3229.

Amagase, H., and J. Milner. "Impact of various sources of garlic and their constituents on 7-12-dimethylbenz[a]anthracene binding to mammary cell DNA." *Carcinogenesis* Vol. 14. (1993): 1627–1631.

Chandra-Kuntal, K., J. Lee, and S. Singh. "Critical role for reactive oxygen species in apoptosis induction and cell migration inhibition by diallyl trisulfide, a cancer chemopreventive component of garlic." *Breast Cancer Research and Treatment* Vol. 138. (Feb 2013): 69–71.

Dong, Y., D. Lisk, E. Block, et al. "Characterization of the biological activity of gamma-glutamyl-Se-methylselesnocysteine: a novel, naturally occurring anticancer agent from garlic." *Cancer Research* Vol. 61. (Apr 1, 2001): 2923–2928.

Galeone, C., C. Pelucchi, F. Levi, et al. "Onion and garlic use and human cancer." *American Journal of Clinical Nutrition* Vol. 84. (Nov 2006): 1027–1032.

Gapter, L., O. Yuin, and K. Ng. "S-allylcysteine reduces breast tumor cell adhesion and invasion." *Biochemical and Biophysical Research Communications* Vol. 367. (Mar 2008): 446–451.

Gued, L.R., R.D. Thomas, and M. Green. "Diallyl sulfide inhibits diethylstilbestrol-induced lipid peroxidation in breast tissue of female ACI rats: Implications in breast cancer prevention." *Oncology Report* Vol. 10. (May-Jun 2003): 739–743.

Hirsch, K., M. Danilenko, J. Giat, et al. "Effect of purified allicin, the major ingredient of freshly crushed garlic, on cancer cell proliferation." *Nutrition & Cancer* Vol. 38. (Issue 2, 2000): 245–254.

Horner, C., M.D. "Garlic: a common herb with uncommon benefits." *Channelcincinnati.com*. (2002).

Ip, C., D.J. Lisk, and H.J. Thompson. "Selenium-enriched garlic inhibits the early stage but not the late stage of mammary carcinogenesis." *Carcinogenesis* Vol. 17. (Sept 1996): 1979–1982.

Lei, X., S. Yao, X. Zu, et al. "Apoptosis induced by diallyl disulfide in human breast cancer cell line MCF-7." *Acta Pharmacologica Sinica* Vol. 29. (Oct 2008): 1233–1239.

Lin, J., J. Milner, et al. *Carcinogenesis* Vol. 13. (1992a): 1847–1851.

Milner, J., J. Liu. *First World Congress on the Health Significance of Garlic and Garlic Constituents*. (1990): 25.

Malki, A., M. El-Saadani, and A. Sultan. "Garlic constituent diallyl trisulfide induced apoptosis in MCF7 human breast cancer cells." *Cancer Biology & Therapy* Vol. 8. (Nov 2009): 2174–2184.

Modem, S., S. DiCarlo, and T. Reddy. "Fresh garlic extract induces growth arrest and morphological differentiation of MCF7 breast cancer cells." *Genes & Cancer* Vol. 3. (Feb 2012): 177–186.

Na, Hye-Kyung, E., M. Choi, J. Park, et al. "Diallyl trisulfide induces apoptosis in human breast cancer cells through ROS-mediated activation of JNK and AP-1." *Biochemical Pharmacology* Vol. 84. (Nov 2012): 1241–1250.

Nakagawa, H., K. Tsuta, K. Kiuchi, et al. "Growth inhibitory effects of diallyl disulfide on human breast cancer cell lines." *Carcinogenesis* Vol. 22. (Jun 2001): 891–897.

Nian, H., E. Ho, and R. Dashwood. "Modulation of histone deacetylase activity by dietary isothio-cyanates and allyl sulfides: studies with sulforaphane and garlic organosulfur compounds." *Environmental and Molecular Mutagenesis* Vol. 50. (Apr 2009): 213–221.

Nkrumah-Elie, Y., J. Reuben, A. Hudson, et al. "The attenuation of early benzo (a) pyrene-induced carcinogenic insults by diallyl disulfide (DADS) in MCF-10A Cells." *Nutrition and Cancer* Vol. 64. (Sept 2012): 1112–1121.

Pinto, J.T., and R.S. Rivlin. "Antiproliferative effects of allium derivatives from garlic." *Journal of Nutrition* Vol. 131. (Mar 2001): 1058S–1060S.

Pinto, J., and R. Rivlin. "Recent advances on the nutritional benefits accompanying the use of garlic as a supplement." Newport Beach, CA: Nov 15–17, 1998.

Tiwari, R., J. Pinto, et al. *Breast Cancer Research & Treatment* Vol. 27. (Issue 1-2, 1993): 80.

Tsubura, A., Y. Lai, M. Kuwata, et al. "Anticancer effects of garlic and garlic-derived compounds for breast cancer control." *Anti-cancer Agents in Medicinal Chemistry* Vol. 11. (Mar 2011): 249–253.

Seaweed

Aceves, C., B. Anguiano, G. Delgado. "Is iodine a gatekeeper of the integrity of the mammary gland." *Journal of Mammary Gland Biology and Neoplasia* Vol. 10. (April 2005): 189–196.

Aceves, C., P. García-Solís, O. Arroyo-Helguera, et al. "Antineoplastic effect of iodine in mammary cancer: participation of 6-iodolactone (6-IL) and peroxisome proliferator-activated receptors (PPAR)." *Molecular Cancer* Vol. 8. (June 2009): 33.

Altman, M., M. Flynn, R. Nishikawa, et al. "The potential of iodine for improving breast cancer diagnosis and treatment." *Medical Hypotheses* Vol. 80. (Jan 2013): 94–98.

Cann, S.A., J.P. van Netten, and C. van Netten. "Hypothesis: iodine, selenium and the development of breast cancer." *Cancer Causes and Control* Vol. 11. (Feb 2000): 121–127.

Chatterjee, S., R. Malhotra, F. Varghese, et al. "Quantitative immunohistochemical analysis Rreveals association between sodium iodide symporter and estrogen receptor expression in breast cancer." *PloS One* Vol. 8. (Jan 2013): e54055.

Funahashi, H., T. Imai, T. Mase, et al. "Seaweed prevents breast cancer?" *Japanese Journal of Cancer Research* Vol. 92. (May 2001): 483–487.

Kilbane, M.T., R.A. Ajjan, A.P. Weetman, et al. "Tissue iodine content and serum mediated 125I uptake-blocking activity in breast cancer." *Journal* of Clinical Endocrinology & Metabolism Vol. 85. (Mar 2000): 1245–1250.

Nunez-Anita, R.E., M. Cajero-Juárez, and C. Aceves. "Peroxisome proliferator-activated receptors: role of isoform gamma in the antineoplastic effect of iodine in mammary cancer." Current Cancer Drug Targets Vol. 11. (Sept 2011): 775–786.

Sekiya, M., H. Funahashi, K. Tsukamura, et al. "Intracellular signaling in the induction of apoptosis in a human breast cancer cell line by water extract of mekabu." International Journal of Clinical Oncology Vol. 10. (Apr 2005): 122–126.

Shamsabadi, F., A. Khoddami, S. Ghasemi Fard, et al. "Comparison of tamoxifen with edible seaweed (Eucheuma cottonii L.) extract in suppressing breast tumor." Nutrition and Cancer Vol. 65. (Feb 2013): 255–262.

Singh, P., M. Godbole, G. Rao, et al. "Inhibition of autophagy stimulate molecular iodine-induced apoptosis in hormone independent breast tumors." Biochemical and Biophysical Research Communications Vol. 415 (Nov 2011): 181–186.

Smyth, P.P. "The thyroid and breast cancer: a significant association?" Annals of Medicine Vol. 29. (Jun 1997): 189–191.

Soriano, O., G. Delgado, B. Anguiano, et al. "Antineoplastic effect of iodine and iodide in dimethylbenz [a] anthracene-induced mammary tumors: association between lactoperoxidase and estrogen-adduct production." Endocrine-Related Cancer Vol. 8. (July 2011): 529–539.

Tasebay, U.H., I.L. Wapnir, O. Levy, et al. "The mammary gland iodine transporter is expressed during lactation and in breast cancer." Natural Medicine Vol. 6. (Aug 2000): 871–878.

Teas, J., T. Hurley, J. Hebert, et al. "Dietary seaweed modifies estrogen and phytoestrogen metabolism in healthy postmenopausal women." The Journal of Nutrition Vol. 139. (May 2009): 939–944.

Updhyay, G., R. Singh, G. Agarwal, et al. "Functional expression of sodium iodide symporter (NIS) in human breast cancer tissue." Breast Cancer Research & Treatment Vol. 77. (Jan 2003): 157–165.

Yang, Y., S. Nam, G. Kong, et al. "A case–control study on seaweed consumption and the risk of breast cancer." British Journal of Nutrition Vol. 103. (May 2010): 1345–1353.

Rosemary, Licorice, Black Cohosh, Vitex, Hops, and Chinese Herbs

Amato, P., S. Christophe, and P.L. Mellon. "Estrogenic activity of herbs commonly used as remedies for menopausal symptoms." Menopause Vol. 9. (Mar-Apr 2002): 145–150.

Arpornsuwan, T., Punjanon, T. "Tumor cell-selective antiproliferative effect of the extract from Morinda citrifolia fruits." Phytotherapy Research Vol. 20. (June 2006): 515–517.

Bilinski, K, and J. Boyages. "Association between 25-hydroxyvitamin D concentration and breast cancer risk in an Australian population: an observational case-control study." Breast Cancer Research and Treatment Vol. 137. (Jan 2013): 599–607.

Bodinet, C., and J. Freudenstein. "Influence of marketed herbal menopause preparations on MCF-7 cell proliferation." Menopause Vol. 11. (May-Jun 2004): 281–289.

Campbell, M.J., B. Hamilton, M. Shoemaker, et al. "Antiproliferative activity of Chinese medicinal herbs on breast cancer cells in vitro." Anticancer Research Vol. 22. (Nov-Dec 2002): 3843–3852.

Dixon-Shanies, D., and N. Shaikh. "Growth inhibition of human breast cancer cells by herbs and phytoestrogens." Oncology Report Vol. 6. (Nov-Dec 1999): 1383–1387.

Duda, R.B., B. Taback, B. Kessel, et al. "pS2 expression induced by American ginseng in MCF-7 breast cancer cells." Annals of Surgical Oncology Vol. 3. (Nov 1996): 515–520.

Duda, R.B., Y. Zhong, V. Navas, et al. "American ginseng and breast cancer therapeutic agents synergistically inhibit MCF-7 breast cancer cell growth." Journal of Surgical Oncology Vol. 72. (Dec 1999): 230–239.

Duda, R.B., S. Kang, S.Y. Archer, et al. "American ginseng transcriptionally activates p21 mRNA in breast cancer cell lines." Journal of Korean Medical Science Vol. 16 Suppl. (Dec 2001): S54–S60.

Eibond, L.S., H. Wu, R Kashiwazaki, et al. "Carnosic acid inhibits the growth of ER-negative human breast cancer cells and synergizes with curcumin." Fitoterapia Vol. 83 (Oct 2012): 1160–1168

Einbond, L.S., M. Shimizu, D. Xiao, et al. "Growth inhibitory activity of extract and purified components of black cohosh on human breast cancer cells." Breast Cancer Research & Treatment Vol. 83. (Feb 2004): 221–231.

Hiramatsu, T., Imoto, M., Koyano, T., et al. "Induction of normal phenotypes in ras-transformed cells by damnacanthal from Morinda citrifolia." Cancer Letters Vol. 73. (Sept 30, 1993): 161–166.

Hornick, C.A., Meyers, A., Sadowska-Krowicka, H., et al. "Inhibition of angiogenic initiation and disruption of newly established human vascular networks by juice from Morinda citrifolia (noni)." *Angiogenesis* Vol. 6. (2003): 143–149.

Hostanska, K., T. Nisslein, J. Freudenstein, et al. "Cimicifuga racemosa extract inhibits proliferation of estrogen receptor-positive and negative human breast carcinoma cell line by induction of apoptosis." *Breast Cancer Research & Treatment* Vol. 84. (Mar 2004): 151–160.

Jo, E.H., H.D. Hong, N.C. Ahn, et al. "Modulation of the Bcl-2/Bax family were involved in the chemopreventative effects of licorice root (Glycyrrhiza uralensis Fisch) in MCF-7 human breast cancer cell." *Journal of Agricultural and Food Chemistry* Vol. 52. (Mar 24, 2004): 1715–1719.

Lee, Y.J., Y.R. Jin, W.C. Lim, et al. "Ginsenoside-Rb1 acts as a weak phytoestrogen in MCF-7 human breast cancer cells." *Archives of Pharmaceutical Research* Vol. 26. (Jan 2003): 58–63.

Li, X.K., M. Motwani, W. Tong, et al. "Huanglian, A Chinese herbal extract, inhibits cell growth by suppressing the expression of cyclin B1 and inhibiting CDC2 kinase activity in human cancer cells." *Molecular Pharmacology* Vol. 58. (Dec 2000): 1287–1293.

Lupu, R., I. Mehmi, E. Atlas, et al. "Black cohosh, a menopausal remedy, does not have estrogenic activity and does not promote breast cancer cell growth." *International Journal of Oncology* Vol. 23. (Nov 2003): 1407–1412.

Maggiolini, M., G. Statti, A. Vivacqua, et al. "Estrogenic and antiproliferative activities of isoliquiritigenin in MCF7 breast cancer cells." *Journal of Steroid Biochemistry & Molecular Biology* Vol. 82. (Nov 2002): 315–322.

Miranda, C.L., J.F. Stevens, A. Helmrich, et al. "Antiproliferative and cytotoxic effects of prenylated flavonoids from hops (Humulus lupulus) in human cancer cell lines." *Food and Chemical Toxicology* Vol. 37. (Apr 1999): 271–285.

Oh, M.S., Y.H. Choi, H.Y. Chung, et al. "Anti-proliferative effects of ginsenoside RH2 on MCF-7 human breast cancer cells." *International Journal of Oncology* Vol. 14. (May 1999): 869–875.

Plouzek, C.A., H.P. Ciolino, R. Clarke, et al. "Inhibition of P-glycoprotein activity and reversal of multidrug resistance by in vitro rosemary extract." *European Journal of Cancer* Vol. 35. (Oct 1999): 1541–1545.

Rong, H., T. Boterberg, J. Maubach, et al. "8-Prenyl-naringenin, the phytoestrogen in hops and beer, upregulates the function of E-cadherin/catenin complex in human mammary carcinoma cells." *Eu-*

ropean Journal of Cell Biology Vol. 80. (Sept 2001): 580–585.

Singletary, K., C. MacDonald, and M. Wallig. "Inhibition of rosemary and carnosol of 7,12-dimethylbenz[a] anthracene (DMBA)-induced rat mammary tumorigenesis and in vivo DMBA-DNA adduct formation." *Cancer Letters* Vol. 104. (Jun 24, 1996): 43–48.

Singletary, K., et al. "Inhibition of 7,12-dimethylbenz[a] anthracene (DMBA)-induced mammary tumorigenesis and in vivo formation of mammary DMBA-DNA adduct by rosemary extract." *Cancer Letters* Vol. 60. (Nov 1991): 169–175.

Sliva, D., M. Sedlak, V. Slivova, et al. "Biologic activity of spores and dried powder from Ganoderma lucidum for inhibition of highly invasive breast and prostate cancer cells." *Journal of Alternative & Complementary Medicine* Vol. 9. (Aug 2003): 491–497.

Sun, J., Hai Liu, R. "Cranberry phytochemical extracts induce cell cycle arrest and apoptosis in human MCF-7 breast cancer cells." *Cancer Letters* Vol. 241. (Sept 8, 2006): 124–134.

Tagliaferri, M., M.D., I. Cohen, O.M.D., L.Ac., D. Tripathy, M.D. *Breast Cancer: Beyond Convention.* New York: Atria Books, 2002.

Tamir, S., M. Eizenberg, D. Somjen, et al. "Estrogenic and antiproliferative properties of glabridin from licorice in human breast cancer cells." *Cancer Research* Vol. 60. (Oct 15, 2000): 5704–5709.

Vacek J.L., S. R. Vanga, M. Good M, et al. "Vitamin D deficiency and supplementation and relation to cardiovascular health." *American Journal of Cardiology* Vol. 109 (Feb 2012): 359–363.

Zierau, O., C. Bodinet, S. Kolba, et al. "Antiestrogenic activity of Cimicifuga racemosa extracts." *Journal of Steroid Biochemistry & Molecular Biology* Vol. 80. (Jan 2002): 125–130.

Ginkgo

An, G., J. Gallegos, M. Morris. "The bioflavonoid kaempferol is an Abcg2 substrate and inhibits Abcg2-mediated quercetin efflux." *Drug Metabolism and Disposition* Vol. 39. (Mar 2011): 426–432.

Barton, D., K. Burger, P. Novotny, et al. "The use of Ginkgo biloba for the prevention of chemotherapy-related cognitive dysfunction in women receiving adjuvant treatment for breast cancer, N00C9." *Supportive Care in Cancer* Vol. 21. (Apr 2013): 1185–1192.

DeFeudis, F.V., Papadopoulos, V., Drieu, K. "Ginkgo biloba extracts and cancer: a research area in its infancy." *Fundamental & Clinical Pharmacology* Vol. 17. (Aug 2003): 405–417.

Kim, J., Y. Park, K. Chung, et al. "The inhibitory effects of the standardized extracts of Ginkgo biloba on aromatase activity in JEG-3 human choriocarcinoma cells." *Phytotherapy Research* (Jan 2013): doi: 10.1002/ptr.4927.

Li, W., Pretner, E., Shen, L., et al. "Common gene targets of Ginkgo biloba extract (EGb 761) in human tumor cells: relation to cell growth." *Cellular and Molecular Biology* Vol. 48. (Sept 2002): 655–662.

Park, J., M. Kim, H. Kim, et al. "Chemopreventive effects of Ginkgo biloba extract in estrogen-negative human breast cancer cells." *Archives of Pharmacal Research* Vol. 36. (Jan 2013): 102–108.

Oh, J., I. Hyun Hwang, C.Hong, et al. "Inhibition of fatty acid synthase by ginkgolic acids from the leaves of Ginkgo biloba and their cytotoxic activity." *Journal of Enzyme and Medicinal Chemistry* Vol. 28 (Jun 13): 565–568.

Oh, S.M., Chung, K.H. "Antiestrogenic activities of Ginkgo biloba extracts." *The Journal of Steroid Biochemistry and Molecular Biology* Vol. 100. (Aug 2006): 167–176.

Papadopoulos, V., Kapsis, A., Li, H., et al. "Drug-induced inhibition of the peripheral-type benzodiazepine receptor expression and cell proliferation in human breast cancer cells." *Anticancer Research* Vol. 20. (Sept-Oct 2000): 2835–2847.

Pertner, E., Amri, H., Li, W., et al. "Cancer-related overexpression of the peripheral-type benzodiazepine receptor and cytostatic anticancer effects of Ginkgo biloba extract (EGb 761)." *Anticancer Research* Vol. 26. (Jan-Feb 2006): 9–22.

Yi, S., K. Nan, S. Chen. "Effect of extract of Ginkgo biloba on doxorubicin-associated cardiotoxicity in patients with breast cancer." *Journal of Integrated Traditional and Western* Vol. 28. (Jan 2008): 68–70.

Ginseng

Bao, P., W. Lu, Y. Cui, et al. "Ginseng and Ganoderma lucidum use after breast cancer diagnosis and quality of life: a report from the Shanghai Breast Cancer Survival Study." *PloS One* Vol. 7. (June 2012): e39343.

Choi, S., T. Kim, S. Singh. "Ginsenoside Rh2-mediated G1 phase cell cycle arrest in human breast cancer cells is caused by p15 Ink4B and p27 Kip1-dependent inhibition of cyclin-dependent kinases." *Pharmaceutical Research* Vol. 26. (Oct 2009): 2280–2288.

Cui, Y., Shu, X.O., Gao, Y.T., et al. "Association of ginseng use with survival and quality of life among breast cancer patients." *American Journal of Epidemiology* Vol. 163. (April 1, 2006): 645–653.

Duda, R.B., Kang, S.S., Archer, S.Y., et al. "American ginseng transcriptionally activates p21 mRNA in breast cancer cell lines." *Journal of Korean Medical Science* Vol. 16. (Dec 2001): S54–60.

Duda, R.B., Taback, B., Kessel, B., et al. "pS2 expression induced by American ginseng in MCF-7 breast cancer cells." *Annals of Surgical Oncology* Vol. 3. (Nov 1996): 515–520.

Duda, R.B., Zhong, Y., Navas, V., et al. "American ginseng and breast cancer therapeutic agents synergistically inhibit MCF-7 breast cancer cell growth." *Journal of Surgical Oncology* Vol. 72. (Dec 1999): 230–239.

Jia, W.W., Bu, X., Philips, D., et al. "Rh2, a compound extracted from ginseng, hypersensitizes multidrug-resistant tumor cells to chemotherapy." *Canadian Journal of Physiology and Pharmacology* Vol. 82. (July 2004): 431–437.

Jin, J., Shahi, S., Kang, H.K., et al. "Metabolites of ginsenosides as novel BCRP inhibitors." *Biochemical and Biophysical Research Communications* Vol. 345. (July 14, 2006):1308–1314.

Kang, J., K. Song, J. Woo, et al. "Ginsenoside Rp1 from Panax ginseng exhibits anti-cancer activity by down-regulation of the IGF-1R/Akt pathway in breast cancer cells." *Plant Foods for Human Nutrition* Vol. 66. (Sept 2011): 298–305.

Kim, D., K. Ah Kang, R. Zhang, et al. "Ginseng saponin metabolite induces apoptosis in MCF-7 breast cancer cells through the modulation of AMP-activated protein kinase." *Environmental Toxicology and Pharmacology* Vol. 30. (Sept 2010): 134–140.

Kim, J. "Protective effects of Asian dietary items on cancers—soy and ginseng." *Asian Pacific Journal Cancer Prevention* Vol. 9. (Oct-Dec 2008): 543–548.

King, M.L., Adler, S.R., Murphy, L.L. "Extraction-dependent effects of American ginseng (Panax quinquefolium) on human breast cancer cell proliferation and estrogen receptor activation." *Integrative Cancer Therapies* Vol. 5. (Sept 2006): 236–243.

Lau, W., R. Yat-Kan Chan, D. Guo, et al. "Ginsenoside Rg1 exerts estrogen-like activities via ligand-independent activation of ERα pathway." *The Journal of Steroid Biochemistry and Molecular Biology* Vol. 108. (Jan 2008): 64–71.

Lee, Y.J., Jin, Y.R., Lim, W.C., et al. "Ginsenoside-Rb1 acts as a weak phytoestrogen in MCF-7 human breast cancer cells." *Archives of Pharmacal Research* Vol. 26. (Jan 2003): 58–63.

Lee, Y., Jin, Y., Ji, S., et al. "A ginsenoside-Rh1, a

component of ginseng saponin, activates estrogen receptor in human breast carcinoma MCF-7 cells." *The Journal of Steroid Biochemistry and Molecular Biology* Vol. 84. (March 2003): 463–480.

Lo, L., C. Chen, S. Chen, et al. "Therapeutic efficacy of traditional Chinese medicine, Shen-Mai San, in cancer patients undergoing chemotherapy or radiotherapy: study protocol for a randomized, double-blind, placebo-controlled trial." *Trials* Vol. 13. (Dec 2012): 232.

Loo, W.T., Cheung, M.N., Chow, L.W. "The inhibitory effect of a herbal formula comprising ginseng and carthamus tinctorius on breast cancer." *Life Sciences* Vol. 76. (Nov 26, 2004): 191–200.

Ma, H., J. Sullivan-Halley, A. Smith, et al. "Estrogenic botanical supplements, health-related quality of life, fatigue, and hormone-related symptoms in breast cancer survivors: a HEAL study report." *BMC Complementary and Alternative Medicine* Vol. 11. (Nov 2011): 109.

Mantle, D., Lennard, T.W., Pickering, A.T. "Therapeutic applications of medicinal plants in the treatment of breast cancer: a review of their pharmacology, efficacy, and tolerability." *Adverse Drug Reactions and Toxicological Reviews* Vol. 19. (Aug 2000): 223–240.

Oh, M., Choi, S., Chung, H., et al. "Anti-proliferative effects of ginsenoside-Rh2 on MCF-7 human breast cancer cells." *International Journal of Oncology* Vol. 14. (May 1999): 869–875.

Peralta, E., L. Murphy, J. Minnis, et al. "American ginseng inhibits induced COX-2 and NFKB activation in breast cancer cells." *Journal of Surgical Research* Vol. 157. (Dec 2009): 261–267.

Pokharel, Y., N. Kim, H. Han, et al. "Increased ubiquitination of multidrug resistance 1 by ginsenoside Rd." *Nutrition and Cancer* Vol. 62. (Jan 2010): 252–259.

Wang, C., H. Aung, B. Zhang, et al. "Chemopreventive effects of heat-processed Panax quinquefolius root on human breast cancer cells." *Anticancer Research* Vol. 28. (Oct 2008): 2545–2551.

Wang, W., X. Zhang, J. Qin, et al. "Natural product ginsenoside 25-OCH3-PPD inhibits breast cancer growth and metastasis through down-regulating MDM2." *PloS One* Vol. 7. (July 2012): e41586.

Yim, H.W., Jong, H.S., Kim, T.Y., et al. "Cyclooxygenase-2 inhibits novel ginseng *metabolite-mediated apoptosis.*" *Cancer* Research Vol. 65. (March 2005): 1952–1960.

Coffee

Anderson, L.F., Jacobs, D.R. Jr., Carlsen, M.H., et al.

"Consumption of coffee is associated with reduced risk of death attributed to inflammatory and cardiovascular disease in the Iowa Women's Study." *American Journal of Clinical Nutrition* Vol. 83. (May 2006): 1039–1046.

Ascherio, A., Chen, H., Schwarzschild, M.A., et al. "Caffeine, postmenopausal estrogen, and risk of Parkinson's disease." *Neurology* Vol. 60. (March 11, 2003): 790–795.

Baker, J.A., Beehler, G.P., Sawant, A.C., et al. "Consumption of coffee, but not black tea, is associated with decreased risk of premenopausal breast cancer." *Journal of Nutrition* Vol. 136. (Jan 2006): 166–171.

Boggs, D., J. Palmer, M. Stampfer, et al. "Tea and coffee intake in relation to risk of breast cancer in the Black Women's Health Study." *Cancer Causes & Control* Vol. 21. (Nov 2010): 1941–1948.

Downey, M. "Discovering coffee's unique health benefits." *Life Extension* (Mar 2012): 39–49.

Freedman, N., J. Everhart, K. Lindsay, et al. "Coffee intake is associated with lower rates of liver disease progression in chronic hepatitis C." *Hepatology* Vol. 50. (Nov 2009): 1360–1369.

Ganmaa, D., W. Willett, T. Li, et al. "Coffee, tea, caffeine and risk of breast cancer: a 22-year follow-up." *International Journal of Cancer* Vol. 122. (May 2008): 2071–2076.

Gierach, G., N. Freedman, A. Andaya, et al. "Coffee intake and breast cancer risk in the NIH-AARP diet and health study cohort." *International Journal of Cancer* Vol. 131. (July 2012): 452–460.

Gronwald, J., Byrski, T., Huzaarski, T., et al. "Influence of selected lifestyle factors on breast and ovarian cancer risk in BRCA1 mutation carriers from Poland." *Breast Cancer Research and Treatment* Vol. 95. (Jan 2006): 105–109.

Hayashi, M., Tsuchiya, H., Tamamotot, N., et al. "Caffeine-potentiated chemotherapy for metastatic carcinoma and lymphoma of bone and soft tissue." *Anticancer Research* Vol. 25. (May-June 2005): 2399–2405.

Higdon, J., B. Frei. "Coffee and health: a review of recent human research." *Critical Reviews in Food Science and Nutrition* Vol. 46. (2006): 101–123.

Hirvonen, T., Mennen, L.I., de Bree, A., et al. "Consumption of antioxidant-rich beverages and risk for breast cancer in French women." *Annals of Epidemiology* Vol. 16. (July 2006): 503–508.

Holick, C., S. Smith, E. Giovannucci, et al. "Coffee, tea, caffeine intake, and risk of adult glioma in three prospective cohort studies." *Cancer Epidemiology Biomarkers & Prevention* Vol. 19. (Jan 2010): 39–47.

Huxley, R., C. Man Ying Lee, F. Barzi, et al. "Coffee, decaffeinated coffee, and tea consumption in relation to incident type 2 diabetes mellitus: a systematic review with meta-analysis." *Archives of Internal Medicine* Vol. 169. (Dec 2009): 2053–2063.

Ishitani, K., J. Lin, J. Manson, et al. "Caffeine consumption and the risk of breast cancer in a large prospective cohort of women." *Archives of Internal Medicine* Vol. 168. (Oct 2008): 2022–2031.

Jacobsen, B., E. Bjelke, G. Kvåle, et al. "Coffee drinking, mortality, and cancer incidence: results from a Norwegian prospective study." *Journal of the National Cancer Institute* Vol. 76. (May 1986): 823–831.

Jiang, W., Y. Wu, X. Jiang. "Coffee and caffeine intake and breast cancer risk: an updated dose-response meta-analysis of 37 published studies." *Gynecologic Oncology* Vol. 129. (June 2013):620–629.11.

Klug, T.L., Bageman, E., Ingvar, C., et al. "Moderate coffee consumption improves the estrogen metabolite profile in adjuvant treated breast cancer patients: A pilot study comparing pre- and post-operative levels." *Molecular Genetics and Metabolism* Vol. 89. (Dec 2006): 381–389.

Kotsopoulos, J., A. Eliassen, S. Missmer, et al. "Relationship between caffeine intake and plasma sex hormone concentrations in premenopausal and postmenopausal women." *Cancer* Vol. 115. (Jun 2009): 2765–2774.

Kotsopoulos, J., P. Ghadirian, A. El-Sohemy, et al. "The CYP1A2 genotype modifies the association between coffee consumption and breast cancer risk among BRCA1 mutation carriers." *Cancer Epidemiology Biomarkers & Prevention* Vol. 16. (May 2007): 912–916.

Lee, W.J., Zhu, B.T. "Inhibition of DNA methylation by caffeic acid and chlorogenic acid, two common catechol-containing coffee polyphenols." *Carcinogenesis* Vol. 27. (Feb 2006): 269–277.

Li, J., P. Seibold, J. Chang-Claude, et al. "Coffee consumption modifies risk of estrogen-receptor negative breast cancer." *Breast Cancer Research* Vol. 13. (May 2011): R49.

Li, X., Z. Ren, J. Qin, et al. "Coffee consumption and risk of breast cancer: an up-to-date meta-analysis." *PloS One* Vol. 8. (Jan 2013): e52681.

Lopez-Garcia, E., F. Rodriguez-Artalejo, K. Rexrode, et al. "Coffee consumption and risk of stroke in women." *Circulation* Vol. 119. (Mar 2009): 1116–1123.

Michels, K., L. Holmberg, L. Bergkvist, et al. "Coffee, tea, and caffeine consumption and breast cancer incidence in a cohort of Swedish women." *Annals of Epidemiology* Vol. 12. (Jan 2002): 21–26.

Michels, K., W. Willett, C. Fuchs, et al. "Coffee, tea, and caffeine consumption and incidence of colon and rectal cancer." *Journal of the National Cancer Institute* Vol. 97. (Feb 2005): 282–292.

Modi, A., J. Feld, Y. Park, et al. "Increased caffeine consumption is associated with reduced hepatic fibrosis." *Hepatology* Vol. 51. (Jan 2010): 201–209.

Nagata, C., Kabuto, M., Shimizu, H. "Association of coffee, green tea, and caffeine intakes with serum concentrations of estradiol and sex hormone-binding globulin in premenopausal Japanese women." *Nutrition and Cancer* Vol. 30. (1998): 21–24.

Natarajan, T.G., Ganesan, N., Cater-Nolan, P., et al. "gamma-Radiation-induced chromosomal mutagen sensitivity is associated with breast cancer risk in African-American women: caffeine modulates the outcome of mutagen sensitivity assay." *Cancer, Epidemiology, Biomarkers and Prevention* Vol. 15. (March 2006): 437–442.

Nilsson, L., I. Johansson, P. Lenner et al. "Consumption of filtered and boiled coffee and the risk of incident cancer: a prospective cohort study." *Cancer Causes & Control* Vol. 21. (Oct 2010): 1533–1544.

Nkondjock, A., Ghadirian, P., Kotsopoulos, J., et al. "Coffee consumption and breast cancer risk among BRCA1 and BRCA2 mutation carriers." *International Journal of Cancer* Vol. 118. (April 2006): 103–107.

Oleaga, C., V. Noé, M. Izquierdo-Pulido. "Coffee polyphenols change the expression of STAT5b and ATF-2 modifying cyclin D1 levels in cancer cells." *Oxidative Medicine and Cellular Longevity* 2012 (May 2012): 390385.

Pereia, M.A., Parker, E.D., Folsom, A.R. "Coffee consumption and risk of type 2 diabetes mellitus: an 11-year prospective study of 28,812 postmenopausal women." *Archives of Internal Medicine* Vol. 166. (June 2006): 1311–1316.

Sääksjärvi, K., P. Knekt, H. Rissanen, et al. "Prospective study of coffee consumption and risk of Parkinson's disease." *European Journal of Clinical Nutrition* Vol. 62. (Jul 2008): 908–915.

Simonsson, M., V. Söderlind, M. Henningson, et al. "Coffee prevents early events in tamoxifen-treated breast cancer patients and modulates hormone receptor status." *Cancer Causes & Control* Vol. 24.(May 2013): 929–940.

Tavani, A., A. Pregnolato, C. La Vecchia, et al. "Coffee consumption and the risk of breast cancer." *European Journal of Cancer Prevention* Vol. 7. (Feb 1998): 77–82.

Tavani, A., C. La Vecchia. "Coffee, decaffeinated coffee, tea and cancer of the colon and rectum: a review of epidemiological studies, 1990-2003." *Cancer Causes & Control* Vol. 15. (Oct 2004): 743–757.

Van Dam, R., F. Hu. "Coffee consumption and risk of type 2 diabetes : a systematic review." *JAMA: the Journal of the American Medical Association* Vol. 294. (July 2005): 97–104.

Yu, X., Z. Bao, J. Zou, et al. "Coffee consumption and risk of cancers: a meta-analysis of cohort studies." *BMC Cancer* Vol. 11. (Mar 2011): 96.

Chapter 12: Mighty Micronutrients

Folate

Branda, R.F., J.P. O'Neill, D. Jacobson-Kram. "Factors influencing mutation at the hprt locus in T-lymphocytes: studies in normal women and women with benign and malignant breast masses." *Environmental and Molecular Mutagenesis* Vol. 19. (Issue 4, 1992): 274–281.

Castillo-L., C., J.A. Tur, R. Uauy. "Folate and breast cancer risk: a systemic review." *Revista médica de Chile* Vol. 140. (Feb 2012):251-60

Chou, Y.C., Wu, M.H., Yu, J.C., et al. "Genetic polymorphisms of the methylenetetrahydrofolate reductase gene, plasma folate levels and breast cancer susceptibility: a case-control study in Taiwan." *Carcinogenesis* Vol. 27. (Nov 2006): 2295–2300.

Harris, H. R., L. Bergkvist, A. Wolk. "Folate intake and breast cancer mortality in a cohort of Swedish women." *Breast Cancer Research and Treatment* Vol. 132(1). (Feb 2012): 243–250.

Kim, Y.I. "Does a high folate intake increase the risk of breast cancer?" *Nutrition Reviews* Vol. 64. (Oct 2006); 468–475.

Kotsopoulos, J., Y. I. Kim, S. A. Narod. "Folate and breast cancer: what about high-risk women?" *Cancer Causes & Control* Vol. 23(9). (Sept 2012): 1405–1420.

Lajous, M., Lazcano-Ponce, E., Hernandez-Avila, M., et al. "Folate, vitamin B(6), and vitamin B(12) intake and the risk of breast cancer among Mexican women." *Cancer, Epidemiology, Biomarkers and Prevention* Vol. 15. (March 2006): 443–448.

Larsson, S.C., Giovannucci, E., Wolk, A. "Folate and risk of breast cancer: a meta-analysis." *Journal of the National Cancer Institute* Vol. 99. (Jan 2007): 64–76.

Laux, M. "Breast Cancer and Nutritional Supplements." www.ATDonline.org

Lee, Y., S. A. Lee, J. Y. Choi, et al. "Prognosis of breast cancer is associated with one-carbon metabolism related nutrients among Korean women." *Nutrition Journal* Vol. 11. (Aug 2012): 59.

Lewis, S.J., Harbord, R.M., Harris, R., et al. "Meta-analyses of observational and genetic association studies of folate intakes or levels and breast cancer risk." *Journal of the National Cancer Institute* Vol. 98. (Nov 15, 2006): 1607–1622.

Lubecka-Pietruszewska, L., A. Kaufman-Szymczyk, B. Stefanska, et al. "Folic acid enforces DNA methylation-mediated transcriptional silencing of PTEN, APC and RARbeta2 tumour suppressor genes in breast cancer." Biochemical and *Biophysical Research Communications* Vol. 430(2). (Jan 2013): 623–628.

Mohammad, N.S., R. Yedluri, P. Addepalli, et al. "Aberrations in one-carbon metabolism induce oxidative DNA damage in sporadic breast cancer." *Molecular and Cellular Biochemistry* Vol. 349(1-2). (Mar 2011): 159–167.

Naushad, S.M., A. Pavani, Y. Rupasree, et al. "Association of aberrations in one-carbon metabolism with molecular phenotype and grade of breast caner." *Molecular Carcinogenesis* Vol. 51. (Oct 2012): E32–41.

Sellars, T.A., Kushi, L.H., Cerhan, J.R., et al. "Dietary folate intake, alcohol, and risk of breast cancer in a prospective study of postmenopausal women." *Epidemiology* Vol. 12. (July 2001): 420–428.

Shrubsole, M.J., F. Jin, Q. Dai, et al. "Dietary folate intake and breast cancer risk: results from the Shanghi Breast Cancer Study." *Cancer Research* Vol. 61. (2001): 7136–7141.

Stolzenberg-Solomon, R.Z., Chang, S.C., Leitzmann, M.F., et al. "Folate intake, alcohol use, and postmenopausal breast cancer risk in the Prostate, Lung, Colorectal, and Ovarian Cancer Screening Trial." *American Journal of Clinical Nutrition* Vol. 83. (April 2006): 895–904.

Tavani, A., S. Malerba, C. Pelucchi, et al. "Dietary folates and cancer risk in a network of case-control studies." *Annals of Oncology: Official Journal of the European Society for Medical Oncology* Vol. 23(10). (Oct 2012). 2737–2742.

Zhang, S., D.J. Hunter, and S.E. Hankinson. "A prospective study of folate intake and the risk of breast cancer." *Journal of the American Medical Association* (*JAMA*) Vol. 281. (May 5, 1999):

1632–1637.

Zhang, S.M., W.C. Willett, J. Selhub, et al. "Plasma folate, vitamin B$_6$, vitamin B$_{12}$, homocysteine, and the risk of breast cancer." *Journal of the National Cancer Institute* Vol. 95. (Mar 5, 2003): 373–380.

Zhang, C.X., S.C. Ho, Y.M. Chen, et al. "Dietary folate, vitamin B6, vitamin B12 and methionine intake and the risk of breast cancer by oestragen and progesterone receptor status." *The British Journal of Nutrition* Vol. 106(6). (Sept 2011): 936–943.

Vitamin B$_{12}$

Choi, S.W. "Vitamin B$_{12}$ deficiency: a new risk factor for breast cancer?" *Nutrition Reviews* Vol. 57. (1999): 250–253.

Zhang, S.M., W.C. Willett, J. Selhub, et al. "Plasma folate, vitamin B$_6$, vitamin B$_{12}$, homocysteine, and the risk of breast cancer." *Journal of the National Cancer Institute* Vol. 95. (Mar 5, 2003): 373–380.

Vitamin D

Abbas, S., J. Linseisen, T. Slanger, et al. "Serum 25-hydroxyvitamin D and risk of post-menopausal breast cancer—results of a large case-control study." *Carcinogenesis* Vol. 29(1). (Jan 2008): 93–99

Bertone-Johnson, E. R. "Vitamin D and breast cancer." *Annals of Epidemiology* Vol. 19(7). (Jul 2009): 462–467.

Bortman, P., M.A. Folgueira, M.L. Katayama, et al. "Antiproliferative effects of 1,25-dihydrocyvitamin D$_3$ on breast cells: a mini review." *Brazil Journal of Medical & Biological Research* Vol. 35. (Jan 2002): 1–9.

Chen, P., M. Li, X. Gu. "Higher blood 25(OH)D level may reduce the breast cancer risk: evidence from a Chinese population based case-control study and meta-analysis of the observational studies." *PloS One* Vol. 8(1). (2013):e49312.

Ding C., D. Gao, J. Wilding, et al. "Vitamin D signaling in adipose tissue." *British Journal of Nutrition* Vol. 108. (Dec 2012): 1915–1923

Diorio, C., S. Berube, C. Byrne, et al. "Influence of insulin-like growth factors on the strength of the relation of vitamin D and calcium intakes to mammographic breast density." *Cancer Research* Vol. 66. (Jan 1, 2006): 588–597.

Garland, C.F., F.C. Garland, and E.D. Gorham. "Calcium and vitamin D. Their potential roles in colon and breast cancer prevention." *Annals of the N Y Academy of Science* Vol. 889. (1999): 107–119.

Lazzeroni, M., S. Gandini, M. Puntoni, et al. "The

science behind vitamins and natural compounds for breast cancer prevention. Getting the most prevention out of it." *Breast (Edinburgh, Scotland)* Suppl. (2011 Oct):S36–41.

Lipkin, M., and H.L. Newmark. "Vitamin D Calcium and prevention of breast cancer: a review." *Journal of the American College of Nutrition* Vol. 18. (Oct 1999; 5 Suppl): 392S–397S.

Mehta, R.G., E.A. Hussin, R.R. Mehta, et al. "Chemoprevention of mammary carcinogenesis by 1 alpha-hydrocyvitamin D$_5$, a synthetic analog of Vitamin D." *Mutation Research* Vol. 523–524. (Feb-Mar 2003): 253–264.

Shao, T., P. Klein, M. L. Grossbard. "Vitamin D and breast cancer." *The Oncologist* Vol. 17(1). (Jan 2012):36–45.

Shin, M.H., M.D. Holmes, S.E. Hankinson, et al. "Intake of dairy products, calcium, and vitamin D and risk of breast cancer." *Journal of the National Cancer Institute* Vol. 94. (Sept 4, 2002): 1301–1311.

Schöttker, B., U. Haug, L. Schomburg, et al. "Strong associations of 25-hydroxyvitamin D concentrations with all-cause, cardiovascular, cancer, and respiratory disease mortality in a large cohort study." *American Journal of Clinical Nutrition* Vol. 97 (April 2013): 782–793.

Standahl, O., C. Rylander, M. Brustad, et al. "Plasma 25 hydroxyvitamin D level and blood gene expression profiles: a cross-sectional study of Norwegian Women and Cancer Post-genome Cohort." *European Journal of Clinical Nutrition* (March 2013) DOI: 10.1038/ejcn.2013.53

van der Rhee, H., J.W. Coebergh, E. de Vries. "Is prevention of cancer by sun exposure more than just the effect of vitamin D? A systematic review of epidemiological studies." *European Journal of Cancer* Vol. 49(6). (Apr 2013):1422–1436.

van der Rhee, H., J.W. Coebergh, E. de Vries. "Sunlight, vitamin D and the prevention of cancer: a systematic review of epidemiological studies." *European Journal of Cancer Prevention: the Official Journal of the European Cancer Prevention Organization* Vol. 18(6). (Nov 2009): 458–475.

Welsh, J., J. A. Wietzke, G. M. Zinser. "Vitamin D-3 receptor as a target for breast cancer prevention." *The Journal of Nutrition* Suppl 7. (Jul 2003): 2425S–2433S.

Yin, L., N. Grandi, E. Raum. "Meta-analysis: serum vitamin D and breast cancer risk." *European Journal of Cancer* Vol. 46(12). (Aug 2010): 2196–2205.

Vitamin E

Ambrosone, C.B., J.R. Marshall, J.E. Vena, et al. "Interaction of family history of breast cancer and dietary antioxidants with breast cancer risk." *Cancer Causes and Control* Vol. 6. (Sept 1995): 407–415.

Chamras, H., Barsky, S.H., Ardashian, A., et al. "Novel interaction of vitamin E and estrogen in breast cancer." *Nutrition and Cancer* Vol. 52. (2005): 43–48.

Dabrosin, C., and K. Ollinger. "Protection by alpha-tocopherol but not ascorbic acid from hydrogen peroxide induced cell death in normal human breast epithelial cells in culture." *Free Radical Research* Vol. 29. (Sept 1998): 227–234.

Ju, J., S.C. Picinich, Z. Yang, et al. "Cancer-preventive activities of tocopherols and tocotrienols." *Carcinogenesis* Vol. 31(4). (Apr 2010): 533–542.

Kline, K., W. Yu, B.G. Sanders. "Vitamin E and breast caner." *The Journal of Nutrition* Suppl. 12. (Dec 2004):3458S–3462S.

Malfa, M.P., and L.T. Neitzel. "Vitamin E succinate promotes breast cancer tumor dormancy." *Journal of Surgical Research* Vol. 93. (Sept 2000): 163–170.

Schwenke, D.C. "Does lack of tocopherols and tocotrienols put women at increased risk of breast cancer?" *Journal of Nutrition & Biochemistry* Vol. 13. (Jan 2002): 2–10.

Smolarek, A.K., N. Suh. "Chemopreventive activity of vitamin E in breast cancer: a focus on γ tocopherol." *Nutrients* Vol. 3(11). (Nov 2011): 962–986.

Smolarek, A.K., J.Y. So, B. Burgess, et al. "Dietary administration of - and -tocopherol inhibits tumourigenesis in the animal model of estrogen receptor-positive, but not HER-2 breast cancer." *Cancer Prevention Research* Vol. 5(11). (Nov 2012): 1310–1320.

Viola, V., S. Ciffolilli, S. Legnaioli, et al. "Mitochondrial-dependent anticancer activity of -tocotrienol and its synthetic derivatives in HER-2/neu overexpressing breast adenocarcinoma cells." *BioFactors* (Jan 2013):

Wada, S. "Cancer preventive effects of vitamin E." *Current Pharmaceutical Biotechnology* Vol. 13(1). (Jan 2012):156–164.

Yu, W., M. Simmons-Menchaca, A. Gapor, et al. "Induction of apoptosis in human breast cancer cells by tocopherols and tocotrienols." *Nutrition & Cancer* Vol. 33. (Issue 1, 1999): 26–32.

Vitamin A

Andrade, F.O., M.K. Nagamine, A.D. Conti. "Efficacy of the dietary histone deacetylase inhibitor butyrate alone or in combination with vitamin A against proliferation of MCF-7 human breast cancer cells." *Brazilian Journal of Medical and Biological Research* Vol. 45(9). (Sept 2012):841–850.

Chen, Q., A.C. Ross. "All-trans-retinoic acid and the glycolipid -galactosylceramide combined reduce breast tumor growth and lung metastasis in a 4T1 murine breast tumor model." *Nutrition and Cancer* Vol. 64(8). (2012):1219–1227.

Ciolino, H.P., Z. Dai, V. Nair. "Retinol inhibits aromatase activity and expression in vitro." *The Journal of Nutritional Biochemistry* Vol. 22(6). (June 2011): 522–526.

Crowe, D.L., R.A. Chandraratna. "A retinoid X receptor (RXR)-selective retinoid reveals that RXR-alpha is potentially a therapeutic target in breast cancer cell lines, and that it potentiates antiproliferative and apoptotic responses to peroxisome proliferator-activated receptor ligands." *Breast Cancer Research* Vol. 6(5). (2004): R546–555.

Fitzgerald, P., M. Teng, R. A. Chandraratna, et al. "Retinoic acid receptor alpha expression correlates with retinoid-induced growth inhibition of human breast cancer cells regardless of estrogen receptor status." *Cancer Research* Vol. 57(13). (1997): 2642–2650.

Formelli, F., E. Meneghini, E. Cavadini, et al. "Plasma retinol and prognosis of postmenopausal breast cancer patients." *Cancer Epidemiology, Biomarkers & Prevention* Vol. 18(1). (Jan 2009): 42–48.

Fulan, H., J. Changxing, W. Y. Baina, et al. "Retinol, vitamins A, C, and E and breast cancer risk: a meta-analysis and meta-regression." *Cancer Causes & Control* Vol. 22(10). (Oct 2011): 1383–1396.

Ginstier, C., J. Wicinski, N. Cervera, et al. "Retinoid signaling regulates breast cancer stem cell differentiation." *Cell Cycle* Vol. 8(20). (Oct 2009): 3297–3302.

Hua, S., R. Kittler, K. P. White. "Genomic antagonism between retinoic acid and estrogen signaling in breast cancer." *Cell* Vol. 137(7). (Jun 2009): 1259–1271.

Kabat, G. C., M. Kim, L. L. Adams-Campbell, et al. "Longitudinal study of serum carotenoid, retinol, and tocopherol concentrations in relation to breast cancer risk among postmenopausal women." *The American Journal of Clinical Nutrition* Vol. 90(1). (Jul 2009): 162–169.

Koay D. C., C. Zerillo, M. Narayan, et al. "Anti-tumor effects of retinoids combined with trastuzumab or tamoxifen in breast cancer cells: induction of apoptosis by retinoid/trastuzumab combinations." *Breast Cancer Research* Vol. 12(4). (2010):R62.

Li, R. J., X. Ying, Y. Zhang, et al. "All-trans retinoic acid stealth liposomes prevent the relapse of breast cancer arising from the cancer stem cells." *Journal of Controlled Release: Official Journal of the Controlled Release Society* Vol. 149(3). (Feb 2011):281–291.

Margheri, M., N. Pacini, A. Tani, et al. "Combined effects of melatonin and all-trans retinoic acid and somatostatin on breast cancer cell proliferation and death: molecular basis for the anticancer effect of these molecules." *European Journal of Pharmacology* Vol. 681(1–3). (Apr 2012): 34–43.

Phipps, S.M., W.K. Love, T. White, et al. "Retinoid-induced histone deacetylation inhibits telomerase activity in estrogen receptor-negative breast cancer cells." *Anticancer Research* Vol. 29(12). (Dec 2009): 4959–4964.

Stefanska, B., K. Rudnicka, A. Bednarek, et al. "Hypomethylation and induction of retinoic acid receptor beta 2 by concurrent action of adenosine analogues and natural compounds in breast cancer cells." *European Journal of Pharmacology* Vol. 638(1-3). (Jul 2010):47–53.

Stefanska, B., P. Salame, A. Bednarek. "Comparative effects of retinoic acid, vitamin D and resveratrol alone and in combination with adenosine analogues on methylation and expression of phosphatase and tensin homologue tumour suppressor gene in breast cancer cells." *The British Journal of Nutrition* Vol. 107(6). (Mar 2012):781–790.

Stoll, B. A. "Linkage between retinoid and fatty acid receptors: implications for breast cancer prevention." *European Journal of Cancer Prevention* Vol. 11(4). (Aug 2002):319–325.

Tang, X.H., and L.J. Gudas. "Retinoids, retinoic acid receptors, and cancer." *Annual Review of Pathology* Vol. 6. (2011):345–364.

Methylation

Craig, S.A. "Betamine in human nutrition 1'2." *American Society for Clinical Nutrition* Vol. 80(3). (Sept 2004): 539–549.

Ferguson, L.R., A.L. Tatham, Z. Lin, et al. "Epigenetic regulation of gene expression as an anticancer drug target." *Current Cancer Drug Targets* Vol. 11(2). (Feb 2011):199–212.

Khan, S.I., P. Aumsuwan, I.A. Khan, et al. "Epigenetic events associated with breast cancer and their prevention by dietary components targeting the epigenome." *Chemical Research in Toxicology* Vol. 25(1). (Jan 2012):61–73.

LeBeau, C., M. Konlee. "Beets and other methyl donors inhibit interleukin-6. Beets used to treat cancer, MS, nerve damage. Methyl donors used for HIV, chronic fatigue, joint pain, candidiasis, cancer, and heart disease." *Journal of Immunity* Vol. 3(2). (Apr 2005)

Li, Y., T. O. Tolledsbol. "Impact on DNA methylation in cancer prevention and therapy by bioactive dietary components." *Current Medicinal Chemistry* Vol. 17(20). (2010): 2141–2151.

Ong, T.P., F.S. Moreno, S.A. Ross. "Targeting the epigenome with bioactive food components for cancer prevention." *Journal of Nutrigenetics and Nutrigenomics* Vol. 4(5). (2011): 275–292.

Stefanska, B., H. Karlic, F. Varga, et al. "Epigenetic mechanisms in anti-cancer actions of bioactive food components—the implications in cancer prevention." *British Journal of Pharmacology* Vol. 167(2). (Sept 2012): 279–297.

Vo, A.T., R.M. Millis. "Epigenetics and breast cancer." *Obstetrics and Gynecology Int'l* (2012).

Chapter 13: Defense Shields

Austin, S. "Antioxidants and chemotherapy-a rebuttal." *Healthnotes Review of Complementary & Integrative Medicine (HNR)* Vol. 6. (Issue 4, 1999): 234– 236.

Ching, S., D. Ingram, R. Hahnel, et al. "Serum levels of micronutrients, antioxidants and total antioxidant status predict risk of breast cancer in a case control study." *Journal of Nutrition* Vol. 132. (Feb 2002): 303–306.

Lamson, D.W., and M. Brignall. "Antioxidants in cancer therapy; their actions and interactions with oncologic therapies." *Alternative Medicine Review* Vol. 4. (Issue 5, 1999): 304–329.

Prasad, K.N., A. Kumar, V. Kochupillai, et al. "High dose of multiple antioxidant vitamins: essential ingredient in improving the efficacy of standard cancer therapy." *Journal of the American College of Nutrition* Vol. 18. (Issue 1, 1999): 13–25.

Simon, M.S., Z. Djuric, B. Dunn, et al. "An evaluation of plasma antioxidant levels and the risk of breast cancer: a pilot case control study." *Breast Journal* Vol. 6. (Nov 2000): 388–395.

Selenium

Cann, S.A., J.P. van Netten, and C. van Netten. "Hypothesis: iodine, selenium and the development of breast cancer." *Cancer Causes and Control* Vol. 11. (Feb 2000): 121–127.

Clark, L.C., G.F. Combs, B.W. Turnball, et al. "Effects of selenium supplementation for cancer prevention in patients with carcinoma of the skin. A randomized controlled trial. Nutritional Prevention of Cancer Study Group." *Journal of the American Medical Association (JAMA)* Vol. 276. (Dec 25, 1997): 1957–1963.

Dong, Y., D. Lisk, E. Block, et al. "Characterization of the biological activity of gamma-glutamyl-Se-methylselesnocysteine: a novel, naturally occurring anticancer agent from garlic." *Cancer Research* Vol. 61. (Apr 1, 2001): 2923–2928.

Dziaman, T., T. Huzarski, D. Gackowski. "Selenium supplementation reduced oxidative damage in adnexectomized BRCA1 mutation carriers. Cancer Epidemiology, Biomarkers and Prevention Vol. 18. (Nov 2009): 2923–2928.

Gao, R., L. Zhao, X. Liu. "Methylseleninic acid is a novel suppressor of aromatase expression." *The Journal of Endocrinology* Vol. 212(2). (Feb 2012):199–205.

Hamdy, S.M., A.K. Latif, E.A. Drees. "Prevention of rat breast cancer by genistin and selenium." *Toxicology and Industrial Health* Vol. 28(8). (Sept 2012):746–757.

He, N., X. Shi, Y. Zhao, et al. "Inhibitory effects and molecular mechanisms of selenium-containing tea polysaccharides on human breast cancer mcf-7 cells." *Journal of Agricultural and Food Chemistry* Vol. 61(3). (Jan 2013):579–588.

Harris, H. R., L. Bergkvist, A. Wolk. "Selenium intake and breast cancer mortality in a cohort of Swedish." *Breast Cancer Research and Treatment* Vol. 134(3). (Aug 2012):1269–1277.

Horner, C., M.D. "Trace minerals: selenium." Channelcincinati.com. (Feb 23, 2002).

Ip, C., M. Birringer, E. Block, et al. "Chemical speciation influences comparative activity of selenium-enriched garlic and yeast in mammary cancer prevention." *Journal of Agricultural and Food Chemistry* Vol. 48 (Jun 2000): 2062–2070.

Ip, C., D.J. Lisk, and H.J. Thompson. "Selenium-enriched garlic inhibits the early stage but not the late stage of mammary carcinogenesis." *Carcinogenesis* Vol. 17. (Sept 1996): 1979–1982.

Jiang, C., W. Jiang, C. Ip, et al. "Selenium-induced inhibition of angiogenesis in mammary cancer at chemopreventative levels of uptake." *Molecular Carcinogenesis* Vol. 26. (Dec 1999): 213–225.

Okuno, T., K. Miura, F. Sakazaki, et al. "Methylseleninic acid (MSA) inhibits 17 -estradiol-induced cell growth in breast cancer T47D cells via enhancement of the antioxidative thioredoxin/thioredoxin reductase system." *Biomedical Research* Vol. 33(4). (2012): 201–210.

Sinha, R., E. Unni, H.E. Ganther, et al. "Methylseleninic acid, a potent growth inhibitor of synchronized mouse mammary epithelial tumor cells in vitro." *Biochemical Pharmacology* Vol. 61. (Feb 1, 2001): 311–317.

Susana, S., B.G. Cham, G. Ahmad Rohi, et al. "Relationship between selenium and breast cancer: a case-control study in the Klang Valley." *Singapore Medical Journal* Vol. 50(3). (2009): 265–269.

Vadgama, J.V., Y. Wu, D. Shen, et al. "Effect of selenium in combination with Adriamycin and Taxol on several different cancer cells." *Anticancer Research* Vol. 20. (May-Jun 2000): 1391–1414.

Vadgama, J.V., Y. Wu, S. Hsia, et al. "Anti-neoplastic properties of selenium in various cancers." *Proceedings of the American Association of Cancer Research.* (Mar 1999): 40.

Yazdi, M.H., M. Mahdavi, E. Kheradmand, et al. "The preventive oral supplementation of a selenium nanoparticle-enriched probiotic increases the immune response and lifespan of 4T1 breast cancer bearing mice." *Arzneimittel-Forschung* Vol. 62(11). (Nov 2012): 525–531.

CoQ$_{10}$

Bahar, M., S. Khaghani, P. Pasalar, et al. "Exogenous coenzyme Q$_{10}$ modulates MMP-2 activity in MCF-7 cell line as a breast cancer cellular model." *Nutrition Journal* Vol. 9. (Nov 2010): 62.

Chai, W., R. V. Cooney, A. A. Franke, et al. "Plasma coenzyme Q10 levels and postmenopausal breast cancer risk the multiethnic cohort study." *Cancer Epidemiology, Biomarkers & Prevention* Vol. 19(9). (Sept 2010): 2351–2356.

Cooney, R. V., Q. Dai, Y. T. Gao, et al. "Low plasma coenzyme Q(10) levels and breast cancer risk in Chinese women." *Cancer Epidemiology, Biomarkers & Prevention* Vol. 20(6). (Jun 2011): 1124–1130.

Greenlee, H., J. Shaw, Y. K. Lau, et al. "Lack of effect of coenzyme q10 on doxorubicin xytoxicity in breast cancer cell cultures." *Integrative Cancer Therapies* Vol. 11(3). (Sept 2012): 243–250.

Folkers, K., A. Osterborg, M. Nylander, et al. "Activities of vitamin Q10 in animal models and a serious deficiency in patients with cancer." *Biochemical and Biophysical Research Communications* Vol. 234. (May 19, 1997): 296–299.

Hertz, N., R. E. Lister. "Improved survival in patients with end-stage cancer treated with coenzyme Q(10) and other antioxidants: a pilot study." *The Journal of International Medical Research* Vol. 37(6). (Nov-Dec 2009): 1961–1971.

Horner, C., M.D. "CoQ$_{10}$." Channelcincinnati.com. (Apr 5, 2001).

Lockwood, K., S. Moesgaard, and K. Folkers. "Partial and complete regression of breast cancer in patients in relation to dosage of coenzyme Q$_{10}$." *Biochemical and Biophysical Research Communications* Vol. 199. (Mar 30, 1994): 1504–1508.

Lockwood, K., S. Moesgaard, and K. Folkers. "Apparent partial remission of breast cancer in 'high risk' patients supplemented with nutritional antioxidants, essential fatty acids and coenzyme Q$_{10}$." *Molecular Aspects of Medicine* Vol. 15. (1994; Suppl): S231– S240.

Lockwood, K., S. Moesgaard, T. Yamamoto, et el. "Progress on therapy of breast cancer with vitamin Q$_{10}$ and the regression of metastases." *Biochemical and Biophysical Research Communications* Vol. 212. (Jul 6, 1995): 172–177.

Perumal, S.S., P. Shanthi, P. Sachdanandam. "Combined efficacy of Tamoxifen and coenzyme Q10 on the status of lipid peroxidation and antioxidants in DMBA induced breast cancer." *Molecular and Cellular Biochemistry* Vol. 273. (May 2005): 151–160.

Portakal, O., O. Ozkaya, et al. "Coenzyme Q$_{10}$ concentrations and antioxidant status in tissues of breast cancer patients." *Clinical Biochemistry* Vol. 33. (Issue 4, 2000): 279–284.

Premkumar, V.G., S. Yuvaraj, P. Shanthi, et al. "Coenzyme Q$_{10}$, riboflavin and niacin supplementation on alteration of DNA repair enzyme and DNA methylation in breast cancer patients undergoing tamoxifen therapy." *The British Journal of Nutrition* Vol. 100(6). (Dec 2008): 1179–1182.

Premkumar, V.G., S. Yuvaraj, S. Sathish, et al. "Anti-angiogenic potential of coenzymeQ$_{10}$, riboflavin and niacin in breast cancer patients undergoing tamoxifen therapy." *Vascular Pharmacology* Vol. 48(4-6). (Apr-Jun 2008):191–201.

Sachdanandam, P. "Antiangiogenic and hypolipidemic activity of coenzyme Q$_{10}$ supplementation to breast cancer patients undergoing tamoxifen thera-py." *BioFactors* Vol. 32(1-4). (2008): 151–159.

Amrit Kalash

Dileepan, K.N., S.T. Varghese, et al. "Enhanced lymphoproliferative response, macrophage mediated tumor cell killing and nitric oxide production after ingestion of an Ayurvedic drug." *Biochemistry Archives* Vol. 9. (1993): 365–374.

Dwivedi, C., Agrawal, P., Natarajan, K., et al. "Antioxidant and protective effects of Amrit Nectar tablets on adriamycin- and cisplatin-induced toxicities." *Journal of Alternative and Complementary Medicine* Vol. 11. (Feb 2005): 143–148.

Horner, C., M.D. "Amrit Kalash." *Channelcincinnati.com.* (Mar 24, 2001).

Misra, N.C., H.M. Sharma, A. Chaturvedi, et al. "Antioxidant adjuvant therapy using a natural herbal mixture (MAK) during intensive chemotherapy: reduction in toxicity." *Proceedings of the XVI International Cancer Congress, Italy.* (1994): 3099–3102.

Sharma, H., D. Chandradhar, B. Satter, et al. "Antineoplastic properties of Maharishi Amrit Kalash, an Ayurvedic food supplement against 7,12- dimethylbenz[a]anthracene-induced mammary tumors in a rat." *Journal of Research & Education in Indian Medicine* Vol. 3. (Jul-Sept 1991): 1–8.

Sharma, H., B. Dwivedi, C. Satter, et al. "Antineoplastic properties of Maharishi-4 against DMBA-induced mammary tumors in rats." *Pharmacology, Biochemistry, and Behavior* Vol. 35. (1990): 767–773.

Srivastava, A., V. Samiya, P. Taranikanti, et al. "Maharishi Amrit (MAK) reduces chemotherapy toxicity in breast cancer patients." The *FASEB Journal* Vol. 14. (Issue 4, 2000; Abstract): A720.

Chapter 14: Smothering the Flames

Abou-Issa, H.M., G.A. Alshafie, K. Seibert, et al. "Dose-response effects of the COX-2 inhibitor, celecoxib, on the chemoprevention of mammary carcinogenesis." *Anticancer Research* Vol. 21. (Sept-Oct 2001): 3425–3432.

Badawi, A.F., and M.Z. Badr. "Chemoprevention of breast cancer by targeting cyclooxygenase-2 and peroxisome proliferators-activated receptor-gamma (Review)." *International Journal of Oncology* Vol. 20. (Jun 2002): 1109–1122.

Badawi, A.F., and M.Z. Badr. "Expression of cyclooxygenase-2 and peroxisome proliferator-activated receptor-gamma and levels of prostaglandin

E2 and 15-deoxy-elta 12,14-prostaglandin J2 in human breast cancer and metastasis." *International Journal of Cancer* Vol. 103. (Jan 1, 2003): 84–90.

Bardia, A., J.E. Olson, C.M. Vachon, et al. "Effect of aspirin and other NSAIDs on postmenopausal breast cancer incidence by hormone receptor status: results from a prospective cohort study." *Breast Cancer Research and Treatment* Vol. 126(1). (Feb 2011): 149–155.

Bing, R.J., M. Miyataka, K.A. Rich, et al. "Nitric oxide, prostanoids, Cyclooxygenase, and angiogenesis in colon and breast cancer." *Clinical Cancer Research* Vol. 7. (Nov 2001): 3385–3392.

Bocca, C., F. Bozzo, A. Bassignana, et al. "Antiproliferative effect of COX-2 inhibitor celecoxib on human breast cancer cell lines." Molecular and Cellular Biochemistry Vol. 350(1-2). (Apr 2011):59–70.

Brasky, T.M., M.R. Bonner, K.B. Moysich, et al. "Genetic variants in COX-2, non-steroidal anti-inflammatory drugs, and breast cancer risk : the Western New York Exposures and Breast Cancer (WEB) Study." *Breast Cancer Research and Treatment* Vol. 126(1). (Feb 2011): 157–165.

Costa, C., R. Soares, J.S. Reis-Filho, et al. "Cyclooxygenase 2 expression is associated with angiogenesis and lymph node metastasis in human breast cancer." *Journal of Clinical Pathology* Vol. 55. (Jun 2002): 429–434.

Davies, G., L.A. Martin, N. Sacks, et al. "Cyclooxygenase-2 (COX-2), aromatase and breast cancer: a possible role for COX-2 inhibitors in breast cancer chemoprevention." *Annals of Oncology* Vol 13. (May 2002): 669–678.

Glover, J.A., C.M. Hughes, M.M. Cantwell, et al. "A systematic review to establish the frequency of cyclooxygenase-2 expression in normal breast epithelium, ductal carcinoma in situ, microinvasive carcinoma of the breast and invasive breast cancer." *British Journal of Cancer* Vol. 105(1). (Jun 2011): 13–17.

Harris, R.E., Beebe-Donke, J., Alshafie, G.A. "Reduction in the risk of human breast cancer by selective cyclooxygenase-2 (COX-2) inhibitors." *BMC Cancer* Vol. 6. (Jan 2006):27.

Howe, L.R., and A.J. Dannenberg. "A role for cyclooxygense-2 inhibitors in the prevention and treatments of cancer." *Seminars in Oncology* Vol. 29. (Jun 2002; Suppl 11): 111–119.

Kang, J.H., K.H. Song, K.C. Jeong, et al. "Involvement of Cox-2 in the metastatic potential of chemotherapy-resistant breast cancer cells." *BMC Cancer* Vol. 11. (Aug 2011): 334.

Kryzystyniak, K.L. "Current strategies for anti-cancer chemoprevention and chemoprotection." *Acta poloniae Pharmaceutica* Vol. 59. (Nov-Dec 2002): 473–478.

Kundu, N., M.J. Smyth, L. Samsel, et al. "Cyclooxygenase inhibitors block cell growth, increase ceramind and inhibit cell cycle." *Breast Cancer Research & Treatment* Vol. 76. (Nov 2002): 57–64.

Lee, K. Y., Y. J. Kim, H. Yoo, et al. "Human brain endothelial cell-derived COX-2 facilitates extravasation of breast cancer cells across the blood-brain barrier." *Anticancer Research* Vol. 31(12). (Dec 2011): 4307–4313.

Lu, S., X. Zhang, A.F. Badawi, et al. "Cyclooxygenase-2 inhibitor celecoxib inhibits promotion of mammary tumorigenesis in rats fed a high fat diet rich in n-polyunsaturated fatty acids." *Cancer Letters* Vol. 184. (Oct 8, 2002): 7–12.

Michael, M.S., M.Z. Badr, and A.F. Badawi. "Inhibition of cyclooxygense-2 and activation of peroxisome proliferator-activated receptor-gamma synergistically induces apoptosis and inhibits growth in human breast cancer cells." *International Journal of Molecular Medicine* Vol. 11. (Jun 2003): 733–736.

Miglietta, A., M. Toselli, N. Ravarino, et al. "COX-2 expression in human breast carcinomas: correlation with clinicopathological features and prognostic molecular markers." *Expert Opinion on Therapeutic Targets* Vol. 14(7). (Jul 2010): 655–664.

Nassar, A., A. Radhakrishnan, I.A. Cabrero, et al. "COX-2 expression in invasive breast cancer: correlation with prognostic parameters and outcome." *Applied Immunohistochemistry & Molecular Morphology* Vol. 15(3). (Sept 2007): 255–259.

Singh, B., A. Lucci, et al. "Role of Cyclooxygenase-2 in breast cancer." *Journal of Surgical Research* Vol. 108. (Nov 2002): 173–179.

Singh, B., J.A. Berry, A. Shoher, et al. "COX-2 overexpression increases motility and invasion of breast cancer cells." *International Journal of Oncology* Vol. 26(5). (May 2005): 1393–1399.

Singh, B., K.R. Cook, L. Vincent, et al. "Role of COX-2 in tumorospheres derived from a breast cancer cell line." *The Journal of Surgical Research* Vol. 168(1). (Jun 2011): e39–49.

Spizzo, G., G. Gasti, D. Wolf, et al. "Correlation of COX-2 and Ep-CAM overexpression in human invasive breast cancer and its impact on survival." *The*

British Journal of Cancer Vol. 88. (Feb 24, 2003): 574–578.

Xin, X., M. Majumder, G.V. Girish, et al. "Targeting COX-2 and EP4 to control tumor growth, angiogenesis, lymphangiogenesis and metastasis to the lungs and lymph nodes in a breast cancer model." *Laboratory Investigation* Vol. 92(8). (Aug 2012): 1115–1128.

Zhao, Y.S., S. Zhu, X.W. Li, et al. "Association between NSAIDs use and breast cancer risk : a systematic review and meta-analysis." *Breast Cancer Research and Treatment* Vol. 1117(1). (Sept 2009): 141–150.

Zyflamend

Bemis, D.L., Capodice, J.L., Anastasiadis, A.G., et al. "Zyflamend, a unique herbal preparation with nonselective COX inhibitory activity, induces apoptosis of prostate cancer cells that lack COX-2 expression." *Nutrition and Cancer* Vol. 52. (2005): 202–212.

Bernis, D.L., K.A. Kozakowski, B.C. Anastasiadis, et al. "Zyflamend, an herbal COX-2 inhibitor with *in vitro* anti-prostate cancer activity." Center for Holistic Urology Columbia University. (2003).

Capodice, J.L., P. Gorroochurn, A.S. Cammack, et al. "Zyflamend in men with high-grade prostatic intraepithelial neoplasia: results of a phase I clinical trial." *Journal of the Society for Integrative Oncology* Vol. 7(2). (Spring 2009): 43–51.

Ekmekcioglu, S., C. Chattopadhyay, U. Akar, et al. "Zyflamend mediates therapeutic induction of autophagy to apoptosis in melanoma cells." *Nutrition and Cancer* Vol. 63(6). (2011): 940–949.

Huang, E.C., M.F. McEntee, J. Whelan. "Zyflamend, a combination of herbal extracts, attenuates tumor growth in murine xenograft models of prostate cancer." *Nutrition and Cancer* Vol. 64(5). (2012): 749–760.

Huang, E.C., G. Chen, S.J. Baek, et al. "Zyflamend reduces the expression of androgen receptor in a model of castrate-resistant prostate cancer." *Nutrition and Cancer* Vol. 63(8). (Nov 2011): 1287–1296.

Kim, J.H., B. Parl, S.C. Gupta, et al. "Zyflamend sensitized tumor cells to TRAIL-induced apoptosis through up-regulation of death receptors and down-regulation of survival proteins: role of ROS-dependent CCAAT/enhancer-binding protein-homologous protein pathway." *Antioxidants & Redox Signaling* Vol. 16(5). (Mar 2012): 413–427.

Kunnumakkara, A.B., B. Sung, J. Ravindran, et al. "Zyflamend suppresses growth and sensitizes human pancreatic tumors to gemcitabine in a orthotopic mouse model through modulation of multiple targets." *International Journal of Cancer* Vol. 131(3). (Aug 2012): E292–303.

Rafailove, S., S. Cammack, B.A. Stone, et al. "The role of Zyflamend, an herbal anti-inflammatory, as a potential chemopreventive agent against prostate cancer: a case report." *Integrative Cancer Therapies* Vol. 6(1). (Mar 2007): 74–76.

Sandur, S.K., K.S. Ahn, H. Ichikawa, et al. "Zyflamend, a polyherbal preparation, inhibits invasion, suppresses osteoclastogenesis, and potentiates apoptosis through down-regulation of NF-kappa B activation and NF-kappa B-regulated gene products." *Nutrition and Cancer* Vol. 57(1). (2007): 78–87.

Weil, A. "Breast cancer: beating the odds?" www.DrWeil.com. (2003).

Yan, J., B. Xie, J.L. Capodice, et al. "Zyflamend inhibits the expression and function of androgen receptor and acts synergistically with bicalutimide to inhibit prostate cancer cell growth." *The Prostate* Vol. 72(3). (Feb 2012): 244–252.

Yang, P., C. Cartwright, D. Chan, et al. "Zyflamend-mediated inhibition of human prostate cancer PC3 cell proliferation: effects on 12-LOX and Rb protein phosphorylation." *Cancer Biology & Therapy* Vol. 6(2). (Feb 2007): 228–236.

Barberry

Fukuda, K., Y. Hibiya, M. Mutoh, et al. "Inhibition by berberine of Cyclooxygenase-2 transcriptional activity in human colon cancer cells." *Journal of Ethnopharmacology* Vol. 66. (Aug 1999): 227–233.

Feverfew

Hwang, D., N. Fischer, B. Jang, et al. "Inhibition of the expression of inducible Cyclooxygenase and proinflammatory cytokines by sesquiterpene lactones in macrophages correlates with inhibition of MAP kinase." *Biochemical and Biophysical Research Communications* Vol. 226. (1996; article 1433): 810–818.

Ginger

Liang, Y.C., Y.T. Huang, and S.H. Tsai. "Suppression of inducible cyclooxygenase and inducible nitric oxide synthase by apigenin and related flavonoids in mouse macrophages." *Carcinogenesis* Vol. 20. (Oct 1999): 1945–1952.

Green Tea

Noreen, Y., G. Serrano, P. Perera, et al. "Flavan-3-ols isolated from some medicinal plants inhibiting COX-1 and COX-2 catalyzed by prostaglandin biosynthesis." *Planta Medica* Vol. 64. (Aug 1998): 520–524.

Hops

Yamamoto, K., J. Wang, and S. Yamamoto. "Suppression of cyclooxygenase-2 gene transcription by humulon of beer hop extract studied in reference to glucocorticoid." *FEBS Letters* Vol. 465. (Jan 14, 2000): 103–106.

Huzhang

Subbaramaiah, K., W.J. Chung, P. Michaluart, et al. "Resveratrol inhibits cyclooxygenase-2 transcription and activity in phorbol ester-treated human mammary epithelial cells." *Journal of Biology & Chemistry* Vol. 273. (Aug 21, 1998): 21875–21882.

Holy Basil (Oscimum Sanctum)

Kelm, M.A., M.G. Nair, G.M. Strasburg, et al. "Antioxidant and Cyclooxygenase inhibitory phenolic compounds from Oscimum sanctum." *Phytomedicine* Vol. 7. (Mar 2000): 7–13.

Rosemary

Ringbom, T., L. Segura, Y. Noreen, et al. "Ursolic acid from Plantago major, a selective inhibitor of cyclooxygenase-2 catalyzed prostaglandin biosynthesis." *Journal of Natural Products* Vol. 61. (Oct 1998): 1212–1215.

Scutellariae

Sanchez, T., and J.J. Moreno. "Role of prostaglandin H synthase isoforms in murine ear edema induced by phorbol ester application on skin." *Prostaglandins & Other Lipid Mediators* Vol. 57. (May 1999): 199–231.

Turmeric

Zhang, F., N.K. Altorki, and J.R. Mestre. "Curcumin inhibits cyclooxygenase-2 transcription in bile-acid and phorbol ester-treated human gastrointestinal epithelial cells." *Carcinogenesis* Vol. 20. (Mar 1999): 45–51

Chapter 15: The Perils of Red Meat

Alexander, D., L. Morimoto, P. Mink, et al. "A review and meta-analysis of red and processed meat consumption and breast cancer." *Nutrition Research Reviews* Vol. 23. (Dec 2010): 349–365.

"Artificial hormones in U.S. beef linked to breast, prostate cancer." *NaturalNews.com* (Jul2006). Website: www.newstarget.com/019557.html.

Aune, D., E. De Stefani, A. Ronco, et al. "Meat consumption and cancer risk: a case-control study of Uruguay." *Asian Pacific Journal of Cancer Prevention* Vol. 10. (Jul-Sept 2009): 429–436.

Cho, E., Chen, W.Y., Hunter, D.J., et al. "Red meat intake and risk of breast cancer among premenopausal women." *Archives of Internal Medicine* Vol. 166. (Nov 2006): 2253–2259.

Dai, Q., X.O. Shu, F. Jin, et al. "Consumption of animal foods, cooking methods, and risk of breast cancer." *Cancer Epidemiology, Biomarkers & Prevention* Vol. 11. (Sept 2002): 801–808.

De Stefani, E., A. Ronco, and M. Mendilaharsu. "Meat intake, heterocyclic amines, and the risk of breast cancer: a case-control study in Uruguay." *Cancer Epidemiology, Biomarkers & Prevention* Vol. 6. (Aug 1997): 573–581.

Delfino, R.J., R. Sinha, and C. Smith. "Breast cancer, heterocyclic aromatic amines from meat and N-acetyltransferace 2 genotype." *Carcinogenesis* Vol. 21. (Apr 2000): 607–615.

Ferrucci, L., A. Cross, B. Graubard, et al. "Intake of meat, meat mutagens, and iron and the risk of breast cancer in the Prostate, Lung, Colorectal, and Ovarian Cancer Screening Trial." *British Journal of Cancer* Vol. 101. (Jul 2009): 178–184.

Fu, Z., S. Deming, A. Fair, et al. "Well-done meat intake and meat-derived mutagen exposures in relation to breast cancer risk: the Nashville Breast Health Study." *Breast Cancer Research and Treatment* Vol. 129. (Oct 2011): 919–928.

Genkinger, J., E. Friberg, R. Goldbohm, et al. "Long-term dietary heme iron and red meat intake in relation to endometrial cancer risk." *The American Journal of Clinical Nutrition* Vol. 96. (Oct 2012): 848–854.

Giacosa, A., R. Barale, L. Bavaresco, et al. "Cancer prevention in Europe: the Mediterranean diet as a protective choice." *European Journal of Cancer Prevention* Vol. 22. (Jan 2013): 90–95.

Herman, S., J. Linseisen, J. Chang-Claude, et al. "Nutrition and breast cancer risk by age 50: a population-based case-control study in Germany." *Nutrition & Cancer* Vol. 44. (Issue 1, 2002): 22–34.

Holmes, M.D., G.A. Colditz, D.J. Hunter, et al. "Meat, fish and egg intake and risk of breast cancer." *International Journal of Cancer* Vol. 140. (Mar 20, 2003): 221–227.

Lauber, S., and N. Gooderham. "The cooked meat derived genotoxic carcinogen 2-amino-3-methylimidazo [4,5-b]pyridine has potent hormone-like activity: mechanistic support for a role in breast cancer." *Cancer Research* Vol. 67. (Oct 2007): 9597–9602.

Linos, E., W. Willett, E. Cho, et al. "Adolescent diet in relation to breast cancer risk among premenopausal women." *Cancer Epidemiology, Biomarkers and Prevention* Vol. 19. (Mar 2010): 689–696.

Linos, E., W. Willett, E. Cho, et al. "Red Meat consumption during adolescence among premenopausal women and risk of breast cancer." *Cancer Epidemiology, Biomarkers and Prevention* Vol. 17. (Aug 2008): 2146–2151.

Kruk, J. "Association of lifestyle and other risk factors with breast cancer according to menopausal status: a case-control study in the region of Western Pomerania (Poland)." *Asian Pacific Journal of Cancer Prevention* Vol. 8. (Oct-Dec 2007): 513–524.

Kulp, K., M. Knize, C. Malfatti, et al. "Identification of urine metabolites of 2-amino-1-methyl-6-phenylimidazo[4,5-b]pyridine following consumption of a single cooked chicken meal by humans." *Carcinogenesis* Vol. 21. (Nov 2000): 2065–2072.

Pan A., Q. Sun, A. Bernstein, et al. "Red meat consumption and mortality: results from 2 prospective cohort studies." *Archives of Internal Medicine* Vol. 172. (April 2012): 556–563.

Ronco, R., E. De Stefani, and H. Deneo-Pellegrino. "Risk factors for premenopausal breast cancer: a case-control study in Uruguay." *Asian Pacific Journal of Cancer Prevention* Vol. 13. (2012): 2879–2886.

Shannon, J., L.S. Cook, and J.L. Stanford. "Dietary intake and risk of postmenopausal breast cancer (United States)." *Cancer Causes and Control* Vol. 14. (Feb 2003): 19–27.

Sinha, R. "An epidemiologic approach to studying heterocyclic amines." *Mutation Research* Vol. 506-507. (Sept 30, 2002): 197–204.

Taylor, E., V. Burley, D. Greenwood, et al. "Meat consumption and risk of breast cancer in the U.K. Women's Cohort Study." *British Journal of cancer* Vol. 96. (Apr 2007): 1139–1146.

Taylor, V., M. Misra, and S. Mukherjee. "Is red meat intake a risk factor for breast cancer among premenopausal women?" *Breast Cancer Research and Treatment* Vol. 117. (Sept 2009): 1–8.

Tseng, M., T. Olufade, K. Evers, et al. "Adolescent lifestyle factors and adult breast density in U.S. Chinese immigrant women." *Nutrition and Cancer* Vol. 63. (2011): 342–349.

Zhang, C., S. Ho, Y. Chen, et al. "Meat and egg consumption and risk of breast cancer among Chinese women." *Cancer Causes and Control* Vol. 20. (Dec 2009): 1845–1853.

Zhang, W., and S. Lee. "Well-done meat intake, heterocyclic amine exposure, and cancer risk." *Nutrition and Cancer* Vol. 61. (2009): 437–446.

Zheng, W., A.C. Deitz, D.R. Campbell, et al. "N-acetyltransfrace 1 genetic polymorphism, cigarette smoking, well-done meat intake, and breast cancer risk." *Cancer Epidemiology, Biomarkers & Prevention* Vol. 8. (Mar 1999): 233–239.

Zheng, W., D. Xie, J.R. Cerhan, et al. "Sulfotransferase 1a1 polymorphism, endogenous estrogen exposure, well-done meat intake, and breast cancer risk." *Cancer Epidemiology, Biomarkers & Prevention* Vol. 10. (Feb 2001): 89–94.

Chapter 16: Dangerous Foe in a Sweet Disguise

Dong, J., and L. Qin. "Dietary glycemic index, glycemic load, and risk of breast cancer: meta-analysis of prospective cohort studies." *Breast Cancer Research and Treatment* Vol. 2. (Apr 2011): 287–294.

Esfahani, A., J. Wong, A. Mirrahimi, et al. "The glycemic index: physiology significance." *Journal of American College of Nutrition* (Aug 2009): 439S–445S.

Hamelers, I.H., and P.H. Steenbergh. "Interactions between estrogen and insulin-like growth factor signaling pathways in human breast tumor cells." *Endocrine-Related Cancer* Vol. 10. (Jun 2003): 331–345.

Hu, J., C. La Vecchia, L. Augustin, et al. "Glycemic index, glycemix load and cancer risk." *Annals of Oncology* Vol. 1. (Jan 2013): 245–251.

Lajous, M., M. Boutron-Ruault, A. Fabre, et al. "Carbohydrate intake, glycemic index, glycemic load, and risk of postmenopausal breast cancer in a prospective student of French women." *The American Journal of Clinical Nutriton* Vol. 5. (May 2008): 1384–1391.

Larsson, S., L. Bergkvist, and A. Wolk. "Glycemic load, glycemic index and breast cancer risk in a prospective cohort of Swedish women." *International Journal of Cancer* Vol. 1. (Jul 2009): 153–157.

McCann, S., W. McCann, C. Hong, et al. "Dietary

patterns related to glycemic index and load and risk of premenopausal and postmenopausal breast cancer in the Western New York Exposure and Breast Cancer Study." *The American Journal of Clinical Nutrition* Vol. 2. (Aug 2007): 465–471.

Michels, K.B., C.G. Solomon, F.B. Hu, et al. "Type 2 diabetes and subsequent incidence of breast cancer in Nurses' Health Study." *Diabetes Care* Vol. 26. (Jun 2003): 1752–1758.

Muti, P., T. Quattrin, B.J. Grant, et al. "Fasting glucose is a risk factor for breast cancer: a prospective study." *Cancer Epidemiology, Biomarkers & Prevention* Vol. 11. (Nov 2002): 1361–1368.

Potischman, N., R.J. Coates, C.A. Swanson, et al. "Increased risk of early-stage breast cancer related to consumption of sweet foods among women less than age 45 in the United States." *Cancer Causes and Control* Vol. 13. (Dec 2002): 937–946.

Romieu, I., and M. Lajous. "The role of obesity, physical activity and dietary factors on the risk for breast cancer: Mexican experience." *Salud Publica de Mexico* Vol. 51. (Jan 2009): s172–180.

Romieu, I., P. Ferrari, S. Rinaldi, et al. "Dietary glycemic index and glycemic load and breast cancer risk in European Prospective Investigation into Cancer and Nutrition (EPIC)." *The American Journal of Clinical Nutrition* Vol. 2. (Aug 2012): 345–355.

Sieri, S., V. Pala, F. Brighenti, et al. "Dietary glycemic index, glycemic load, and the risk of breast cancer in an Italian prospective cohort study." *The American Journal of Clinical Nutrition* Vol. 4. (Oct 2007): 1160–1166.

Sieri, S., V. Pala, F. Brighenti, et al. "High glycemic diet and breast cancer occurrence in the Italian EPIC cohort." *Nutrition, Metabolism and Cardiovascular Diseases* (Apr 2012).

Tavani, A., L. Giodano, S. Gallus, et al. "Consumption of sweet foods and breast cancer risk in Italy." *Annals of Oncology* Vol. 2. (Feb 2006): 341–345.

Wed, W., X. Shu, H. Li, et al. "Dietary carbohydrates, fiber, and breast cancer risk in Chinese Women." *The American Journal of Clinical Nutrition* Vol. 1. (Jan 2009): 283–289.

Stevia

Boonkaewwan, C., Toskulkao, C., Vongsakul, M. "Anti-inflammatory and immunomodulatory activities of Stevioside and its metabolite steviol on THP-1 calls." *Journal of Agricultural and Food Chemistry* Vol. 54. (Feb 8, 2006): 785–789.

Cardelo, H.M., M.A. Da Silva, and M.H. Famasio. "Measurement of the relative sweetness of Stevia extract, aspartame and cyclamate/saccharin blend as compared to sucrose at different concentrations." *Plant Foods for Human Nutrition* (*Dordrecht, Netherlands*) Vol. 54. (Issue 2, 1999): 119–130.

Chan, P., B. Tomlinson, Y.J. Chen, et al. "A double-blinded placebo-controlled study of effectiveness and tolerability of oral stevioside in human hypertension." *British Journal of Clinical Pharmacology* Vol. 50. (Sept 2000): 215–220.

Chang, J.C., M.C. Wu, I.M. Liu, et al. "Increase of insulin sensitivity by stevioside in fructose-rich chow fed rats." *Hormone and Metabolic Research* Vol. 37. (Oct 2005): 601–616.

Chen, T.H., Chen, S.C., Chan, P., et al. "Mechanism of the hypoglycemic effect of stevioside, a glycoside of Stevia rebaudiana." *Planta Medica* Vol. 71. (Feb 2005): 108–113.

Cohen, J. "The effects of different storage temperatures on the taste and chemical composition of Diet Coke." (1997). www.suewidemark.freeservers.com/ aspartame-formaldehyde.htm.

Curi, R., M. Alveraz, R.B. Bazotte, et al. "Effects of Stevia rebaudiana on glucose tolerance in normal adult humans." *Brazilian Journal of Medical and Biological Research* Vol. 19. (Issue 6, 1986): 771–774.

Ferri, L.A., Alves-Do-Prado, W., Yamada, S.S., et al. "Investigation of the antihypertensive effect of oral crude stevioside in patients with mild essential hypertension." *Phytotherapy Research* Vol. 20. (Sept 2006): 732–736.

Gregersen, S., Jeppesen, P.B., Holst, J.J., et al. "Antihyperglycemic effects of stevioside in type 2 diabetic subjects." *Metabolism* Vol. 53. (Jan 2004): 73–76.

Horner, C., M.D. "300 times sweeter—a plant from Paraguay." Channelcincinnati.com. (Mar 14, 2002).

Jeppesen, P.B., S. Gregersen, C.R. Poulsen, et al. "Stevioside acts directly on pancreatic beta cells to secrete insulin: actions independent of cyclic adenosine monophosphate and adenosine triphosphate-sensitive K+- channel activity." *Metabolism* Vol. 49. (Feb 2000): 208–214.

Lailerd, N., Saengsirisuwan, V., Sloniger, J.A., et al. "Effects of stevioside on glucose transport activity in insulin-sensitive and insulin resistant rat skeletal muscle." *Metabolism* Vol. 53. (Jan 2004): 101–107.

Lee, C.N., K.L. Wong, J.C. Liu, et al. "Inhibitory effects of steviocide on calcium influx to produce antihypertension." *Planta Medica* Vol. 67. www

.ncbi.nlm.nih.gov/entrez/query.fcgi?cmd=Retrieve &db=journals&list_uids=6480&dopt=full (Dec 2001): 769.

Melis, M.S. "A crude extract of Stevia rebaudiana increases the renal plasma flow of normal and hypertensive rats." *Brazilian Journal of Medical and Biological Research* Vol. 29. (May 1996): 69–75.

Melis, M.S. "Chronic administration of aqueous extract of Stevia rebaudiana in rats: renal effects." *Journal of Ethnopharmacology* Vol. 47. (Jul 28, 1995): 129–134.

Oyama, Y., H. Sakai, T. Arata, et al. "Cytotoxic effect of methanol, formaldehyde, and formate on dissociated rat thrombocytes: a possibility of aspartame toxicity." *Cell Biology & Toxicology* Vol. 18. (Issue 1, 2002): 43–50.

Patel, R.M., Sarma, R., Grimsley, E. "Popular sweetener sucralose as a migraine trigger." *Headache* Vol. 46. (Sept 2006): 1303–1304.

Takahashi, K., M. Matsuda, K. Ohashi, et al. "Analysis of anti-rotavirus activity of extract from Stevia rebaudiana." *Antiviral Research* Vol. 49. (Jan 2001): 15–24.

Tomita, T., N. Sato, T. Arai, et al. "Bacteriocidal activity of a fermented hot-water extract from Stevia rebaudiana Bertoni towards enterohemorrhagic Escherichia coli O157:H7 and other food-borne pathogenic bacteria." *Microbiology & Immunology* Vol. 41. (Issue 12, 1997): 1005–1009.

Trocho, C., R. Pardo, I. Rafecas, et al. "Formaldehyde derived from dietary aspartame binds to tissue components in vivo." *Life Sciences* Vol. 63. (Issue 5, 1998): 337–349.

Xylitol

Isokangas, P., et al. "Xylitol chewing gum in caries prevention. A field study in children." *Journal of the American Dental Association* Vol. 117. (Aug 1988): 315–320.

Peldyak, J., Makinen, K.K. "Xylitol for caries prevention." *Journal of Dental Hygiene* Vol. 76. (Fall 2002): 276–285.

Pierini, C., "Xylitol: A sweet alternative." Vitamin Research Products website: www.vrp.com/library/735742.html.

Soderling, E., Makinen, K.K., Chen, C-Y., Pape, Jr., H.R., Makinen, P-L. "Effect of sorbitol, xylitol and xylitol/sorbitol chewing gums on dental plaque." *Journal of Dental Research* Vol. 67. (Special Issue, Abstract 1988): 1334.

Svanberg, M., Knuuttila, M. "Dietary xylitol prevents ovariectomy-induced changes of bone inorganic fraction in rats." *Bone and Mineral* Vol. 26. (July 1994): 81–88.

Chocolate

Aimoosawi, S., L. Fyfe, C. Ho, et al. "The effect of polyphenol-rich dark chocolate on fasting capillary whole blood glucose, total cholesterol, blood pressure and glucocorticoids in healthy overweight and obese subjects." *British Journal of Nutrition* Vol. 6. (Mar 2010): 842–850.

Carnesecchi, S., Y. Schneider, S. Lazarus, et al. "Flavanols and procyanidins of cocoa and chocolate inhibit growth and polyamine biosynthesis of human colonic cancer cells." *Cancer Letters* Vol. 2. (Jan 2002): 147–55.

Ferrazzano, G., I. Amato, A. Ingenito, et al. "Anticariogenic effects of polyphenols from plant stimulant beverages (cocoa, coffee, tea)." *Fitoterapia* Vol. 5. (Jul 2009): 255–262.

Metformin

Bo, S., A. Benso, M. Durazzo, et al. "Does use of metformin protect against cancer in Type 2 diabete mellitus?" *Journal of Endocrinological Investigation* Vol. 2. (Feb 2012): 231–235.

Bonanni, B., M. Puntoni, M. Cazzanagi, et al. "Dual effect of metformin on breast cancer proliferation in a randomized presurgical trial." *Journal of Clinical Oncology* Vol. 21. (Jul 2012): 2593–2600.

Chlebowski, R., A. McTiernan, J. Wactawski-Wende, et al. "Diabetes, metformin, and breast cancer in postmenopausal women." *Journal of Clinical Oncology* Vol. 23. (Aug 2012): 2844–2852.

Corominas-Faja, B., R. Quirantes-Pine, C. Olivera-Ferraros, et al. "Metabolic fingerprint reveal that metformin impairs one-carbon metabolism in a manner similar to the anti-folate class of chemotherapy drug." *Archive of Aging (Albany NY)* Vol. 7. (Jul 2012): 480–498.

Dowling, R., P. Goodwin, and W. Stambolic. "Understanding the benefit of metformin use in cancer treatment." *BMC Medicine* Vol. 9. (April 2011).

Decensi, A., M. Puntoni, P. Goodwin, et al. "Metformin and cancer risk in diabetic patients: a systematic review and meta-analysis." *Cancer Prevention Research* Vol. 11. (Nov 2011): 1451–1461.

He, X., F. Esteva, G. Hortobagyi, et al. "Metformin and thiazolidinediones are associated with improved breast cancer-specific survival of diabetic women with HER2+ breast cancer." *Annals of Oncology* Vol. 7. (Jul 2012): 1771–1780.

Hirsh, H., D. Iliopoulos, and K. Struhl. "Metformin inhibits the inflammatory response associated with cellular transformation and cancer stem cell growth." *Proceedings of the National Academy of Science of the United States of America* Vol. 3. (Jan 2013): 972–977.

Jung, J., S. Park, S. Lee, et al. "Metformin represses self-renewal of the human breast carcinoma stem cell via inhibition of estrogen receptor-mediated OCT4 expression." *PLoS One* Vol. 11. (2011): e28068.

Koh, M., J. Lee, C. Min, et al. "A novel metformin derivative, HL010183, inhibit proliferation and invasion of triple-negative breast cancer cells." *Bioorganic and Medical Chemistry* Vol. 13.(Feb 2013): s0968–0896.

Niraula, S., R. Dowling, M. Ennis, et al. "Metformin in early breast cancer: a prospective window of opportunity neoadjuvant study." *Breast Cancer Research and Treatment* Vol. 3. (Oct 2012): 821–830.

Noto, H., A. Goto, T. Tsujimoto, et al. "Cancer risk in diabetic patients treated with metformin: a systematic review and meta-analysis." *PLoS One* Vol. 3. (2012): e33411.

Sanchez-Alvarez, R., U. Martinez-Outschoorn, R. Lamb, et al. "Mitochondrial dysfunction in breast cancer cells prevents tumor growth: understanding chemoprevention with metformin." *Cell Cycle* Vol. 1. (Jan 2013): 172–182.

Song, C., H. Lee, R. Dings, et al. "Metformin kills and radiosensitizes cancer cells and preferentially kill cancer stem cells." *Scientific Reports* Vol. 2. (2012).

Chapter 17: Losing Your Goddess-Like Figure

Alokail, M., N. Al-Daghri, A. Abdulkareem, et al. "Metabolic syndrome biomarkers and early breast cancer in Saudi women: evidence for the presence of a systemic stress response and/or a pre-existing metabolic syndrome-related neoplasia risk?" *BMC Cancer* (Feb 2013): 54.

Amadou, A., P. Hainaut, and I. Romieu. "Role of obesity in the risk of breast cancer: lessons from anthropometry." *Journal of Oncology* (Feb 2013): 906495.

Anderson, G., and M. Neuhouser. "Obesity and the risk for premenopausal and postmenopausal breast cancer." *Cancer Prevention Research* Vol. 4. (Apr 2012): 515–521.

Baillie-Hamilton, P. "Chemical toxins: a hypothesis to explain global obesity epidemic." *Journal of Alternative & Complementary Medicine* Vol. 8. (Issue 2, 2002): 185–192.

Brown, K., and E. Simpson. "Obesity and breast cancer: mechanisms and therapeutic implications." *Frontiers in Bioscience (Elite Edition)* (Jun 2012): 2515–2524.

Brown, K., and E. Simpson. "Obesity and breast cancer: progress to understanding the relationship." *Cancer Research* Vol. 1. (Jan 2010): 4–7.

Carpenter, C., K. Duvall, P. Jardack, et al. "Weight loss reduces breast ductal fluid estrogen in obese postmenopausal women: a single arm intervention pilot study." *Nutrition Journal* (Dec 2012): 102.

Crujeiras, A., A. Diaz-Lagares, M. Carreira, et al. "Oxidative stress associated to dysfunctional adipose tissue: a potential link between obesity, type 2 diabetes mellitus and breast cancer." *Free Radical Research* Vol. 4. (Apr 2013): 243–256.

Dal Maso, L., A. Zucchetto, R. Talamini, et al. "Effect of obesity and other lifestyle factors on mortality in women with breast cancer." *International Journal of Cancer* Vol. 9. (Nov 2008): 2188–2194.

Eliassen, A.H., G.A. Colditz, B. Rosner, et al. "Adult weight change and risk of postmenopausal breast cancer." *Journal of the American Medical Association* Vol. 296. (July 12, 2006): 193–201.

Flegal, K., M. Carrol, C. Ogdan, et al. "Prevalence and trends in obesity among U.S. adults, 1999–2000." *Journal of the American Medical Association (JAMA)* Vol. 288. (Oct 9, 2002): 1723–1732.

Franceschi, S., A. Favero, C. La Vecchia, et al. "Body size indices and breast cancer risk before and after menopause." *International Journal of Cancer* Vol. 67. (Jul 1996): 181–186.

Frazier, A.L., C.T. Ryan, H. Rockett, et al. "Adolescent diet and risk of breast cancer." *Cancer Causes and Control* Vol. 15. (Feb 2004): 73–82.

Gastelu, Daniel, and Fred Hatfield, Ph.D. *Dynamic Nutrition for Maximum Performance.* Garden City Park, NY: Avery Publishing Group, 1997.

Ghosh, S., and K. Ashcraft. "An IL-6 link between obesity and cancer." *Frontiers in Bioscience (Elite Edition)* (Jan 2013): 461–478.

Gilbert, C., and J. Slingerland. "Cytokines, obesity, and cancer: new insights on mechanisms linking obesity to cancer risk and progression." *Annual Review of Medicine* (2013): 45–57.

Giles, E., E. Wellberg, D. Astling, et al. "Obesity and overfeeding affecting both tumor and systemic metabolism activates the progesterone receptor to contribute to postmenopausal breast cancer." *Cancer Research* Vol. 24. (Dec 2012): 6490–6501.

Go, A., D. Mozaffarian, V. Roger, et al. "Heart disease and stroke statistics—2013 update: a report from the American Heart Association." *Circulation* (2013): e6–e245.

Grossmann, M., A. Ray, J. Nkhata, et al. "Obesity and breast cancer: status of leptin and adiponectin in pathological processes." *Cancer and Metastasis Reviews* Vol. 4. (Dec 2012): 641–653.

Gu, J., E. Young, S. Patterson, et al. "Postmenopausal obesity promotes tumor angiogenesis and breast cancer progression in mice." *Cancer Biology and Therapy* Vol. 10. (May 2011): 910–917.

Harvie, M., L. Hooper, and A. Howell. "Central obesity and breast cancer risk: a systematic review." *Obesity Reviews* Vol. 3. (Aug 2003): 157–173.

Hauner, H. and D. Hauner. "The Impact of nutrition on the development and prognosis of breast cancer." *Breast Care (Basel)* Vol. 6. (2010): 377–381.

Haus, E., and M. Smolensky. "Shift work and cancer risk: potential mechanistic role of circadian disruption, light at night, and sleep deprivation." *Sleep Medicine Reviews* Vol. 12. (Nov 2012): 00098–6.

Horner, C., M.D. "300 times as sweet as sugar: the shrub from Paraguay." Channelcincinnati. com. (Mar 14, 2002).

Huang, Z., S.E. Hankinson, G.A. Colditz, et al. "Avoiding adult weight gain helps women reduce breast cancer risk." *Journal of the American Medical Association (JAMA)* Vol. 278. (Nov 5, 1997): 1407– 1411.

Jernstrom, H., and E. Barret-Conner. "Obesity, weight change, fasting insulin, proinsulin, C-peptide, and insulin-like growth factor-1 levels in women with and without breast cancer: the Rancho Bernardo Study." *Journal of Women's Health & Gender Based Medicine* Vol. 8. (Dec 1999): 1265–1272.

Lahmann, P.H., L. Lissner, B. Gullberg, et al. "A prospective study of adiposity and postmenopausal breast cancer: the Malmo Diet and Cancer Study." *International Journal of Cancer* Vol. 103. (Jan 10, 2003): 246–252.

Ligibel, J. "Obesity and breast cancer." *Oncology (Williston Park)* Vol. 11. (Oct 2012): 994–1000.

McTiernan, A. "Behavioral risk factors in breast cancer: can risk be modified?" *Oncologist* Vol. 8. (Issue 4, 2003): 326–334.

Macchio, A., C. Madeddu, and G. Mantovani. "Adi-

pose tissue as target organ in the treatment of hormone-dependent breast cancer: new therapeutic perspectives." *Obesity Reviews* Vol. 6. (Nov 2009): 660–670.

Maccio, A., and C. Madeddu. "Obesity, inflammation, and postmenopausal breast cancer: therapeutic implications." *The Scientific World Journal* (2011): 2020–2036.

Mokdad, A., E. Ford, B. Bowman, et al. "Prevalence of obesity, diabetes, and obesity-related risk factors, 2001." *Journal of the American Medical Association (JAMA)* Vol. 289. (Jan 2003): 75–79.

Mokdad, A., E. Ford, B. Bowman, et al. "The continuing epidemic of obesity and diabetes in the United States." *Journal of the American Medical Association (JAMA)* Vol. 286. (Sept 12, 2001): 1195– 1200.

Nogueira, L., J. Lavigne, G. Chandramouli, et al. "Dose-dependent effects of calorie restriction on gene expression, metabolism, and tumor progression are partially mediated by insulin-like growth factor-1." *Cancer Medicine* Vol. 2. (Oct 2012): 275–288.

Palmer, J., L. Adams-Campbell, D. Boggs, et al. "A prospective study of body size and breast cancer in black women." *Cancer Epidemiology, Biomarkers and Prevention* Vol. 9. (Sept 2007): 1795–1802.

Patterson, R., C. Rock, J. Kerr, et al. "Metabolism and breast cancer risk: frontiers in research and practice." *Journal of the Academy of Nutrition and Dietetics* Vol. 2. (Feb 2013): 288–296.

Pierobon, M., and C. Frankenfeld. "Obesity as a risk factor for triple-negative breast cancers: a systematic review and meta-analysis." *Breast Cancer Research and Treatment* Vol. 1. (Jan 2013): 307–314.

Protani, M., M. Coory, and J. Martin. "Effect of obesity on survival of women with breast cancer: systematic review and meta-analysis." *Breast Cancer Research and Treatment* Vol. 3. (Oct 2010): 627–635.

Rock, C., C. Pande, S. Flatt, et al. "Favorable changes in serum estrogens and other biological factors after weight loss in breast cancer survivors who are overweight or obese." *Clinical Breast Cancer* Vol. 12. (Jan 2013): 00295–00299

Rock, C., T. Byers, W. Demark-Wahnefried, et al. "Reducing breast cancer recurrence with weight loss, a vanguard trial: The Exercise and Nutrition to Enhance Recovery and Good Health for You (ENERGY) Trial." *Contemporary Clinical Trials* Vol. 2. (Mar 2013): 282–295.

Rose, D., and L. Vona-Davis. "Interaction between menopausal status and obesity in affecting breast cancer risk." *Maturitas* Vol.1. (May 2010): 33–38.

Sauter, E., S. Scott, J. Hewett, et al. "Biomarkers associated with breast cancer are associated with obesity." *Cancer Detection and Prevention Journal* Vol. 2. (2008): 149–155.

Schernhammer, E., S. Tworoger, A. Eliassen, et al. "Body shape throughout life and correlations with IGFs and GH." *Endocrine-Related Cancer* Vol. 3. (Sept 2007): 721–732.

Steohensin, G.D., and D.P. Rose. "Breast cancer and obesity: an update." *Nutrition & Cancer* Vol. 45. (Issue 1, 2003): 1–16.

Suzuki, R., M. Iwasaki, M. Inoue, et al. "Body weight at age 20 years, subsequent weight change and breast cancer risk defined by estrogen and progesterone receptor status—the Japan public health center-based prospective study." *International Journal of Cancer* Vol. 5. (Sept 2011): 1214–1224.

Trentham-Dietz, A., Newcomb, P., Nichols, H.B., et al. "Breast cancer risk factors and second primary malignancies among women with breast cancer." *Breast Cancer Research and Treatment* (Dec 21, 2006) [Epud ahead of print]

Vrieling, A., K. Buck, R. Kaaks, et al. "Adult weight gain in relation to breast cancer risk by estrogen and progesterone receptor status: a meta-analysis." *Breast Cancer Research and Treatment* Vol. 3. (Oct 2010): 641–649.

Xu, X., A. Dailey, M. Peoples-Sheps, et al. "Birth weight as a risk factor for breast cancer: a meta-analysis of 18 epidemiological studies." *Journal of Women's Health* Vol. 8. (Jan 2009): 1169–1178.

Xue, F., and K. Michels. "Diabetes, metabolic syndrome, and breast cancer: a review of the current evidence." *The American Journal of Clinical Nutrition* Vol. 3. (Sept 2007): s823–835.

Chapter 18: A Drink Not to Drink

Bagnardi, V., M. Rota, E. Botteri, et al. "Light alcohol drinking and cancer." *Annals of Oncology: Official Journal of the European Society for Medical Oncology / ESMO* Vol. 24. (2013): 301–308.

Bissonauth, V., B. Shatenstein, E. Fafard, et al. "Risk of breast cancer among French-Canadian women, noncarriers of more frequent BRCA 1/2 mutations and consumption of total energy, coffee, and alcohol." *The Breast Journal* Vol. 15. (Sept-Oct 2009): 1524–4741.

Breslow, R., C. Chiung, B. Graubard, et al.

"Prospective study of alcohol consumption quantity and frequency and cancer-specific mortality in the U.S. population." *American Journal of Epidemiology* Vol. 179. (Nov 2011): 1044–1053.

Chen, W., B. Rosner, S. Hankinson, et al. "Moderate alcohol consumption during adult life, drinking patterns, and breast cancer risk." *The Journal of the American Medical Association* Vol. 306. (Nov 2011): 1884–1890.

Chen, W.Y., G.A. Colditz, and B. Rosner. "Use of postmenopausal hormones, alcohol, and risk for invasive breast cancer." *Annals of Internal Medicine* Vol. 137. (Nov 19, 2002): 798–804.

Dorgan, J.F., D.J. Baer, and P.S. Albert. "Serum hormones and the alcohol-breast cancer association in postmenopausal women." *Journal of the National Cancer Institute* Vol. 93. (May 2, 2001): 710–715.

Eng, E.T., J. Ye, D. Williams, et al. "Suppression of estrogen biosynthesis by procyanidin dimers in red wine and grape seeds." *Cancer Research* Vol. 63. (Dec 1, 2003): 8516–8522.

Flatt, S., C. Thomson, E. Gold, et al. "Low to moderate alcohol intake is not associated with increased mortality after breast cancer." *Cancer Epidemiology, Biomarkers & Prevention* Vol. 19. (Mar 2010): 681–688.

Friedenreich, C.M., G.R. Howe, A.B. Miller, et al. "A cohort study of alcohol consumption and risk of breast cancer." *American Journal of Epidemiology* Vol. 137. (Mar 1, 1993): 512–520.

Garvin, S., Ollinger, K., Dabrosin, C. "Resveratrol induces apoptosis and inhibits angiogenesis in human breast cancer xenografts in vivo." *Cancer Letters* Vol. 231. (January 8, 2006): 113–122.

Gaspstur, S.M., J.D. Potter, C. Dinkard, et al. "Synergistic effects between alcohol and estrogen replacement therapy on the risk of breast cancer differ by estrogen/progesterone receptor status in the Iowa Women's Health Study." *Cancer Epidemiology, Biomarkers & Prevention* Vol. 4. (Issue 4, 1995): 313–318.

Hamajima, N., K. Hirose, K. Tajima, et al. "Alcohol, tobacco, and breast cancer—collaborative reanalysis of individual data from 53 epidemiological studies including 58,515 women with breast cancer and 95,067 women without the disease." *The British Journal of Cancer* Vol. 87. (Nov 18, 2002): 1234–1245.

Harris, H., L. Bergkvist, A. Wolk. "Alcohol intake and mortality among women with invasive breast cancer." *British Journal of Cancer* Vol. 106. (Jan

2012): 592–595.

Jain, M.G., R.G. Ferrace, J.T. Rehm, et al. "Alcohol and breast cancer mortality in a cohort study." *Breast Cancer Research & Treatment* Vol. 64. (Nov 2001): 201–209.

Kotha, A., Sekharam, M., Cilenti, L., et al. "Resveratrol inhibits Src and Stat3 signaling and induces the apoptosis of malignant cells containing activated Stat3 protein." *Molecular Cancer Therapeutics* Vol. 5. (March 2006): 621–629.

Lew, J., N. Freedman, M. Leitzmann, et al. "Alcohol and risk of breast cancer by histologic type and hormone receptor status in postmenopausal women: the NIH-AARP Diet and Health Study." *American Journal of Epidemiology* Vol. 170. (Aug 2009): 308–317.

Li, C., et al. "Alcohol consumption and risk of postmenopausal breast cancer by subtype: the Women's Health Initiative Observational Study." *Journal of the National Cancer Institute* Vol.102. (Sept 2012): 1422–1431.

Li, C., R. Chlebowski, M. Freiberg, et al. "Alcohol consumption and risk of postmenopausal breast cancer by subtype: the women's health initiative observational study." *Journal of the National Cancer Institute* Vol. 102. (Sept 2013): 1422–1431.

Longnecker, M.P. "Alcohol beverage consumption in relation to risk of breast cancer: meta-analysis and review." *Cancer Causes and Control* Vol. 5. (Jan 1994): 73–82.

Muti, P., M. Trevisan, A. Micheli, et al. "Alcohol consumption and total estradiol in premenopausal women." *Cancer Epidemiology, Biomarkers & Prevention* Vol. 7. (Mar 1998): 189–193.

Oyesanmi, O., D. Snyder, N. Sullivan, et al. "Alcohol consumption and cancer risk: understanding possible causal mechanisms for breast and colorectal cancers." *Evidence Report/technology Assessment* Vol. 197. (Nov 2010): 1–151.

Rohan, T.E., M. Jain, G.R. Howe, et al. "Alcohol consumption and risk of breast cancer: a cohort study." *Cancer Causes and Control* Vol. 11. (Mar 2000): 239–247.

Schatzkin, A., and M.P. Longnecker. "Alcohol and breast cancer: Where are we now and where do we go from here?" *Cancer* Vol. 74. (Aug 1, 1994; Suppl 3): 1101–1111.

Sharma, G., A.K. Tyagi, R.P. Singh, et al. "Synergistic anti-cancer effects of grape seed extract and conventional cytotoxic agent doxorubicin against human breast carcinoma cells." *Breast Cancer Research*

& Treatment Vol. 85. (May 2004): 1–12.

Smith-Warner, S.A., D. Spiegelman, S.S. Yaun, et al. "Alcohol and breast cancer in women: a pooled analysis of cohort studies." *Journal of the American Medical Association (JAMA)* Vol. 279. (Feb 18, 1998): 535–540.

Suzuki, R., W. Ye, T. Rylander-Rudqvist, et al. "Alcohol and postmenopausal breast cancer risk defined by estrogen and progesterone receptor status: a prospective cohort study." *Journal of the National Cancer Institute* Vol. 97. (Nov 2005): 1601–1608.

Thomas, D.B. "Alcohol as a cause of cancer." *Environmental Health Perspectives* Vol. 103. (Nov 1995; Suppl 8): 153–160.

Wang, Y., K.W. Lee, F.L. Chan, et al. "The red wine polyphenols resveratrol displays bilevel inhibition on aromatase in breast cancer cells." *Toxicological Sciences* Vol. 92. (July 2006): 71–77.

Wu, A., C. Vigen, P. Razavi, et al. "Alcohol and breast cancer risk among Asian-American women in Los Angeles County." *Breast Cancer Research* Vol. 14. (Nov 2012): 151.

Ye, X., R.L. Krohn, W. Liu, et al. "The cytotoxic effects of a novel IH636 grape seed proanthocyanidin extract on cultured human cancer cells." *Molecular & Cell Biochemistry* Vol. 196. www.ncbi.nlm.nih.gov /entrez/query.fcgi?cmd=Retrieve&db=journals&list_uids=5915&dopt=full (Jun 1999): 99–108.

Resveratrol

Aires, V., E. Limagne, A. Cotte, et al. "Resveratrol metabolites inhibit human metastatic colon cancer cells progression and synergize with chemotherapeutic drugs to induce cell death." *Molecular Nutrition & Food Research* (Mar 2013): doi: 10.1002/mnfr.201200766.

Aravindan, S., M. Natarajan, T. Herman, et al. "Molecular basis of 'hypoxic' breast cancer cell radio-sensitization: phytochemicals converge on radiation induced Rel signaling." *Radiation Oncology Journal* Vol. 8. (Mar 2013): 46.

Brown, V., K. Patel, M. Viskaduraki, et al. "Repeat dose study of the cancer chemopreventive agent resveratrol in healthy volunteers: safety, pharmacokinetics, and effect on the insulin-like growth factor axis." *Cancer Research* Vol. 70. (Nov 2010): 9003–9011.

Ferraz da Costa, D., F. Casanova, J. Quarti, et al. "Transient transfection of a wild-type p53 gene triggers resveratrol-induced apoptosis in cancer cells." *PloS One* Vol. 7. (2012): e48746.

Gescher A., W. Steward. "Relationship between mechanisms, bioavailability, and preclinical chemopreventive efficacy of resveratrol: a conundrum." *Cancer Epidemiology, Biomarkers & Prevention:* Vol.12. (Oct 2003): 953–957.

Gomez, L., P. Zancan, M. Marcondes, et al. "Resveratrol decreases breast cancer cell viability and glucose metabolism by inhibiting 6-phosphofructo-1-kinase." *Biochimie* Vol. S0300–9084. (Feb 2013): 00070–9.

Khan, M., H. Chen, X. Wan, et al. "Regulatory effects of resveratrol on antioxidant enzymes: A mechanism of growth inhibition and apoptosis induction in cancer cells." *Molecules and Cells* Vol. 35. (Mar 2013): 219–225.

Lee H., A. Ha, W. Kim. "Effect of resveratrol on the metastasis of 4T1 breast cancer cells in vitro and in vivo." *Nutrition Research and Practice* Vol. 6. (Aug 2012): 294–300.

Lee, H., P. Zhang, A. Herrmann, et al. "Acetylated STAT3 is crucial for methylation of tumor-suppressor gene promoters and inhibition by resveratrol results in demethylation." *Proceedings of the National Academy of Sciences of the United States of America* Vol. 109. (May 2012): 7765–7769.

Leon-Galicia I., J. Diaz-Chavez, E. Garcia-Villa, et al. "Resveratrol induces downregulation of DNA repair genes in MCF-7 human breast cancer cells." *European Journal of Cancer Prevention* Vol. 22. (Jan 2013): 11–20.

Liu, M., Y. Huang, J. Wang. "Developing phytoestrogen for breast cancer prevention." *Anti-cancer Agents in Medicinal Chemistry* Vol. 12. (Dec 2012): 1306–1313.

Maccario C., M. Savio, D. Ferraro, et al. "The resveratrol analog 4, 4'–dihydroxy-trans-stilbene suppresses transformation in normal mouse fibroblasts and inhibits proliferation and invasion of human breast cancer cells." *Carcinogenesis* Vol. 33. (Nov 2012): 2172–2180.

Pandey P., F. Xing, S. Sharma, et al. "Elevated lipogenesis in epithelial stem-like cell confers survival advantage in ductal carcinoma in situ of breast cancer." *Oncogene* (Dec 2013).

Patel, K., V. Brown, D. Jones, et al. "Clinical pharmacology of resveratrol and its metabolites in colorectal cancer patients." *Cancer Research* Vol. 70. (Oct 2010): 7392–7399.

Osman, A., H. Bayoumi, S. Al-Harthi, et al. "Modulation of doxorubicin cytotoxicity by resveratrol in human breast cancer cell line." *Cancer Cell International* Vol. 12. (Nov 2012): 47.

Scott, E., W. Steward, A. Gescher, et al. "Resveratrol in human cancer chemoprevention—choosing the 'right' dose." *Molecular Nutrition & Food Research* Vol. 56. (Jan 2012): 7–13.

Singh, N., D. Zaidi, H. Shyam, et al. "Polyphenols sensitization potentiates susceptibility of MCF-7 and MDA MB-231 cells to centchroman." *PloS One* Vol. 7. (Jun 2012):e37736.

Wietzke, J., J. Welsh. "Phytoestrogen regulation of a vitamin D3 receptor promoter and 1,25-dihydroxyvitamin D3 actions in human breast cancer cells." *The Journal of Steroid Biochemistry and Molecular Biology* Vol. 84. (Feb 2003): 149–157.

Grapeseed Extract

Chen, C., C. Liu, J. Zhang, et al. "[Grape seed extract inhibit proliferation of breast cancer cell MCF-7 and decrease the gene expression of surviving]." *Zhongguo Zhong Yao Za Zhi* Vol. 34. (Feb 2009): 433–437.

"Grape Seed Extract." www.usana-nutritionals.com/research/USNUSUPPINGREDIE_19499.html

Lu, J., K. Zhang, S. Chen, et al. "Grape seed extract inhibits VEGF expression via reducing HIF-1alpha protein expression." *Carcinogenesis* Vol. 30. (Apr 2009): 636–644.

Song, X., N. Siriwardhana, K. Rathore, et al. "Grape seed proanthocyanidin suppression of breast cell carcinogenesis induced by chronic exposure to combined 4-(methylhitrosamino)-1-(3-pyridyl)-1-butanone and benzo[a]pyrene." *Molecular Carcinogenesis* Vol. 49. (May 2010): 450–463.

Wen, W., J. Lu, K. Zhang, et al. "Grape seed extract inhibits angiogenesis via suppression of the vascular endothelial growth factor receptor signaling pathway." *Cancer Prevention Research (Philadelphia, Pa.)* Vol. 1. (Dec 2008): 554–561.

Chapter 19: Sir Walter Raleigh's Folly

Ahern, T., T. Lash, K. Egan, et al. "Lifetime tobacco smoke exposure and breast cancer incidence." *Cancer Causes & Control* Vol. 20. (Dec 2009):1837–1844.

Ambrosone C., S. Kropp, J. Yang, et al. "Cigarette smoking, N-acetyltransferase 2 genotypes, and breast cancer risk: pooled analysis and meta-analysis." *Cancer Epidemiology, Biomarkers & Prevention* Vol. 17. (Jan 2008):15–26.

Anderson, L., M. Cotterchio, L. Mirea, et al. "Passive cigarette smoke exposure during various periods of life, genetic variants, and breast cancer risk among never smokers." *American Journal of Epidemiology* Vol. 175. (Feb 2012): 289–301.

Band, P.R., N.D. Le, R. Fang, et al. "Carcinogenic and endocrine disrupting effects of cigarette smoke and risk of breast cancer." *The Lancet* Vol. 360. (Oct 5, 2002): 1044–1049.

Baumgartner K., T. Schlierf, D. Yang, et al. "N-acetyltransferase 2 genotype modification of active cigarette smoking on breast cancer risk among Hispanic and non-hispanic white women." *The Journal of Toxicological Sciences* Vol. 112. (Nov 2009): 211–220.

Betts K. "Secondhand suspicions: breast cancer and passive smoking." *Environmental Health Perspectives* Vol. 115. (Mar 2007): A136–A143.

Butler, L., E. Gold, S. Conroy, et al. "Active, but not passive cigarette smoking was inversely associated with mammographic density." *Cancer Causes & Control* Vol. 21. (Feb 2010): 301–311.

CalEPA study www.komen.org

Chang-Claude, J., S. Kropp, B. Jager, et al. "Differential effect of NAT2 on the association between active and passive smoking exposure and breast cancer risk." *Cancer Epidemiology, Biomarkers & Prevention* Vol. 11. (Aug 2002): 698–704.

Conlon, M., K. Johnson, M. Bewick, et al. "Smoking (active and passive), N-acetyltransferase 2, and risk of breast cancer." *Cancer Epidemiology* Vol. 34. (Apr 2010):142–149.

Egan, K.M., P.A. Newcomb, L. Titus-Ernstoff, et al. "Association of NAT2 and smoking in relation to breast cancer incidence in a population-based control study (United States)." *Cancer Causes and Control* Vol. 14. (Feb 2003): 43–51.

Gaudet M., S. Gapstur, J. Sun, et al. "Active smoking and breast cancer risk: original cohort data and meta-analysis." *Journal of the National Cancer Institute* Vol. 105.(Apr 2013): 515–525.

Hamajima, N., K. Hirose, K. Tajima, et al. "Alcohol, tobacco, and breast cancer—collaborative reanalysis of individual data from 53 epidemiological studies including 58,515 women with breast cancer and 95,067 women without the disease." *The British Journal of Cancer* (Nov 18, 2002): 1234–1245.

Jacobs, E., C. Thomson, S. Flatt, et al. "Correlates of 25-hydroxyvitamin d and breast cancer stage in the women's healthy eating and living study." *Nutrition and Cancer* Vol. 65. (Feb 2013):188–194.

Johnson, K., A. Miller, N. Collishaw, et al. "Active

smoking and secondhand smoke increase breast cancer risk: the report of the Canadian Expert Panel on Tobacco Smoke and Breast Cancer Risk (2009)." *Tobacco Control* Vol. 20. (Jan 2011): e2 doi: 10.1136/tc.2010.035931.

Johnson, K., S. Glantz. "Evidence secondhand smoke causes breast cancer in 2005 stronger than for lung cancer in 1986." *Preventive Medicine* Vol. 46. (Jun 2008): 492–496.

Knight, J., L. Bernstein, J. Largent, et al. "Alcohol intake and cigarette smoking and risk of a contralateral breast cancer: the Women's Environmental Cancer and Radiation Epidemiology Study." *American Journal of Epidemiology* Vol. 169. (Apr 2009): 962–968.

Kropp, S., and J. Chang-Claude. "Active and passive smoking and risk of breast cancer by age 50 years among German women." *American Journal of Epidemiology* Vol. 156. (Oct 1, 2002): 616–626.

Lin, Y., K. Tamakoshi, K. Wakai, et al. "Active smoking, passive smoking, and breast cancer risk: findings from the Japan Collaborative Cohort Study for Evaluation of Cancer Risk." *American Journal of Epidemiology* Vol. 18. (2008): 77–83.

"List of smoking-related diseases expanded: surgeon general warns of other cancer, pneumonia, cataracts and more." *Associated Press* Release. (May 27, 2004).

"New stats show heart diseases still America's No. 1 Killer, stroke No.3." American Heart Association Journal Report. (Jan 1, 2004). www.americanheart.org/presenter.jhtml?identifier=3018015.

Luo, J., K. Margolis, J. Wactawski-Wende, et al. "Association of active and passive smoking with risk of breast cancer among postmenopausal women: a prospective cohort study." *BMJ (Clinical researched.)* Vol. 342. (Mar 2011): d1016.

McCarty K., R. Santella, S. Steck, et al. "PAH-DNA adducts, cigarette smoking, GST polymorphisms, and breast cancer risk." *Environmental Health Perspectives* Vol. 117. (Apr 2009): 552–558.

Miller, D., M. Marty, R. Broadwin, et al. "The association between exposure to environmental tobacco smoke and breast cancer: a review by the California Environmental Protection Agency." *Preventive Medicine* Vol. 44. (Feb 2007): 93–106.

Pirie, K., V. Beral, R. Peto, et al. "Passive smoking and breast cancer in never smokers: prospective study and meta-analysis." *International Journal of Epidemiology* Vol. 37. (Oct 2008): 1069–1079.

Reynolds, P., D. Goldberg, S. Hurley, et al. "Passive Smoking and Risk of Breast Cancer in the California Teachers Study." *Cancer Epidemiology, Biomarkers & Prevention* Vol. 18. (Dec 2009): 2389–3398.

Ritter, John. "Secondhand smoke causes breast cancer, study says." www.usatoday.com/news/health/2005-03-08-smoking-breastcancer_x.htm.

Sadri, G., and H. Mahjub. "Passive or active smoking, which is more relevant to breast cancer." *Saudi Medical Journal* Vol. 28. (Feb 2007): 254–258

Slattery M., K. Curtin, A. Guiliano, et al. "Active and passive smoking, IL6, ESR1, and breast cancer risk." *Breast Cancer Research and Treatment* Vol. 109. (May 2008): 101–111.

Stephenson, N., L. Beckmann, J. Chang-Claude. "Carcinogen metabolism, cigarette smoking, and breast cancer risk: a Bayes model averaging approach." *Epidemiologic Perspectives & Innovation* Vol. 7. (Nov 2010): 7.

Terry, P., M. Thun, T. Rohan. "Does tobacco smoke cause breast cancer?" *Women's Health* Vol. 7. (July 2011): 405–408.

Terry, P.D., and T.E. Rohan. "Cigarette smoking and the risk of breast cancer in women: a review of the literature." *Cancer Epidemiology, Biomarkers & Prevention* Vol. 11. (Oct 2002; 10 Pt 1): 953–971.

Chapter 20: Fatally Flawed Pharmaceuticals

Haile, R.W., Thomas, D.C., McGuire, V., et al. "BRCA1 and BRCA2 mutation carriers, oral contraceptive use, and breast cancer before age 50." *Cancer Epidemiology, Biomarkers, and Prevention* Vol. 15. (Oct 2006): 1863–1870.

Jernstrom, H., Loman, N., Johannsson, O.T., et al. "Impact of teenage oral contraceptive use in a population-based series of early-onset breast cancer cases who have undergone BRCA mutation testing." *European Journal of Cancer* Vol. 41. (Oct 2005): 2312–2320.

Kahlenborn, C., Modugno, F., Potter, D.M., et al. "Oral contraceptive use as a risk factor for premenopausal breast cancer: a meta-analysis." *Mayo Clinic Proceedings* Vol. 81. (Oct 2006): 1290–1302.

Milne, R.L., Knight, J.A., John, E.M., et al. "Oral contraceptive use and risk of early-onset breast cancer in carriers and noncarriers of BRCA1 and BRCA2 mutations." *Cancer Epidemiology, Biomarkers, and Prevention* Vol. 14. (Feb 2005): 350–356.

Pettypiece, S., Pearson, S. "Wyeth vows to fight all menopause drug suits."

www.iht.com/articles/2006/08/20/bloomberg/bx-drug.php

Tamimi, R.M., Hankinson, S.E., Chen, W.Y., et al. "Combined estrogen and testosterone use and the risk of breast cancer in postmenopausal women." *Archives of Internal Medicine* Vol. 166. (July 24, 2006): 1483–1489.

The Pill and HRT

Beral, V., et al. "Breast cancer and hormone-replacement therapy in the Million Women Study." *Lancet* Vol. 362. (Aug 9, 2003): 419-27.

Chen, W.Y., G.A. Colditz, and B. Rosner. "Use of postmenopausal hormones, alcohol, and risk for invasive breast cancer." *Annals of Internal Medicine* Vol. 137. (Nov 19, 2002): 798–804.

Chen, W.Y., N. Weiss, and P. Newcomb. "Hormone replacement therapy in relation to breast cancer." *Journal of the American Medical Association (JAMA)* Vol. 287. (Feb 13, 2002): 734–741.

Colcitz, G.A., and B. Rosner. "Cumulative risk of breast cancer to age 70 years according to risk factor status: data from the Nurses' Health Study." *American Journal of Epidemiology* Vol. 152. (Nov 15, 2000): 950–964.

Daling, J.R., K.E. Malone, and D.R. Doody. "Relation of regimens of combines hormone replacement therapy to lobular, ductal, and other histologic types of breast cancer." *Cancer* Vol. 95. (Dec 15, 2002): 2455– 2464.

Dolle, D., J. Daling, E. White, et al. "Risk factors for triple-negative breast cancer in women under the age of 45 year." *Cancer Epidemiology, Biomarkers & Prevention* Vol. 18. (Apr 2009): 1157–1166.

Edan, J. "Progestins and cancer." *American Journal of Obstetrics & Gynecology* Vol. 188. (May 2003): 1123– 1131.

Ginsburg, E.S., B.W. Walsh, and B.F. Shea. "Effect of acute ethanol ingestion on prolactin in menopausal women using estradiol replacement." *Gynecologic and Obstetric Investigation* Vol. 39. (Issue 1, 1995): 47–49.

Humphries, K., and S. Gill. "Risks and benefits of hormone replacement therapy: the evidence speaks." *CMAJ: Canadian Medical Association Journal* Vol. 168. (Apr 15, 2003): 1001–1010.

LeBlanc, E., J. Janowsky, and B. Chan. "Hormone replacement therapy and cognition." *Journal of the American Medical Association (JAMA)* Vol. 285. (Mar 2001): 1489–1499.

Leis, H.P., M.M. Black, and S. Sall. "The pill and the

breast." *Journal of Reproductive Medicine* Vol. 16. (Jan 1976): 5–9.

Longman, S.M., and G.C. Buehring. "Oral contraceptives and breast cancer. In vitro effect contraceptive steroids on human mammary growth." *Cancer* Vol. 59. (Jan 15, 1987): 281–287.

Li, C.I., B.O. Anderson, and J.R. Daling. "Trends in incidence rates of invasive lobular and ductal breast carcinoma." *Journal of the American Medical Association (JAMA)* Vol. 289. (Mar 19, 2003): 1421–1424.

Narod, S. "Breast cancer in young women." *Nature Review: Clinical Oncology* Vol. 9. (Jun 2012): 460–470.

Nelson, H., L. Humphrey, et al. "Postmenopausal hormone replacement therapy." *Journal of the American Medical Association (JAMA)* Vol. 288. (Aug 21, 2002): 872–881.

Petitti, D. "Hormone replacement therapy for prevention: more evidence, more pessimism." *Journal of the American Medical Association (JAMA)* Vol. 288. (Jul 3, 2002): 99–100.

Porch, J.V., I.M. Lee, and N.R. Cook. "Estrogen-progestin replacement therapy and breast cancer risk: the Women's Health Study (United States)." *Cancer Causes and Control* Vol. 13. (Nov 2002): 847–854.

Rodriguez, C., A. Patel, and E. Calle. "Estrogen Replacement therapy and ovarian cancer mortality in a large prospective study of US women." *Journal of the American Medical Association (JAMA)* Vol. 285. (Mar 2001): 1460–1465.

Soares R., S. Guerreiro, and M. Botelho. "Elucidating progesterone effects in breast cancer: cross talk with PDGF signaling pathway in smooth muscle cell." *Journal of Cellular Biochemistry* Vol. 100. (Jan 1, 2007): 174–183.

White, E., K. Malone, N. Weiss, et al. "Breast cancer among young U.S. women in relation to oral contraceptive use." *Journal of the National Cancer Institute* Vol. 86. (Apr 1994): 505–514.

Writing group WHI investigators. "Risks and benefits of estrogen plus progestin in healthy postmenopausal women." *Journal of the American Medical Association (JAMA)* Vol. 288. (Jul 17, 2002): 321–333.

Zhu, H., X. Lei, and J. Feng. "Oral contraceptive use and risk of breast cancer: a meta-analysis of prospective cohort studies." *The European Journal of Contraception & Reproductive Health Care* Vol. 17. (Dec 2012): 402–414.

Bio-identical hormones

Adams, J. "Adrenal androgens and human breast cancer: a new appraisal." *Breast Cancer Research and Treatment* Vol. 51. (Sept 1998): 183–188.

Boothby, L., P. Doering. "Bioidentical hormone therapy: a panacea that lacks supportive evidence." *Current Opinion in Obstetrics & Gynecology* Vol. 20. (Aug 2008): 400–407.

Boothby, L., P. Doering, S. Kipersztok. "Bioidentical hormone therapy: a review." *Menopause* Vol. 11. (May-Jun 2004): 356–367.

Campagnoli, C., F. Clavel-Chapelon, R. Kaaks, et al. "Progestins and progesterone in hormone replacement therapy and the risk of breast cancer." *The Journal of Steroid Biochemistry and Molecular Biology* Vol. 96. (July 2005): 95–108.

Cirigliano, M. "Bioidentical hormone therapy: a review of the evidence." *Journal of Women's Health* Vol. 16. (Jun 2007): 600–631.

Files, J., M. Ko, S. Pruthi, et al. "Bioidentical hormone therapy." *Mayo Clinic Proceedings* Vol. 86. (July 2011): 673–680.

Fortner, R., A. Eliassen, D. Spiegelman, et al. "Premenopausal endogenous steroid hormones and breast cancer risk: results from the Nurses' Health Study II." *Breast Cancer Research* Vol. 15. (Mar 2013): R19.

Fournier, A., A. Fabre, S. Mesrine, et al. "Use of different postmenopausal hormone therapies and risk of histology- and hormone receptor-defined invasive breast cancer." *Journal of Clinical Oncology* Vol. 26. (Mar 2008): 1260–1268.

Fournier, A., F. Berrino, E. Riboli, et al. "Breast cancer risk in relation to different types of hormone replacement therapy in the E3N-EPIC cohort." *International Journal of Cancer* Vol. 114. (Apr 2005): 448–454.

Fournier, A., F. Berrino, F. Clavel-Chapelon. "Unequal risks for breast cancer associated with different hormone replacement therapies: results from the E3N cohort study." *Breast Cancer Research and Treatment* Vol. 107. (Jan 2008): 103–111.

Gregoraszczuk, E., T. Milewicz, J. Kolodziejczyk, et al. "Progesterone-induced secretion of growth hormone, insulin-like growth factor I and prolactin by human breast cancer explants." *Gynecological Endocrinology* Vol. 15. (Aug 2001): 251–258.

Hankinson, S., A. Eliassen. "Circulating sex steroids and breast cancer risk in premenopausal women." *Hormones & Cancer* Vol. 1. (Feb 2010): 2–10.

Holtorf, K. "The bioidentical hormone debate: are bioidentical hormones (estradiol, estriol, and progesterone) safer or more efficacious than commonly used synthetic versions in hormone replacement therapy?" *Postgraduate Medicine* Vol. 121. (Jan 2009): 73–85.

Huntley, A. "Compounded or confused? Bioidentical hormones and menopausal health." *Menopause International* Vol. 17. (Mar 2011): 16–18.

Klijin, J., B. Setyono, H. Sander, et al. "Pre-clinical and clinical treatment of breast cancer with antiprogestins." *Human Reproduction* Vol. 1. (Jun 1994): 181–189.

Krzysiek, J., T. Milewicz, K. Augustowska, et al. "The impact of progesterone on simultaneous, local secretion of IGFBP-3 and IGF-1 [IGFBP-3/IGF-1 index] by human malignant and non-malignant breast explants depends on tissue steroid receptor phenotype." *Ginekologia Polska* Vol. 74. (Sept 2003): 767–774.

Lange, C. "Challenges to Defining a Role for Progesterone in Breast Cancer." *Steroids* Vol. 73. (Oct 2008): 914–921.

Lange, C. "Integration of progesterone receptor action with rapid signaling events in breast cancer models." *The Journal of Steroid Biochemistry and Molecular Biology* Vol. 108. (Feb 2008): 203–212.

Lange, C., and D. Yee. "Progesterone and breast cancer." *Women's Health (London, England)* Vol. 4. (Mar 2008): 151–162.

L'hermite, M., T. Simoncini, S. Fuller, et al. "Could transdermal estradiol + progesterone be safer postmenopausal HRT? A review." *Maturitas* Vol. 60. (Jul-Aug 2008): 185–201.

Michna, H., Y. Nishino, G. Neef, et al. "Progesterone antagonists: tumor-inhibiting potential and mechanism of action." *The Journal of Steroid Biochemistry and Molecular Biology* Vol. 41. (Mar 1992): 339–348.

Milewicz, T., E. Gregoraszczuk, K. Augustowska, et al. "Progesterone but not estradiol 17beta potentiates local GH secretions by hormone-dependent breast cancer explants. An in vitro study." *Experimental and Clinical Endocrinology & Diabetes* Vol. 113. (Feb 2005): 127–132.

Miner, J., E. Martini, M. Smith, et al. "Short-term oral progesterone administration antagonizes the effect of transdermal estradiol on endothelium-dependent vasodilation in young healthy women." *American Journal of Physiology, Heart and Circulatory Physiology* Vol. 301. (Oct 2011): H1716–1722.

Missmer, S., A. Eliassen, R. Barberi, et al. "Endogenous estrogen, androgen, and progesterone concentrations and breast cancer risk among postmenopausal women." *Journal of the National Cancer Institute* Vol. 96. (Dec 2004): 1856–1865.

Moskowitz, D. "A comprehensive review of the safety and efficacy of bioidentical hormones for the management of menopause and related health risks." *Alternative Medicine Review* Vol. 11. (Sept 2006): 208–223.

Murkes, D., P. Lalitkumar, K. Leifland, et al. "Percutaneous estradiol/oral micronized progesterone has less-adverse effects and different gene regulations than oral conjugated equine estrogens/medroxyprogesterone acetate in the breasts of healthy women in vivo." *Gynecological Endocrinology* Vol. 28. (Oct 2012): 12–15.

Narod, S. "Hormone replacement therapy and the risk of breast cancer." *Nature Reviews. Clinical Oncology* Vol. 8. (Aug 2011): 669–676.

Pfeifer, S., J. Goldberg, R. Lobo, et al. "Compounded bioidentical menopausal hormone therapy." *Fertility and Sterility* Vol. 98. (Aug 2012): 308–312.

Secreto, G., P. Toniolo, P. Pisani, et al. "Androgens and breast cancer in premenopausal women." *Cancer Research* Vol. 49. (Jan 1989): 471–476.

Secreto, G., P. Toniolo, F. Berrino, et al. "Increased androgenic activity and breast cancer risk in premenopausal women." *Cancer Research* Vol. 44. (Dec 1984): 5902–5905.

Secreto, G., P. Toniolo, F. Berrino, et al. "Serum and urinary androgens and risk of breast cancer in postmenopausal women." *Cancer Research* Vol. 51. (May 1991): 2572–2576.

Simon, J. "What's new in hormone replacement therapy: focus on transdermal estradiol and micronized progesterone." *Climacteric: the journal of the International Menopause Society* Vol. 15. (Apr 2012): 3–10.

Sites, C. "Bioidentical hormones for menopausal therapy." *Women's Health* Vol. 4. (Mar 2008): 163–171.

Soares, R., S. Guerreiro, M. Botelho. "Elucidating progesterone effects in breast cancer: Cross talk with PDGF signaling pathway in smooth muscle cell." *Journal of Cellular Biochemistry* Vol. 100. (Aug 2006): 174–183.

Stahlberg, C., A. Pedersen, E. Lynge, et al. "Increased risk of breast cancer following different regimens of hormone replacement therapy frequently used in Europe." *International Journal of Cancer* Vol. 109. (May 2004): 721–727.

Wang, X., R. Travis, G. Reeves, et al. "Characteristics of the Million Women Study participants who have and have not worked at night." *Scandinavian Journal of Work, Environment & Health* Vol. 38. (Nov 2012): 590–599.

Whelan, A., T. Jurgens, M. Trinacty. "Bioidentical progesterone cream for menopause-related vasomotor symptoms: is it effective?" *The Annals of Pharmacotherapy* Vol. 47. (Jan 2013):112–116.

Wood, C., T. Register, C. Lees, et al. "Effects of estradiol with micronized progesterone or medroxyprogesterone acetate on risk markers for breast cancer in postmenopausal monkeys." *Breast Cancer Research and Treatment* Vol. 101. (Jan 2007): 125–134.

Wurtz, A., A. Tjonneland, J. Christensen, et al. "Serum estrogen and SHBG levels and breast cancer incidence among users and never users of hormone replacement therapy." *Cancer Causes Control* Vol. 23. (Oct 2012): 1711–1720.

Zbuk, K. "Declining incidence of breast cancer after decreased use of hormone-replacement therapy: magnitude and time lags in different countries." *Journal of Epidemiology and Community Health* Vol. 66. (Jan 2012): 1–7.

Antidepressants and Other Pharmaceuticals

Ashbury, J., L. Levesque, P. Beck, et al. "A population-based case-control study of selective serotonin reuptake inhibitors (SSRIs) and breast cancer: the impact of duration of use, cumulative dose and latency." *BMC Medicine* Vol. 8. (Dec 2010): 90.

Ashbury, J., L. Levesque, P. Beck, et al. "Selective serotonin reuptake inhibitor (SSRI) antidepressants, prolactin and breast cancer." *Frontiers in Oncology* Vol. 2. (Dec 2012): 177.

Brandes, L.J., R.J. Arron, R.P. Bogdanovic, et al. "Stimulation of malignant growth in rodents by antidepressant drugs at clinically relevant doses." *Cancer Research* Vol. 52. (Jul 1992): 3796–3800.

Chubak, J., D. Buist, D. Boudreau, et al. "Breast cancer recurrence risk in relation to antidepressant use after diagnosis." *Breast Cancer Research and Treatment* Vol. 112. (Nov 2008): 123–132.

Cosgrove, L., L. Shi, D. Creasey, et al. "Antidepressants and breast and ovarian cancer risk: a review of literature and researchers' financial associations with industry." *PLoS One* Vol. 6. (Apr 2011):

e18210.

Cotterchio, M., N. Kreiger, G. Darlington, et al. "Antidepressant medication use and the risk of breast cancer." *American Journal of Epidemiology* Vol. 151. (May 2000): 951–957.

Davis, S., D. Mirick. "Medication use and the risk of breast cancer." *European Journal of Epidemiology* Vol. 22. (May 2007): 319–325.

Eom, C., S. Park, K. Cho. "Use of antidepressants and the risk of breast cancer: a meta-analysis." *Breast Cancer Research and Treatment* Vol. 136. (Dec 2012): 635–645.

Fulton-Kehoe, D., Rossing, M.A., Rutter, C., et al. "Use of antidepressant medications in relation to the incidence of breast cancer." *British Journal of Cancer* Vol. 94. (April 10, 2006): 1071–1078.

Kurdyak, P.A., W.H. Gnam, and D.L. Streiner. "Antidepressants and the risk of breast cancer." *The Canadian Journal of Psychiatry* Vol. 47. (Dec 2002): 966–970.

Pae, C. "Association between antidepressants and breast/ovarian cancer." *Expert Opinion on Pharmacotherapy* Vol. 13. (Feb 2012): 441–444.

Sharpe, C.R., J.P. Collet, E. Beizile, et al. "The effects of tricyclic antidepressants on breast cancer risk." *The British Journal of Cancer* Vol. 86. (Jan 7, 2002): 92–97.

Undela, K., V. Srikanth, D. Bansal. "Statin use and risk of breast cancer: a meta-analysis of observational studies." *Breast Cancer Research and Treatment* Vol. 135. (Aug 2012): 261–269.

Wernli, K., J. Hampton, A. Trentham-Dietz, et al. "Antidepressant medication use and breast cancer risk." *Pharmacoepidemiology and Drug Safety* Vol. 18. (Apr 2009): 284–290.

Chapter 21: Portrait of an Assassin

"Are pesticides hazardous to our health." *Journal of Pesticide Reform* Vol. 19. (Issue 2, 1999): 4–5.

Buros, M. "Farmed Salmon is said to contain high PCB levels." *The New York Times.* (July 30, 2003).

Bradlow, H.L., D.L. Davis, G. Lin, et al. "Effects of pesticides on the ratio of 16 alpha/2-hydroxyestrone: a biologic marker of breast cancer risk." *Environmental Health Perspectives* Vol. 103. (Oct 1995; Suppl 7): 147–150.

Brotons, J.A., et al. "Environmental Health Issues." *Environmental Health Prospectives* Vol. 103. (1995): 608-612.

Cebbelo, G., A. Juarranz, et al. "Organophospho-

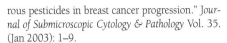

rous pesticides in breast cancer progression." *Journal of Submicroscopic Cytology & Pathology* Vol. 35. (Jan 2003): 1–9.

Chang, J.C., R. Fortmann, et al. "Evaluation of low-VOC latex paint." *Indoor Air* Vol. 9. (Dec 1999): 253–258.

Coco, P., N. Kazerouni, and S.H. Zahm. "Cancer mortality and environmental exposure to DDE in the United States." *Environmental Health Perspectives* Vol. 108. (Jan 2000): 1–4.

Demers, A., P. Ayotte, J. Brisson, et al. "Risk and aggressiveness of breast cancer in relation to plasma organochlorine concentrations." *Cancer Epidemiology, Biomarkers & Prevention* Vol. 9. (Feb 2000): 161–166.

"Environmental estrogens and other hormones." Tulane University website. www.tmc.tulane.edu/ecme/eehome/basics/.

Epstein, S. "Pesticides and Cancer." Transcript of lecture given in 1993.

Franklin, P., P. Dingle, et al. "Raised exhaled nitric oxide in healthy children associated with domestic formaldehyde levels." *American Journal of Critical Care Medicine* Vol. 161. (May 2000): 1757–1759.

Guttes, S., K. Failing, K. Neumann, et al. "Chlororganic pesticides and polychlorinated biphenyls in breast tissue of women with benign and malignant breast disease." *Archives of Environmental Contamination & Toxicology* Vol. 35. (Jul 1998): 140–147.

Horner, C., M.D. "Alternatives to chemical pesticides." Channelcincinnati.com. (May 10, 2001).

Horner, C., M.D. "Hidden toxins in plywood and particle board." *Channelcincinnati.com*. (Jan 5, 2002).

Horner, C., M.D. "Naturally keeping bugs away." Channelcincinnati.com. (May 5, 2001).

Horner, C., M.D. "Nontoxic bedding." *Channel cincinnati.com*. (Mar 16, 2002).

Horner, C., M.D. "Nontoxic paints." *Channelcincinnati. com*. (Jun 10, 2002).

Horner, C., M.D. "Toxic air and household products." *Channelcincinnati.com*. (Jun 21, 2001).

Hoyer, A.P., P. Grandjean, T. Jorgensen, et al. "Organochlorine compounds and breast cancer— is there a connection between environmental pollution and breast cancer." *Ugeskr Laeger* Vol. 162. (Feb 14, 2000): 922–926.

Hoyer, A.P., T. Jorgensen, et al. "Repeated measurements of organochlorine exposure and breast can-

cer risk (Denmark)." *Cancer Causes and Control* Vol. 11. (Feb 2000): 177–184.

Hoyer, A.P., T. Jorgensen, J.W. Brock, et al. "Organochlorine exposure and breast cancer survival." *Journal of Clinical Epidemiology* Vol. 53. (Mar 2000): 323–330.

Jaga, K., and D. Brosius. "Pesticide exposure: human cancers on the horizon." *Reviews on Environmental Health* Vol. 14. (Jan-Mar 1999): 39–50.

Jaga, K., and H. Duvvi. "Risk reduction for DDT toxicity and carcinogenesis through dietary modifications." *Journal of the Royal Society of Health* Vol. 121. (Jun 2001): 107–113.

Krishnan, A.V., et al. "Bisphenol-A: an estrogenic substance is released from polycarbonate flasks during autoclaving." *Endocrinology* Vol. 132. (1993): 2279–2286.

Martin, B. *The Journal of Nature Medicine*. (Aug 2003).

Mather, V., P. Bhatnagar, R.G. Sharma, et al. "Breast cancer incidence and exposure to pesticides among women originating from Jaipur." *Environment International* Vol. 28. (Nov 2002): 331–336.

Meinhert, R., J. Schuz, et al. "Leukemia and non-Hodgkin's lymphoma I childhood exposure to pesticides: results of a register-based case-control study in Germany." *American Journal of Epidemiology* Vol. 15. (Apr 1, 2000): 639–646.

Moysich, K.B., C.B. Ambrosone, P. Mendola, et al. "Exposures associated with serum organochlorine levels among postmenopausal women from western New York State." *American Journal of Independent Indian Medicine* Vol. 41. (Feb 2002): 102–110.

Sonnenschein, C., A.M. Soto. "An updated review of environmental estrogen and androgen mimickers and antagonists." *Journal of Steroid Biochemistry and Molecular Biology* Vol. 65. (Apr 1998): 143–50.

Soto, A.M. et al. "p-Nonyl-phenol: an estrogenic xenobiotic released from "modified" polystyrene." *Environmental Health Perspectives* Vol. 92. (1991): 167–73.

Vaughan, T.L., P.A. Stewart, et al. "Occupational exposure to formaldehyde and wood dust and nasopharyngeal carcinoma." *Occupational & Environmental Medicine* Vol. 57. (Jun 2000): 376–384.

Endocrine Disrupters

Brophy, J.T., M. Keith., A. Watterson, et al. "Breast cancer risk in relation to occupations with exposure to carcinogens and endocrine disruptors: a Canadian case-control study." *Environmental Health* Vol.

11. (Nov 2012): 206–223.

Chen, J., T. Brown., and J. Russo. "Regulation of energy metabolism pathways by estrogens and estrogenic chemicals and potential implications in obesity associated with increased exposure to endocrine disruptors." *Biochimica et Biophysica Acta* Vol. 1793. (Jul 2009): 1128–1143.

Clapp, R.W., M. Jacobs, E. Loechler., et al. "Environmental and occupational causes of cancer new evidence, 2005–2007." *Reviews on Environmental Health* Vol. 23. (Jan-Mar 2008): 1–37.

Crinnion, WJ. "Toxic effects of the easily avoidable phthalates and parabens." *Alternative Medicine Review: A Journal of Clinical Therapeutic* Vol. 15. (Sept 2010): 190–196.

Darbre, P.D., and A.K. Charles. "Environmental oestrogens and breast cancer: evidence for combined involvement of dietary, household and cosmetic xenoestrogens." *Anticancer Research* Vol. 30. (Mar 2010): 815–827.

Darbre, P.D., and P.W. Harvey. "Paraben esters: review of recent studies of endocrine toxicity, absorption, esterase and human exposure, and discussion of potential human health risks." *Journal of Applied Toxicology* Vol. 28. (Jul 2008): 561–578.

Fernandez, S., and J. Russo. "Estrogen and xenoestrogens in breast cancer." *Toxicologic Pathology* Vol. 38. (Nov 2009): 110–122.

"Final amended report on the safety assessment of methylparaben, ethylparaben, propylparaben, isopropylparaben, butylparaben, isobutylparaben, and benzylparaben as used in cosmetic products." *International Journal of Toxicology* Vol. 27. (2008): 1–82.

Fucic, A., M. Gamulin, Z. Ferencic, et al. "Environmental exposure to xenoestrogens and oestrogens related cancers: reproductive system, breast, lung, kidney, pancreas, and brain." *Environmental Health* Vol. 11. (Jun 2012): Suppl 1:S8. doi: 10.1186/1476-069X-11-S1-S8.

Lavicoli, L., L. Fontana, and A. Bergamaschi. "The effects of metals as endocrine disruptors." *Journal of Toxicology and Environmental Health* Vol. 12. (Mar 2009): 206–223.

Newbold, R. "Developmental exposure to endocrine-disrupting chemicals programs for reproductive tract alternations and obesity later in life." *American Journal of Clinical Nutrition* Vol. 94. (Dec 2011): 1939S–1942S.

Newbold, R. "Impact of environmental endocrine disrupting chemicals on the development of obesity." *Hormones* Vol. 9. (2010): 206–217.

Newbold, R., E. Padilla-Banks., and W. Jefferson. "Environmental estrogens and obesity." *Molecular and Cellular Endocrinology* Vol. 304. (May 2009): 84–89.

Shanle, E., and W. Xu. "Endocrine disrupting chemicals targeting estrogen receptor signaling: identification and mechanisms of action." *Chemical Research in Toxicology* Vol. 24. (Jan 2011): 6–19.

Rudel, R., K. Attfield, J. Schifano, et al. "Chemicals causing mammary gland tumors in animals signal new directions for epidemiology, chemicals testing, and risk assessment for breast cancer prevention." *Cancer* Vol. 109. (Jun 2007): 2635–2666.

Tan, S., J. Meiller, and K. Mahaffey. "The endocrine effects of mercury in humans and wildlife." *Critical Reviews in Toxicology* Vol. 39. (2009): 228–269.

Wozniak, M., and M. Murias. "Xenoestrogens: endocrine disrupting compounds." *Ginekologja Polska* Vol. 79. (Nov 2008): 785–790.

Teflon

Chase, R. "Teflon chemical a likely carcinogen, panel says." *Associated Press* (Jan 31, 2006).

Environmental Protection Agency. www.epa.gov/sab/pdf/2006_0120_final_draft_pfoa_report.pdf.

Falalndysz, J., S. Taniyasu, A. Gulkowska, et al. "Is fish a major source of fluorinated surfactants and repellents in humans living on the Baltic Coast?" *Environmental Science & Technology* Vol. 40. (Feb 1, 2006): 748–751.

Gilliliand, F.D., and J.S. Mandel. "Mortality among employees of a perfluorooctanoic acid production plant." *Journal of Occupation Medicine* Vol. 35. (Sept 1993): 950–954.

Kannan, K., L. Tao, E. Sinclair, et al. "Perfluorinated compounds in aquatic organisms at various trophic levels in a Great Lakes food chain." *Archives of Environmental Contamination and Toxicology* Vol. 48. (May 2005): 559–566.

Keller, J.M., K. Kannan, S. Taniyasu, et al. "Perfluorinated compounds in the plasma of loggerhead and Kemp's ridley sea turtles from the southeastern coast of the United States." *Environmental Science and Technology* Vol. 39. (Dec 1, 2005): 9101–9108.

Kannan, K., E. Perrotta, N.J. Thomas. "Association between perfluorinated compounds and pathological conditions in southern sea otters." *Environmental Science and Technology* Vol. 40. (Aug 15, 2006): 4943–4948.

Kennedy, G.L. Jr., J.L Butenhoff, G.W. Olsen, et al. "The toxicology of perfluorooctanoate." *Critical Review of Toxicology* Vol. 34. (Jul-Aug 2004): 351–384.

Kubwabo, C., B. Stewart, J. Shu, et al. "Occurrence of perfluorosulfonates and other perfluorochemicals in dust from selected homes in the city of Ottawa, Canada." *Journal of Environmental Monitoring* Vol. 7. (Nov 2005): 1074–1078.

Nakayama, S., K. Harada, K. Inoue, et al. "Distribution of perfluorooctanoic acid (PFOA) and perfluorooctane sulfonate (PFOS) in Japan and their toxicities." *Environmental Sciences: an International Journal of Environmental Physiology and Toxicology* Vol. 12. (2005): 293–313.

Perfluorooctanoic acid-Wikipedia, the free encyclopedia.   http://en.wikipedia.org/wiki/Perfluorooctanoic_ acid

Scott, B.F., C. Spencer, S.A. Mabury, et al. "Poly and perfluorinated carboxylates in North American precipitation." *Environmental Science & Technology* Vol. 40. (Dec 1, 2006): 7167–7174.

Sinclair, E., D.T. Mayack, K. Roblee, et al. "Occurrence of perfluororalkyl surfactants in water, fish, and birds in New York State." *Archives of Environmental Contamination and Toxicology* Vol. 50. (April 2006): 398–410.

Skutlarek, D., M. Exner, H. Farber. "Perfluorinated surfactants in surface and drinking water." *Environmental Science and Pollution Research International* Vol. 13. (Sept 2006): 299–307.

Smithwick, M., D.C. Muir, S.A. Mabury, et al. "Perfluororalkyl contamination in liver tissue *from East Greenland polar bears (Ursus maritimus).*" *Environmental Toxicology and Chemistry* Vol. 24. (April 2005): 981–986.

Unfair Business Practices: Class Action Lawsuits Filed Against E.I. DuPont De Nemours & Company Over the Manufacture, Advertising, and Sale of "Teflon®" Nonstick Cookware Coating. www.shulaw. com/infair/dupont_main.asp

White, S.S., A. Calafat, Z. Kuklenyik, et al. "Gestational PFOA exposure of mice is associated with altered mammary gland development in dams and female offspring." *Toxicological Sciences* Vol. 96 (2007Nov 28, 2006): 133–144. [Epub ahead of print]

Yamashita, N., K. Kannan, S. Taniyasu, et al. "A global survey of perfluorinated acids in oceans." *Marine Pollution Bulletin* Vol. 51. (2005): 658–668.

Yao, X., and L. Zhong. "Genotoxic risk and oxidative DNA damage in HepG2 cells exposed to perfluorooctanoic acid." *Mutation Research* Vol. 587. (Nov 10, 2005): 38–44.

Plastics/Cosmetics

Balabanic, D., M. Rupnik, and A. Klemencic. "Negative impact of endocrine-disrupting compounds on human reproductive health." *Reproduction, Fertility, and Development* Vol. 23. (2011): 403–416.

Buteau-Lozano, H., G. Velasco, M. Cristofari, et al. "Xenoestrogens modulate vascular endothelial growth factor secretion in breast cancer cells through an estrogen receptor-dependent mechanism." *Journal of Endocrinology* Vol. 196. (Feb 2008): 399–412.

Betancourt, A., J. Wang, S. Jenkins, et al. "Altered carcinogenesis and proteome in mammary glands of rates after prepubertal exposures to the hormonally active chemicals bisphenol A and genistein." *Journal of Nutrition* Vol. 142. (Jul 2012): 1382S–1388S.

Darikee, S., J. Seok, S. Champion, et al. "Bisphenol A induces a profile of tumor aggressiveness in high-risk cells from breast cancer patients." *Cancer Research* Vol. 68. (Apr 2008): 2076–2080.

Doherty, L., J. Bromer, Y. Zhou, et al. "In utero exposure to diethylstilberstrol (DES) or bisphenol-A (BPA) increases EZH2 expression in the mammary gland: an epigenetic mechanism linking endocrine disruptors to breast cancer." *Hormones & Cancer* Vol. 1. (Jun 2010): 146–155.

Dolinoy, D., D. Huang, and R. Jirtle. "Maternal nutrient supplementation counteracts bisphenol A-induced DNA hypomethylation in early development." *Proceedings of the National Academy of Sciences of the United States of America* Vol. 104. (Aug 2007): 13056–13061.

Fernandez, S., Y. Huang, K. Snider, et al. "Expression and DNA methylation changes in human breast epithelial cells after bisphenol A exposure." *International Journal of Oncology* Vol. 41. (Jul 2012): 369–377.

Gray, J., N. Evans, B. Taylor, et al. "State of the evidence: the connection between breast cancer and the environment." *International Journal of Occupational and Environmental Health* Vol. 15. (Jan-Mar 2009): 43–78.

Jenkins, S., A. Betancourt, J. Wang, et al. "Endocrine-active chemicals in mammary cancer causation and prevention." *Journal of Steroid Biochemistry and Molecular Biology* Vol. 129. (Apr 2012): 191–200.

Koo, H.J., and B.M. Lee. "Estimated exposure to phthalates in cosmetics and risk assessment." *Journal of Toxicology and Environmental Health*: Part A Vol. 67. (Dec 2004): 1901–1914.

Olea, N., R. Pulgar, P. Perez, et al. "Estrogenicity of resin-based composites and sealants used in dentistry." *Environmental Health Perspectives* Vol. 104. (March 1996): 298–305.

Kuch, B., F. Kern, J. Metzger, et al. "Effect-related monitoring: estrogen-like substances in groundwater." *Environmental Science and Pollution Research International* Vol. 17. (Feb 2010): 250–260.

LaPensee, E., C. LaPensee, S. Fox, et al. "Bisphenol A and estradiol are equipotent in antagonizing cisplatin-induced cytotoxicity in breast cancer cells." *Cancer Letters* Vol. 290. (Apr 2010): 167–173.

LaPensee, E., T. Tuttle, S. Fox, et al. "Bisphenol A at low nanomolar doses confers chemoresistance in estrogen receptor-alpha-positive and –negative breast cancer cells." *Environmental Health Perspectives* Vol. 117. (Feb 2009): 175–180.

Lee, H., K. Hwang, M. Park, et al. "Treatment with bisphenol A and methoxychlor results in the growth of human breast cancer cells and alteration of the expression of cell cycle-related genes, cyclin D1 and p21, via an estrogen receptor-dependent signaling pathway." *International Journal of Molecular Medicine* Vol. 29. (May 2012): 883–890.

Macon, M., and S. Fenton. "Endocrine disruptors and the breast: early life effects and later life disease." *Journal of Mammary Gland Biology and Neoplasia* Vol. 18. (Mar 2013): 43–61.

Moral, R., R. Wang, I. Russo, et al. "Effect of prenatal exposure to the endocrine disruptor bisphenol A on mammary gland morphology and gene expression signature." *Journal of Endocrinology* Vol. 196. (Jan 2008): 101–112.

Nakaya, M., H. Onda, K. Sasaki, et al. "Effect of royal jelly on bisphenol A-induced proliferation of human breast cancer cells." *Bioscience, Biotechnology, and Biochemistry* Vol. 71. (Jan 2007): 253–255.

Pupo, M., A. Pisano, R. Lappano, et al. "Bisphenol A induces gene expression changes and proliferative effects through GPER in breast cancer cells and cancer-associated fibroblasts." *Environmental Health Perspectives* Vol. 120. (Aug 2012): 1177–1182.

Schlumpf, M., B. Cotton, M. Conscience, et al. "In vitro and in vivo estrogenicity of UV screens." *Environmental Health Prospectives* Vol. 109. (Mar 2001): 239–244.

Sengupta, S., I. Obiorah, P. Maximov, et al. "Molecular mechanism of action of bisphenol and bisphenol-A mediated by estrogen receptor alpha in growth and apoptosis of breast cancer cells." *British Journal of Pharmacology* Vol. 169. (May 2013): 167–178.

Singh, S., and S. Li. "Epigenetic effects of environmental chemicals bisphenol A and phthalates." *International Journal of Molecular Science* Vol. 13. (2012): 10143–10153.

Soto, A., L. Vandenberg, M. Maffini, et al. "Does breast cancer start in the womb?" *Basic & Clinical Pharmacology & Toxicology* Vol. 102. (Feb 2008): 125–133.

Skakkebaek, N., E. Rajpert-De Meyts, and K. Main. "Testicular dysgenesis syndrome: an increasingly common developmental disorder with environmental aspects." *Human Reproduction* Vol. 16. (May 2001): 972–978.

Smith-Bindman, R. "Environmental causes of breast cancer and radiation from medical imaging: findings from the institute of medicine report." *Archives of Internal Medicine* Vol. 172. (Jul 2012): 1023–1027.

Soto, A., M. Maffini, and C. Sonnenschein. "Neoplasia as development gone awry: the role of endocrine disruptors." *International Journal of Andrology* Vol. 31. (Apr 2008): 288–293.

Weber Lozada, K., and R. Keri. "Bisphenol A increases mammary cancer risk in two distinct mouse models of breast cancer." *Biology of Reproduction* Vol. 85. (Sept 2011): 490–497.

Weng, Y., P. Hsu, S. Liyanarachchi, et al. "Epigenetic influences of low-dose bisphenol A in primary human breast epithelial cells." *Toxicology and Applied Pharmacology* Vol. 248. (Oct 2010): 111–121.

Yang, M., J. Ryu, R. Jeon, et al. "Effects of bisphenol A on breast cancer and its risk factors." *Archives of Toxicology* Vol. 83. (Mar 2009): 281–285.

Yu, Z.L., L.S. Zhang, P.Y. Xu, et al. "The effects of three plastic additives on the proliferation of MCF-7 cell." *Zhonghua Yu Fang Yi Xue Za Zhi* Vol. 37. (May 2003): 150–153.

Antiperspirants

Darbre, P.D. "Aluminum, antiperspirants, and breast cancer." *Journal of Inorganic Biochemistry* Vol. 99. (Sept 2005): 1912–1919.

Darbre, P.D. "Underarm antiperspirants/deodorants

and breast cancer." *Breast Cancer Research* Vol. 11. (Dec 2009): Suppl 3:S5. doi: 10.1186/bcr2424

Exley, C., L. Charles, L. Barr, et al. "Aluminum in human breast tissue." *Journal of Inorganic Biochemistry* Vol. 101. (Sept 2007): 1344–1346.

Fakri, S., A. Al-Azzawi, N. Al-Tawil. "Antiperspirant use as a risk factor for breast cancer in Iraq." *Eastern Mediterranean Health Journal* Vol. 12. (May-July 2006): 478–482.

Golden R., J. Gandy, G. Vollmer. "A review of the endocrine activity of parabens and implications for potential risks to human health." *Critical Reviews In Toxicology* Vol. 35 (June 2005) :435–458.

Harvey, P.W., and D.J. Everett. "Significance of detection of esters of p-hydroxybenzoic acid (parabens) in human breast tumours." *Journal of Applied Toxicology* Vol. 24. (Jan-Feb 2004): 1–4.

McGrath, K. "Apocrine sweat gland obstruction by antiperspirants allowing transdermal absorption of cutaneous generated hormones and pheromones as a link to the observed incidence rates of breast and prostate cancer in the 20th century." *Medical Hypotheses* Vol. 72. (Jun 2009): 665–674.

McGrath, K.G. "An earlier age of breast cancer diagnosis related to more frequent use of antiperspirants/deodorants and underarm shaving." *European Journal of Cancer Prevention* Vol. 12. (Dec 2003): 479–485.

Namer, M., E. Luporsi, J. Gligorov, et al. "The use of deodorants/antiperspirants does not constitute a risk factor for breast cancer." *Bull Cancer* Vol. 95. (Sept 2008): 871–880.

Sappino, A., R. Buser, L. Lesne, et al. "Aluminum chloride promotes anchorage-independent growth in human mammary epithelial cells." *Journal of Applied Toxicology* Vol. 32. (Mar 2012): 233–243.

Chapter 22: Invite Friends, Not Foes

Harwood, Barbara. *The Healing House*. Carlsbad, CA: Hay House, 1997.

Horner, C., M.D. "Alternatives to chemical pesticides." Channelcincinnati.com. (May 10, 2001).

Horner, C., M.D. "Hidden toxins in plywood and particle board." Channelcincinnati.com. (Jan 5, 2002).

Horner, C., M.D. "Naturally keeping bugs away." Channelcincinnati.com. (May 5, 2001).

Horner, C., M.D. "Nontoxic bedding." Channel cincinnati.com. (Mar 16, 2002).

Horner, C., M.D. "Nontoxic paints." Channelcincinnati. com. (Jun 10, 2002).

Horner, C., M.D. "Toxic air and household products." Channelcincinnati.com. (Jun 21, 2001).

Marinelli, Janet, and Paul Beirman-Lytle. *Your Natural Home*. Boston, MA: Little Brown & Co., 1995.

Pearson, David. *The Natural House Catalog*. New York, NY: Fireside, 1996.

Pearson, David. *The New Natural House Book*. New York, NY: Fireside, 1998.

Many of the solutions listed are discoveries I made from many different sources over the years in my quest to live a nontoxic life.

Chapter 23: Cellular Housecleaning

Heron, B., and J.B. Fagan. "Effects of Maharishi rejuvenation (Panchakarma) in reducing dangerous environmental toxins." *Alternative Therapies in Health & Medicine* Vol. 8. (Sept-Oct 2002): 93–103.

Horner, C., M.D. "Purification through panchakarma." Channelcincinati.com. (Jan 24, 2002).

Schnare, D.W., M. Ben, and M.G. Shields. "Body Burden reductions of PCBs, PBBs, and chlorinated pesticides in human subjects." *Ambio* Vol. 13. (1991): 37.

Schneider, R.H., K.L. Cavanaugh, et al. "Health promotion with a traditional system of natural health care: Maharishi Ayur-Veda." *Journal of Social Behavior and Personality* Vol. 5. (Issue 3, 1990): 1–27.

Sharma, H. *Freedom from Disease*. Toronto, Canada: Veda Publishing, 1993.

Sharma, H., and C. Alexander. "Improvements in cardiovascular risk factors through Panchakarma purification procedures." *Journal of Research & Education in Indian Medicine* Vol. 12. (Issue 4, 1993): 2–13.

Sharma, H., and C. Clark. *Contemporary Ayurveda*. New York, NY: Churchill Livingstone, 1998.

Waldschutz, R. "Influence of Maharishi Ayur-Veda purification treatment on physiological and psychological health." *Erfhrungsheilkunde-Acta medica empirica* Vol. 11. (1988): 720–729.

Chapter 24: Healing Nectars of the Night

Anisimov, V.N. "The role of pineal gland in breast development." *Critical Reviews in Oncology/Hematology* Vol. 46. (Jun 2003); 221–234.

Antunes, L., R. Levandovski, G. Dantas, et al. "Obesity and shift work: chronobiological aspects." *Nutrition Research Reviews* Vol. 23. (Jun 2010):

155–168.

Bizzarri, M., A. Cucina, M.G. Valente, et al. "Melatonin and vitamin D(3) increase TGF-beta(1) release and induce growth inhibition in breast cancer cell cultures." *Journal of Surgical Research* Vol. 110. (Apr 2003): 332–337.

Blask, D. American Association for Cancer Research 94th Annual Meeting. Washington, DC: Jul 11–14, 2003.

Blask, D.E., R.T. Dauchy, L.A. Sauer. "Putting cancer to sleep at night: the neuroendocrine/circadian melatonin signal." *Endocrine* Vol. 27. (July 2005): 179–188.

Blask, D., S. Hill, R. Dauchy, et al. "Circadian regulation of molecular, dietary, and metabolic signaling mechanisms of human breast cancer growth by the nocturnal melatonin signal and the consequences of its disruption by light at night." *Journal of Pineal Research* Vol. 51. (Oct 2011): 259–269.

Bonde, J., J. Kolstad, S. Mikkelsen, et al."Work at night and breast cancer—report on evidence-based options for preventative actions." *Scandinavian Journal of Work, Environment and Health* Vol. 38. (2012): 380–390

Brudnowska, J., and B. Peplonska. "Night shift work and cancer risk: a literature review." *Medycyna Pracy* Vol. 62. (2011): 323–338.

Davis, S., and D.K. Mirick. "Circadian disruption, shift work and the risk of cancer: a summary of the evidence and studies in Seattle." *Cancer Causes and Control* Vol. 17. (May 2006): 539–545.

Davis, S., D.K. Mirick, and R.G. Stevens. "Night shift work, light at light, and risk of breast cancer." *Journal of the National Cancer Institute* Vol. 93. (Oct 17, 2001): 1557–1562.

Di Bella, G., F. Mascia, L. Gualano, et al. "Melatonin anticancer effects: review." *International Journal of Molecular Sciences* Vol. 14. (Jan 2013): 2410–2430.

Engeda, J., B. Mezuk, S. Ratliff, et al. "Association between duration and quality of sleep and risk of pre-diabetes: evidence from NHANES." *Diabetic Medicine* Vol. 30. (Jun 2013): 676–680.

Franzese, E., and G. Nigri. "Night work as a possible risk factor for breast cancer in nurses. Correlation between the onset of tumors and alterations in blood melatonin levels." *Professioni Infermieristiche* Vol. 60. (Apr-Jun 2007): 89–93.

Froy, O. "Metabolism and circadian rhythms—implications for obesity." *Endocrine Reviews* Vol. 31. (Feb 2010): 1–24.

Girgert, R., V. Hanf, G. Emons, et al. "Membrane-bound melatonin receptor MT1 down-regulates estrogen responsive genes in breast cancer cells." *Journal of Pineal Research* Vol. 47. (Aug 2009): 23–31.

Glickman, G., R. Levin, and G.C. Brainard. "Ocular input for human melatonin regulation: relevance to breast cancer." *Neuroendocrinology Letters* Vol. 23. (Jul 2002; Suppl 2): 17–22.

Greish, K., Sanada, I., Saad, Ael-D., et al. "Protective effect of melatonin on human peripheral blood hematopoeitic cells against doxorubicin cytotoxicity." *Anticancer Research* Vol. 25(6B). (Nov-Dec 2005): 4245–4248.

Hansen, J., and C. Lassen. "Nested case-control study of night shift work and breast cancer risk among women in the Danish military." *Occupational and Environmental Medicine* Vol. 69. (Aug 2012): 551–556.

Haus, E., and M. Smolensky. "Shift work and cancer risk: potential mechanistic roles of circadian disruption, light at night, and sleep deprivation." *Sleep Medicine Reviews* Vol. S1087–0792. (Nov 2012): doi: 10.1016/j.smrv.2012.08.003.

Husse, J., S. Hintze, E. Gregor, et al. "Circadian clock genes per1 and per2 regulate the response of metabolism-associated transcripts to sleep disruption." *PLoS ONE* Vol. 7. (Dec 2012): e52983. doi: 10.1371/journal.pone.0052983

Kaneko, K., T. Yamada, S. Tsukita, et al. "Obesity alters circadian expressions of molecular clock gene sin the brainstem." *Brain Research* Vol. 1263. (Mar 2009): 58–68.

Kiefer, T., P.T. Ram, L. Yuan, et al. "Melatonin inhibits estrogen receptor transactivation and cAMP levels in breast cancer cells." *Breast Cancer Research & Treatment* Vol. 71. (Jan 2002): 37–45.

Kim, C., Kim, N., Joo, H., et al. "Modulation by melatonin of the cardiotoxic and antitumor activities of adriamycin." *Journal of Cardiovascular Pharmacology* Vol. 46. (Aug 2005): 200–210.

Kivimaki, M., G. Batty, C. Hublin, "Shift work as a risk factor for future type 2 diabetes: evidence, mechanism, implications and future research directions." *PLoS Medicine* Vol. 8. (Dec 2011): e1001138

Knower, K., S. To, K. Takagi, et al. "Melatonin suppresses aromatase expression and activity in breast cancer associated fibroblasts." *Breast Cancer Research and Treatment* Vol. 132. (Apr 2012): 765–771.

Kolstad, H. "Nightshift work and risk of breast cancer and other cancers—a critical review of the epidemiologic evidence." *Scandinavian Journal of Work, Environmental & Health* Vol. 34. (Feb 2008): 5–22.

Kovac, J., J. Husse, and H. Oster. "A time to fast, a time to feast: the crosstalk between metabolism and the circadian clock." *Molecules and Cells* Vol. 28. (Aug 2009): 75–80.

Krishan, S. "Sleep like a child." *Total Health Magazine.* (2001).

Kubatka, P., K. Kalick, and M. Chamilova. "Nimesulide and melatonin in mammary carcinogenesis prevention in female Sprague–Dawley rats." *Neoplasma* Vol. 49. (Issue 4, 2002): 255–259.

Lemus–Wilson, A., P.A. Kelly, and D.E. Blask. "Melatonin Blocks the stimulatory effects of prolactin on human breast cancer cell growth in culture." *The British Journal of Cancer* Vol. 72. (Dec 1995): 1435–1440.

Leonardi, G., V. Rapisarda, A. Marconi, et al. "Correlation of the risk of breast cancer and disruption of the circadian rhythm (review)." *Oncology Reports* Vol. 28. (Aug 2012): 418–428.

Lin, Y., T. Hsiao, and P. Chen. "Persistent rotating shift-work exposure accelerates development of metabolic syndrome among middle-aged female employees: a five-year follow-up." *Chronobiology International* Vol. 26. (May 2009): 740–755.

Lissoni, P., S. Barni, and M. Mandala. "Decreased toxicity and increased efficacy of cancer chemotherapy using pineal hormone melatonin in metastatic solid tumor patients with poor clinical status." *European Journal of Cancer* Vol. 35. (Nov 1999): 1688–1692.

Martinez-Campa, C., C. Alonso-Gonzalez, M.D. Mediavilla, et al. "Melatonin inhibits both ER alpha activation and breast cancer cell proliferation induced by metalloestrogen, cadmium." *Journal of Pineal Research* Vol. 40. (May 2006): 291–296.

McMullan, CJ, E. Schernhammer, E. Rimm, et al. "Melatonin secretion and the incidence of type 2 diabetes." Journal of the *American Medical Association* (*JAMA*) Vol. 309. (April 3, 2013): 1388–1396.

Megdal, S.P., C.H. Kroenke, F. Laden, et al. "Night work and breast cancer risk: a systemic review and meta-analysis." *European Journal of Cancer* Vol. 41. (Sept 2005): 2023–2032.

Mosendane, T., T. Mosendane, and F. Raal. "Shift work and its effect on the cardiovascular system." *Cardiovascular Journal of Africa* Vol. 19. (Jul-Aug 2008): 210–215.

Nagata, C., Y. Nagao, C. Shibuya, et al. "Association of vegetable intake and urinary 6-sulfatoxymelatonin level." *Cancer Epidemiology, Biomarkers, and Prevention* Vol. 14. (May 2005): 1333–1335.

Pesch, B., V. Harth, S. Rabstein, et al. "Night work and breast cancer – results from the German GENICA study." *Scandinavian Journal of Work, Environmental &* Health Vol. 36. (Mar 2010): 134–141.

Pukkala, E., M. Ojamo, S.L. Rudanko, et al. "Does incidence of breast cancer and prostate cancer decrease with increasing degree of visual impairment?" *Cancer Causes and Control* Vol. 17. (May 2006): 573– 576.

Puligheddu, M., S. Conti, M. Campagna, et al. "Cancer risk among shift workers: a review." *Giornale Italiano Di Medicina Del Lavoro Ed Ergonomia* Vol. 34. (Jul-Sept 2012): 624–626.

Ram, P.T., J. Dai, and C. Dong. "Involvement of the mt1 melatonin receptor in human breast cancer." *Cancer Letters* Vol. 179. (May 28, 2002): 141–150.

Sanchez-Barcelo, E.J., S. Cos, R. Fernandez. "International congress on hormonal steroids and hormones and cancer: Melatonin and mammary cancer: a short review." *Endocrine-Related Cancer* Vol. 10. (Jun 2003): 153–159.

Sanchez-Barcelo, E.J., S. Cos, D. Mediavilla, et al. "Melatonin-estrogen interactions in breast cancer." *Journal of Pineal Research* Vol. 38. (May 2005): 217–222.

Schernhammer, E.S., C.H. Kroenke, F. Laden, et al. "Night work and risk of breast cancer." *Epidemiology* Vol. 17. (Jan 2006): 108–111.

Schiavo-Cardoz, D., M. Lima, J. Pareja, et al. "Appetite-regulating hormones from the upper gut: disrupted control of xenin and ghrelin in night workers." *Clinical Endocrinology* (Dec 2012): doi: 10.1111/cen.12114.

Shu-qun, S., T. Anasari, O. McGuinness, et al. "Circadian disruption leads to insulin resistance and obesity." *Current Biology* Vol. 23 (Feb 21, 2013): 372–381

Spiegel, K., K. Knutson, R. Leproult, et al. "Sleep loss: a novel risk factor for insulin resistance and type 2 diabetes." *Journal of Applied Physiology* Vol. 99. (Nov 2005): 2008–2019.

Stevens, P. "Working against our endogenous circadian clock: breast cancer and electric lighting in the modern world." *Mutation Research* Vol. 680. (Nov-Dec 2009): 106–108.

Stevens, R.G., S. Davis, D.K. Mirick, et al. "Alcohol consumption and urinary concentration of 6-sulfatoxymelatonin in healthy women." *Epidemiology* Vol. 11. (Nov 2000): 660–665.

"Stress and Insomnia." *Total Health New Online*. Maharishi Ayurveda Products International. (Mar 1, 2001).

Szosland, D. "Shift work and metabolic syndrome, diabetes mellitus and ischaemic heart disease." *International Journal of Occupational Medicine and Environmental Health* Vol. 23. (2010): 287–291.

Viswananthan, A., and E. Schernhammer. "Circulating melatonin and the risk of breast and endometrial cancer in women." *Cancer Letters* Vol. 281. (Aug 2009): 1–7.

Zawilska, J., D. Skene, and J. Arendt. "Physiology and pharmacology of melatonin in relation to biological rhythms." *Pharmacological Reports* Vol. 61. (2009): 383–410.

Zhao, I., F. Bogossian, and C. Turner. "A cross-sectional analysis of the association between night-only or rotating shift work and overweight/obesity among female nurses and midwives." *Journal of Occupational Medicine and Environmental Medicine* Vol. 54. (Jul 2012): 834–840.

Electromagnetic Fields (EMFs)

Beniashvili, D., Avinoach'm, I., Baasov, D., et al. "The role of household electromagnetic fields in the development of mammary tumors in women: clinical case-record observations." *Medical Science Monitor: International Medical Journal of Experimental and Clinical Research* Vol. 11. (Jan 2005): CR10–13.

Caplan, L.S., E.R. Schoenfeld, E.S. O'Leary, et al. "Breast cancer and electromagnetic fields—a review." *Annals of Epidemiology* Vol. 10. (Jan 2000): 31–44.

Carlo George, "The EMF Story." 2006 radio broadcast.

Davis, S., W.Y. Kaune, D.K. Mirick, et al. "Residential magnetic fields, light – at-night, and nocturnal urinary 6-sulfatoxymelatonin concentration in women." *American Journal of Epidemiology* Vol. 154. (Oct 1, 2001): 591–600.

Davis, S., D.K. Mirick, and R.G. Stevens. "Residential magnetic fields and the risk of breast cancer." *American Journal of Epidemiology* Vol. 155. (Mar 1, 2002): 446–454.

Fedrowitz, M., J. Westermann, and W. Losher. "Magnetic field exposure increases cell proliferation but does not affect melatonin levels in the mammary gland of female Sprague-Dawley rats." *Cancer Research* Vol. 62. (Mar 2002): 1356–1363.

Feychting, M., Forssen, U. "Electromagnetic fields and female breast cancer." *Cancer Causes and Control* Vol. 17. (May 2006): 553–558.

Girgert, R., H. Schimming, W. Korner, et al. "Induction of Tamoxifen resistance in breast cancer cells by ELF electromagnetic fields." *Biochemical and Biophysical Research Communications* Vol. 336. (Nov 4, 2004): 1144–1149.

Girgert, R., V. Hanf, G. Emons, et al. "Exposure of MCF-7 breast cancer cells to electromagnetic fields up-regulates the plasminogen activator system." *International Journal of Gynecological Cancer* Vol. 19. (Apr 2009): 334–338.

Girgert, R., V. Hanf, G. Emons, et al. "Signal transduction of the melatonin receptor MT1 is disrupted in breast cancer cells by electromagnetic fields." *Bioelectromagnetics* Vol. 31. (Apr 2012): 237–245.

Hardell, L., and C. Sage. "Biological effects from electromagnetic field exposure and public exposure standards." *Biomedicine & Pharmacotheraphy* Vol. 62. (Feb 2008): 104–109.

Mevissen, M., M. Haussler, and W. Loscher. "Alterations in ornithine decarboxylase activity in the rat mammary gland after different periods of 50Hz magnetic field exposure." *Bioelectromagnetics* Vol. 20. (Sept 1999): 338–346.

Ravindra, T, N. Lakshimi, and Y. Ahuja. "Melatonin in pathogenesis and therapy of cancer." *Indian Journal of Medical Sciences* Vol. 60. (Dec 2006): 523–535.

Stevens, R.G., S. Davis, and D.B. Thomas. "Electric power, pineal function, and the risk of breast cancer." *The FASEB Journal* Vol. 6. (Feb 1, 1992): 853–860.

Chapter 25: The Medicine of Movement

Bryan, A., R. Magnan, A. Hooper, et al. "Physical activity and differential methylation of breast cancer genes assayed from saliva: a preliminary investigation." *Annals of Behavioral Medicine* Vol. 45. (Feb 2013): 89–98.

Carpenter, C.L., R.K. Ross, A. Paganini-Hill, et al. "Effects of family history, obesity, and exercise on breast cancer risk among postmenopausal women." *International Journal of Cancer* Vol. 106. (Aug 10, 2003): 96–102.

Dal Maso, L., A. Zucchetto, R. Talamini, et al. "Effect of obesity and other lifestyle factors on mortality in women with breast cancer." *International Journal of Cancer* Vol. 123. (Nov 2008): 2188–2194.

Friedenreich, C. "Physical activity and breast cancer: review of the epidemiologic evidence and biologic mechanisms." *Recent Results Cancer Research* Vol. 188. (2011): 125–139.

Friedenreich, C. "The role of physical activity in breast cancer etiology." *Seminars in Oncology* Vol. 37. (Jun 2010): 297–302.

Friedenreich, C., and A. Cust. "Physical activity and breast cancer risk: impact of timing, type and dose of activity and population subgroup effects." *British Journal of Sports Medicine* Vol. 42. (Aug 2008): 636–647.

Goh, J., E. Kirk, S. Lee, et al. "Exercise, physical activity and breast cancer: the role of tumor-associated macrophages." *Exercise Immunology Review* Vol. 18. (2012): 158–176.

Hirose, K., N. Hamajima, T. Takezaki, et al. "Physical exercise reduces risk of breast cancer in Japanese women." *Cancer Science* Vol. 94. (Feb 2003): 193–199.

Holmes, M.D., Chen, W.Y., Feskanich, D., et al. "Physical activity and survival after breast cancer diagnosis." *Journal of the American Medical Association* Vol. 293. (May 25, 2005): 2479–2486.

Horner, C., M.D. "Ayurvedic approaches to exercise." Channelcincinnati.com. (Apr 7, 2001).

Jasienska, G., Ziomkiewicz, A., Thune, I., et al." Habitual physical activity and estradiol levels in women of reproductive age." *European Journal of Cancer Prevention* Vol. 15. (Oct 2006): 439–445.

Kapoor, S. "Advantages of exercise in breast cancer patients and survivors in addition to its mitigating effects on chest wall pain." *Current Oncology* Vol. 20. (Feb 2013): e54–e55.

Khan, N., F. Atag, and H. Mukhtar. "Lifestyle as risk factor for cancer: evidence from human studies." *Cancer Letters* Vol. 283. (Jul 2010): 133–43.

Knight, J.A., Thompson, S., Raboud, J.M., et al. "Light and exercise and melatonin production in women." *American Journal of Epidemiology* Vol. 162. (Dec 2005): 1114–1122.

Kruk, J. "Lifetime physical activity and the risk of breast cancer: a case control study." *Cancer Detection and Prevention* Vol. 31. (2007): 18–28.

Lahmann PH, Friedenreich C, et al. "Physical activity and breast cancer risk: the European Prospective Investigation into Cancer and Nutrition." *Cancer, Epidemiology, Biomarkers, and Prevention.* Vol. 16 (December 19, 2006). 36–42.

Lee, I.M., et al. "Physical Activity and coronary artery disease risk in men: does the duration of exercise episodes predict risk?" *Circulation* Vol. 102. (Aug 29, 2000): 981–986.

Ligibel, J. "Lifestyle factors in cancer survivorship." *Journal of Clinical Oncology* Vol. 30. (Oct 2010): 3697–3704.

Lynch, B., H. Nielson, and C. Friedenreich. "Physical activity and breast cancer prevention." Recent Results *Cancer Research* Vol. 186. (2011): 13–42.

Marcus, P. "Exercise/breast cancer connection." *Bottom Line Magazine.* (Jun 15, 1998).

Monninkhof, E., S. Elias, F. Vlems, et al. "Physical activity and breast cancer: a systematic review." *Epidemiology* Vol. 18. (Jan 2007): 137–157.

Moradi, T., O. Nyren, M. Zack, et al. "Breast cancer risk and lifetime leisure-time and occupational physical activity (Sweden)." *Cancer Causes and Control* Vol. 11. (Jul 2000): 523–531.

Neilson, H., C. Friedenreich, N. Brockton, et al. "Physical activity and postmenopausal breast cancer: proposed biologic mechanisms and areas for future research." *Cancer Epidemiology, Biomarkers & Prevention* Vol. 18. (Jan 2009): 11–27.

Peplonska, B., J. Lissowka, T. Hartman, et al. "Adulthood lifetime physical activity and breast cancer." *Epidemiology* Vol. 19. (Mar 2008): 226–236.

Rockhill, B., W.C. Willett, D.J. Hunter, et al. "A prospective study of recreational physical activity and breast cancer risk." *Archives of Internal Medicine* Vol. 159. (Oct 25, 1999): 2290–2296.

Schmidt, M., J. Chang-Claude, A. Vrieling, et al. "Association of pre-diagnosis physical activity with recurrence and mortality among women with breast cancer." *International Journal of Cancer* (Feb 2013); doi:10.1002/ijc.28130.

Scott, E., A. Daley, H. Doll, et al. "Effects of an exercise and hypo caloric healthy eating program on biomarkers associated with long-term prognosis after early-stage breast cancer: a randomized controlled trial." *Cancer Causes Control* Vol. 24. (Jan 2013): 181–191.

Steindorf, K., M. Schmidt, and S. Kropp. "Case-control study of physical activity and breast cancer risk among premenopausal women in Germany." *American Journal of Epidemiology* Vol. 157. (Jan 15, 2003): 121–130.

Van Puymbroeck, M., B. Burk, K. Shinew, et al. "Perceived health benefits from yoga among breast cancer survivors." *American Journal of Health Pro-*

motion Vol. 27. (Feb 2013) 308–315.

Van Uden-Kraan, C., M. Chinapaw, C. Drossaert, et al. "Cancer patients' experiences with and perceived outcomes of yoga: results from focus groups." Support Care Cancer Vol. 21. (Feb 2012): 1861–1870.

Veerloop, J., M.A. Rookus, K. van der Kooy, et al. "Physical activity and breast cancer risk in women aged 20-54 years." Journal of the National Cancer Institute Vol. 92. (Jan 19, 2000): 128–135.

Walsh, N., M. Gleeson, B. Pyne, et al. "Position statement part one: immune function and exercise." Exercise Immunology Review Vol. 17. (2011): 6–63.

Walsh, N., M. Gleeson, B. Pyne, et al. "Position statement part two: maintaining immune health." Exercise Immunology Review Vol. 17. (2011): 64–103.

Wyrick, K.W., and F.D. Wolinsky. "Physical activity, disability, and the risk of hospitalization for breast cancer among older women." The Journals of Gerontology. Series A, Biological Sciences and Medical Sciences Vol. 55. (Jul 2000): M418–M421.

Yaghjyan, L., G. Colditz, and K. Wolin. "Physical activity and mammography breast density: a systematic review." Breast Cancer Research Treatment Vol. 135. (Sept 2012): 367–380.

Yeo, T. "Exercise improves fatigue during and after breast and prostate cancer treatment, with benefits seen for aerobic exercise." Evidence-based Nursing (Feb 2013); doi:10.1136/eb-2012-101198.

Zeng, H., M. Irwin, L. Lu, et al. "Physical activity and breast cancer survival: an epigenetic link through reduced methylation of a tumor suppressor gene L3MBTL1." Breast Cancer Research Treatment Vol. 133. (May 2012): 127–135.

Chapter 26: Emotional Healing

Antonova, L., K. Aronson, and C. Mueller. "Stress and breast cancer: from epidemiology to molecular biology." Breast Cancer Research Vol. 13. (Apr 2011); doi: 10.1186--bcr2836.

Balick, M., and R. Lee. "The role of laughter in traditional medicine and its relevance to the clinical setting: healing with ha!" Alternative Therapies in Health & Medicine Vol. 9. (Jul-Aug 2003): 88–91.

Bennet, M., J. Zeller, and L. Rosenberg. "The effect of mirthful laughter on stress and natural killer cell function." Alternative Therapies in Health & Medicine Vol. 9. (Issue 2, 2003): 38–43.

Berk, L.S., D. Felton, S.A. Tan, et al. "Modulations of immune parameters during the eustress of humor associated with mirthful laughter." Alternative Therapies in Health & Medicine Vol. 7. (Issue 2, 2001): 62–67.

Berk, L.S., S.A. Tan, W.F. Fry, et al. "Neuroendocrine and stress hormones change during mirthful laughter." American Journal of Medical Science Vol. 298. (Issue 6, 1989): 390–396.

Cramer, H., S. Lange, P. Klose, et al. "Yoga for breast cancer patients and survivors: a systematic review and meta-analysis." BioMed Central Cancer Vol. 12. (Sept 2012): 10.1186--1471.

Duijts, S., M. Zeegers, and B. Borne. "The association between stressful life events and breast cancer risk: a meta-analysis." International Journal of Cancer Vol. 107. (Dec 2003): 1023–1029.

Heikkila, K., S. Nyberg, T. Theorell, et al. "Work stress and risk of cancer: meta-analysis of 5700 incident cancer events in 116,000 European men and women." British Medical Journal Vol. 346. (Feb 2013):; doi: 10.1136/bmj.f165.

Hillhouse, J., et al. "Stress, health, and immunity: a review of the literature and implications for the nursing profession." Holistic Nursing Practice Vol. 5. (Jul 1991): 22–31.

Horner, C., M.D. "The healing power of faith." Channelcincinnati.com. (Feb 10, 2001).

Horner, C., M.D. "The power of love and intimacy." Channelcincinnati.com. (Apr 21, 2001).

Myss, Carolyn, Ph.D. Why People Don't Heal. New York, NY: Three Rivers Press, 1997.

Nielson, N., and M. Gronbaek. "Stress and breast cancer: a systematic update on the current knowledge." Nature Clinical Practice Oncology Vol. 3. (Nov 2006): 612–620.

Ornish, Dean, M.D. Love and Survival. New York, NY: Harper Collins, 1995.

Pant, S., and B. Ramaswamy. "Association of major stressors with elevated risk of breast cancer incidence or relapse." Drugs of Today Vol. 25. (2009): S453–S463.

Santos, M., B. Horta, J. Amaral, et al. "Association between stress and breast cancer in women: a meta-analysis." Cadernos de Saude Publica Vol. 25. (2009): S453–S463.

Sharma, Hari, M.D., and Christopher Clark, M.D. Contemporary Ayurveda. New York, NY: Churchill Livingstone, 1998.

Tipping, Colin. Radical Forgiveness: Making Room for the Miracle. Marietta, GA: Global 13 Publications, 1997.

Tolle, Eckhart. *The Power of Now*. Novato, CA: New World Library, 1999.

Wang, L., W. Liao, C. Tsai, et al. "The effects of perceived stress and life style leading to *breast cancer.*" Women Health Vol. 53. (Jan 2013)

Pranayama

Bhargava, R., M.G. Gogate, and J.F. Mascarenhas. "Autonomic responses to breath holding and its variations following pranayama." *Indian Journal of Physiology & Pharmacology* Vol. 32. (Oct-Dec 1998): 257– 264.

Horner, C., M.D. "Pranayama: using the breathing for health." Channelcincinnati.com. (Apr 26, 2001).

Raghuraj, P., R. Nagarathna, et al. "Pranayama increases grip strength without lateralized effects." *Indian Journal of Physiology & Pharmacology* Vol. 41. (Apr 1997): 129–133.

Raju, P.S., K.A. Kumar, S.S. Reddy, et al. "Effects of yoga on exercise tolerance in normal healthy volunteers." *Indian Journal of Physiology & Pharmacology* Vol. 30. (Apr-Jun 1986): 121–132.

Telles, S., R. Nagarantha, and H.R. Nagendra. "Physiological measures of right nostril breathing." *Journal of Alternative & Complementary Medicine* Vol. 2. (Winter 1996): 479–484.

Telles, S., R. Nagarantha, and H.R. Nagendra. "Breathing through a particular nostril can alter metabolism and autonomic activities." *Indian Journal of Physiology & Pharmacology* Vol. 38. (Apr 1994): 133– 137.

Chapter 27: Turning Inward

Alexander, C.N., M.V. Rainforth, and P. Gelderlos. "Transcendental meditation, self-actualization and psychological health: a conceptual overview and statistical meta-analysis." *Journal of Social Behavior and Personality* Vol. 6. (Issue 5, 1991): 189–247.

Alexander, C.N., P. Robinson, et al. "The effects of Transcendental meditation compared to other methods of relaxation and meditation in reducing risk factors, morbidity, and mortality." *Homeostasis* Vol. 35. (1994a): 243–264.

Alexander, C.N., and P. Robinson. "Treating and preventing alcohol, nicotine, and drug abuse through Transcendental meditation: a review and statistical meta-analysis." *Alcohol Treatment Quarterly* Vol. 11. (1994b): 11–84.

Banquet, J.P. "Spectral analysis of the EEG in meditation." *Electroencephalography and Clinical Neurophysiology* Vol. 35. (1973): 145–151.

Dillbeck, M.C., and D.W. Orme-Johnson. "Physiological differences between Transcendental mediation and the rest." *American Physiology* Vol. 42. (1987): 879–881.

Glaser, J.L., J.L. Brind, et al. "Elevated serum dehydroepiandosterone-sulfate levels in practitioner of the Transcendental mediation (TM) and the TM-sidhi programs." *Journal of Behavioral Medicine* Vol. 15. (1992): 327–341.

Heron, R.E., S.L. Hillis, et al. "Impact of the Transcendental mediation program on government payments to physicians in Quebec." *American Journal of Health Promotion* Vol. 10. (Issue 3, 1996): 208–216.

Horner, C., M.D. "TM and cancer." Channelcincinnati.com. (Apr 27, 2002).

Orme-Johnson, D.W. "EEG coherence during transcendental consciousness. *Electroencephalography and Clinical Neurophysiology* Vol. 43. (Issue 4, 1977): 581–582 E 487 (abstract).

Orme-Johnson, D.W. "Medical utilization and the Transcendental mediation program." *Psychosomatic Medicine* Vol. 49. (1987): 493–507.

Orme-Johnson, D.W., and C.T. Haynes. "EEG phase coherence, pure consciousness, creativity, and the TM-Sidhi experience." *International Journal of Neuroscience* Vol. 113. (1981): 211–219.

Sharma, Hari, M.D., and Christopher Clark, M.D. *Contemporary Ayurveda*. New York, NY: Churchill Livingstone, 1998.

Stoll, B. "Dietary supplements of dehydroepiandrosterone in relation to breast cancer risk." *European Journal of Clinical Nutrition* Vol. 53 (Oct 1999): 771--775.

Wallace, R.K., M.C. Dillbeck, et al. "The effects of Transcendental meditation and the TM-Sidhi program on the aging process." *International Journal of Neuroscience* Vol. 16. (1982): 53–58.

Wallace, Robert, Ph.D. *The Neurophysiology of Enlightenment*. Fairfield, IA: Maharishi International University Press, 1991.

Wallace, Robert, Ph.D. *The Physiology of Consciousness*. Fairfield, IA: Maharishi International University Press, 1993.

Index

About the Author

Christine Horner, M.D., F.A.C.S., is a nationally known surgeon, author, and professional speaker residing in San Diego, California. She holds two board certifications: the National Board of Surgery and the National Board of Plastic Surgery. Dr. Horner was recognized as a leader in her field shortly after starting her plastic and reconstructive surgery practice because she successfully ran a national campaign to pass laws requiring insurance companies to pay for breast reconstruction following mastectomy. Her five-year crusade—the Breast Reconstruction Advocacy Project (BRA Project) led to the passage of laws in thirty-five states and a federal bill, which was signed into law by President Clinton on October 21, 1998.

Dr. Horner has been featured in hundreds of national magazines, radio, and televisions shows, including *The Dr. Oz Show, Mercola.com Interviews, Flourish!* with Dr. Christiane Northrup, *CNN Live Saturday*, and *FOX & Friends*. In February 1999, *Glamour* magazine honored her as their "WOW—Woman of the Month." In 2000, Oprah recognized her as part of her "Angel Network" on her television program. In addition to authoring the award-winning book *Waking the Warrior Goddess: Dr. Christine Horner's Program to Protect Against and Fight Breast Cancer*, Dr. Horner has also contributed chapters to several books, including *The Fountain: 25 Experts Reveal Their Secrets of Health and Longevity* and *Chicken Soup for the Soul: Life Lessons for Loving the Way You Live*. A popular keynote speaker, Dr. Horner has traveled across the country and internationally for over ten years and has inspired thousands to achieve better health.

In 1999, Dr. Horner worked to create the first ever syndicated television news segment exclusively focused on complementary and alternative medicine and natural approaches to staying healthy. It aired on WCPO-TV and then WLW-TV in Cincinnati, and in 2001 the segment was syndicated on the WISDOM Television Network reaching 5.5 million households.

In June 2002, Dr. Horner left her plastic surgery practice so that she could dedicate herself full time to writing and teaching about her passion: prevention-oriented medicine and how to become and stay healthy naturally.

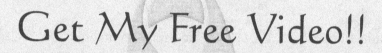

Get My Free Video!!

ACHIEVING AN EXTRAORDINARY STATE OF HEALTH CAN BE SIMPLE.

Dr. Horner is so committed to ending the breast cancer epidemic and helping people to achieve and maintain extraordinary health that she wants you to have a copy of her video with important lifesaving techniques *for free*.

To order your FREE video, simply log on to www.drchristinehorner.com.